The INTERVERTEBRAL DISC

ANTHONY F. DePALMA, M.D.

Professor of Orthopedic Surgery,
Jefferson Medical College, Thomas Jefferson University

RICHARD H. ROTHMAN, M.D., Ph.D.

Associate Professor of Orthopedic Surgery,
Jefferson Medical College, Thomas Jefferson University

With illustrations by Grant Lashbrook

W. B. Saunders Company · Philadelphia · London · Toronto

W. B. Saunders Company: West Washington Square
Philadelphia, Pa. 19105

12 Dyott Street
London, WC1A   1DB

833 Oxford Street
Toronto, Ontario M8Z 5T9, Canada

The Intervertebral Disc   ISBN 0-7216-3035-9

Print No.   9   8   7   6   5   4

Preface

The role of the intervertebral disc in the production of neck and back pain, with or without radiation into one of the extremities, has been the subject of much investigation for many decades. The meticulous painstaking work of Schmorl and Junghanns in the early part of the twentieth century on the human intervertebral disc laid the groundwork for many subsequent studies. The disc has been attacked from every conceivable angle, the most important of which is its biochemical nature and its response to physiologic aging and trauma. In spite of the exhaustive studies recorded in the literature it is alarming to find how little of this knowledge has been acquired by those concerned with neck and back disorders.

This monograph deals with the modern concepts of the biochemical structure of the disc, its functional role and how different phases of alterations in the disc are related to the presenting clinical syndromes. Admittedly, there are many gaps in our knowledge; nevertheless, from the available information a comprehensive concept has evolved, which in a large measure depicts the natural course of disc disease and dictates the kind of management to be instituted.

Over the past 20 years the authors have been fortunate to be able to study a large number of patients with disc disease. In addition, long term results obtained in patients treated conservatively or surgically have been repeatedly analyzed. This, together with the observations noted at the time of operation on intervertebral discs, has permitted us to draw certain conclusions as to the nature and the progressiveness of disc disease and its clinical features, its prognosis and its management.

iii

We are sure that much that is recorded in this book is still very controversial, yet, we believe that our approach to this complex problem will be helpful and rewarding to others.

The preparation, writing and editing of this work has required the loyalty and effort of many persons. In particular we wish to express our gratitude to Miss Gertrude McGowan who typed and edited the many drafts of this book, to Mr. Grant Lashbrook for his fine artwork which exhibits much thought and originality and to the publishers, W. B. Saunders, for their many suggestions, prodding and tolerance.

ANTHONY F. DePALMA, M.D.

RICHARD H. ROTHMAN, M.D., PH.D.

Contents

Chapter 1

ANATOMY 1

Chapter 2

PATHOLOGY... 30

Chapter 3

LUMBAR DISC LESIONS: ANATOMIC AND PATHOLOGIC FEATURES AND
THE CLINICAL SYNDROME 58

Chapter 4

THE CLINICAL SYNDROME OF CERVICAL DISC DISEASE 85

Chapter 5

CONSERVATIVE TREATMENT OF CERVICAL DISC DISEASE..................... 92

Chapter 6

OPERATIVE TREATMENT OF CERVICAL DISC DISEASE......................... 97

Chapter 7

HYPEREXTENSION INJURIES OF THE SOFT TISSUES OF THE
CERVICAL SPINE 134

Chapter 8

COMPLICATIONS AND RESULTS OF OPERATIVE TREATMENT FOR
CERVICAL SPINE DISEASE... 154

Chapter 9

CLINICAL SYNDROME OF THE THORACIC INTERVERTEBRAL DISC 171

Chapter 10

OPERATIVE TREATMENT OF THORACIC DISC DISEASE 176

Chapter 11

SALIENT CLINICAL FEATURES OF LUMBAR DISC LESIONS 181

Chapter 12

CLINICAL MANIFESTATIONS OF LUMBAR DISC SYNDROME 203

Chapter 13

CONGENITAL AND ACQUIRED ABNORMALITIES OF THE LUMBAR SPINE
(Their Relation to Back or Back and Leg Pain) 249

Chapter 14

THE CONSERVATIVE THERAPY OF LUMBAR DISC DISEASE 277

Chapter 15

OPERATIVE TREATMENT OF LUMBAR DISC DISEASE 287

Chapter 16

COMPLICATIONS, FAILURES AND TRAGEDIES OF OPERATIVE
TREATMENT OF LUMBAR DISC DISEASE 324

Chapter 17

RESULTS OF OPERATIVE TREATMENT OF MECHANICAL DISORDERS
OF THE LUMBAR SPINE 354

INDEX 367

Chapter 1

ANATOMY

EMBRYOLOGY

A firm understanding of the developmental processes involved in the embryology of the spine will be a great help in understanding the form and function of the adult spine and deviations from this norm. Many of the congenital anomalies are easily understood when viewed in terms of aberrations of sequential embryologic stages.

The spine is a segmented structure, the precursors of which may be noted as early as the twenty-first day of development. At this time the paraxial mesoderm of the embryo begins to segment into paired cubical masses termed somites. The first somite forms just behind the level of the cephalic end of the notochord and successive somites subsequently differentiate in a caudal direction from the paraxial mesoderm. No somites form beyond the notochord. All together 42 to 44 pairs of somites are found in the human embryo (Fig. 1-1).

As development progresses in the head and tail regions, the somites undergo either degeneration or typical development. In the midportion of the embryo, each typical somite differentiates into three distinct portions: (1) a lateral and superficial mass termed the dermatome, (2) a deeper lateral mass termed the myotome which is destined to become skeletal muscle, and (3) a central medial mass termed the sclerotome. This latter mass will give rise to connective tissue, cartilage and bone. The sclerotome begins to migrate medially and surround the notochord separating it from the neural tube and the gut[18] (Fig. 1-2).

At this stage it should be noted that there is a definite segmental structure with each segment divided by an intersegmental artery. The ultimate segmentation of the spine, however, is shifted one-half segment.

1

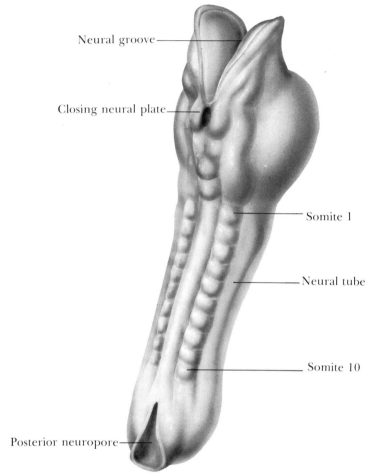

Neural groove

Closing neural plate

Somite 1

Neural tube

Somite 10

Posterior neuropore

Figure 1-1   A 23-day-old embryo showing the ten-somite stage of development.

Each of the original sclerotomes subdivides into a cranial and caudal portion, the cranial half of which fuses with the caudal half of the preceding segment. This accounts for the shift of the original segmentation by one-half segment. Consequently the intersegmental artery is no longer between segments, but in the midportion of a segment that will ultimately become a single vertebra. The segmental muscles that would originally have extended only for the length of a single vertebra now extend between the vertebrae.[24]

The work of Prader has added much to the detailed understanding of this portion of embryologic development. It was his feeling that the earlier explanations over-simplified the development of the vertebral bodies and intervertebral discs.[27] He demonstrated very elegantly that each mass of axial sclerotomic material is composed of a caudal, condensed portion and a cranial, less condensed portion. The area of cellular condensation moves progressively in a cranial direction until it is at the level of the center of the myotome. In this central position this condensed mass then differentiates into the intervertebral disc (Fig. 1-3). Subsequent-

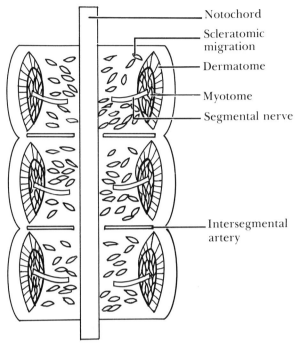

Figure 1-2 Diagrammatic drawing of the three embryonic segments illustrating dermatome, myotome and sclerotome.

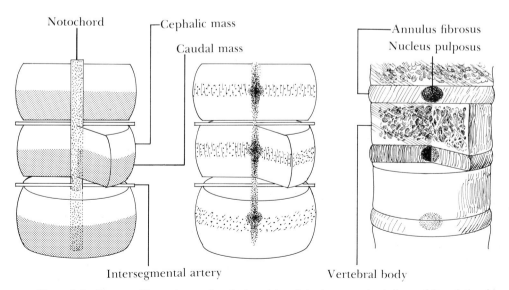

Figure 1-3 Diagram illustrating embryologic origin of the intervertebral disc and its relationship to the intersegmental artery. Note condensation of the notochord to form the nucleus pulposus. Also note cranial migration of condensed mesenchyme to form annulus fibrosus.

ly the caudal portion of the sclerotome and the cephalic portion of the immediately succeeding sclerotome fuse to form the anlage of the vertebral body. Prader's theories concur with the general body of knowledge today in regard to the histogenesis of hyaline cartilage, fibro-cartilage and ligaments (Fig. 1-3).

The notochord becomes less prominent and is gradually extruded into the intervertebral regions as its canal closes. By the end of the tenth embryonic week the notochordal cells are found entirely within that area of the disc termed the nucleus pulposus. It is generally agreed that these cells undergo mucoid degeneration. These notochordal-type cells persist until after birth and then gradually disappear. It is generally agreed that the primitive notochord plays a significant factor as the anlage of the nucleus pulposus.[10] It is also likely that a portion of the nucleus pulposus is formed by mucogelatinous degeneration of the inner portion of the fibrocartilaginous disc.[29, 31]

The annulus fibrosus is formed from the dense condensation of tissue at the intervertebral level. At first the mesodermal cells are round, without specific arrangement, but by the 10 mm. stage have become elongated, showing evidence of concentric arrangement and layering. Subsequently fibers are noted to be present in concentric lamellae, which ultimately assume alternating oblique directions, running a spinal course from one vertebra across the intervertebral space to the next. This peculiar arrangement of fiber layers will subsequently be shown to be of great importance in the physiology of the intervertebral disc.

The annulus fibrosus is the earliest portion of the disc to show a definite cellular arrangement, and it achieves its highly complex architecture long before movement or stress occurs in the vertebral column.[29] Its differentiation is complete by birth.

By the tenth week of embryologic development, the vertebral bodies are composed of typical cartilage cells and ossification centers are present. The remnants of the notochord are marked only by a streak of mucoid material. The ossification center of the vertebral body enlarges, ultimately dividing the cartilaginous anlage of the vertebra into two separate plates covering the adjacent surfaces of the vertebra.[27] These plates contribute by enchondral bone formation to the growth of the vertebra. Cartilaginous plate is comparable to the epiphysis of a long bone; it is thickest at its margins which form the "epiphyseal ring."

In addition to the ossification center present for the body of the vertebra, one is present in the cartilaginous anlage of each side of the neural arch (Fig. 1-4). At the time of birth the vertebra consists of three ossification centers united by cartilage, one piece for the body and the others for the two sides of the neural arch. Subsequently the two sides of the arch will unite and then join the body of the vertebra. Union of the laminae in the midline is accomplished between the first and seventh years of life. The united arch will join the body of the vertebra between the third and seventh years, generally proceeding from a cranial to a caudal direction. Additional ossification centers, referred to as apophyses, appear for the spinous and transverse processes. The previously described epiphyseal rings unite to the body of the vertebra between the seventeenth and twenty-fifth years.[23]

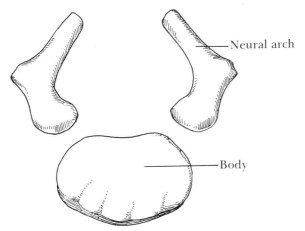

Figure 1-4 Diagrammatic illustration of the three embryologic segments of a typical vertebra. There are two dorsal segments forming the neural arch and one ventral segment forming the body of the vertebra.

THE VERTEBRAL COLUMN

The spine is composed in the human of 33 vertebrae, seven cervical, 12 thoracic, five lumbar, a sacrum of five fused segments and a coccyx of four fused segments. With the exception of the first and second cervical vertebrae the vertebral bodies are separated one from the other by intervertebral discs. One-fourth of the total length of the vertebral column may be accounted for by the discs. During the course of a typical day the length of the spine may shorten because of shrinkage of the disc through dehydration.

The early fetal shape of the vertebral column is essentially that of a letter C with anterior concavity. By the time of parturition a lordosis, which becomes more prominent as the infant begins to hold up his head and to sit, is present in the cervical area. Similarly at a later period the lumbar lordosis becomes evident and progresses as the child begins to stand and walk. The cervical lordosis consolidates at the third month of life, the lumbar lordosis toward the end of the first year[23] (Fig. 1-5).

The typical vertebra consists of a body or centrum and a neural arch. The body and neural arch enclose an area known as the vertebral foramen, through which the spinal cord passes. The arch is composed of two pedicles, which form its sides, and the laminae which form the roof. A spinous process projects dorsally from the midline of the laminae. Extending laterally from the junction of the laminae and pedicles are found the transverse processes. Projecting upward from the junction of the pedicles and the laminae are found the superior articular processes, and, projecting downward, the inferior articular processes which form synovial joints between two adjacent vertebrae. Thus between any two typical vertebrae, articulations are found between their articular processes and the intervertebral disc.

On the lower border of each pedicle is found a deep notch and on the upper border a smaller notch, which together form the intervertebral

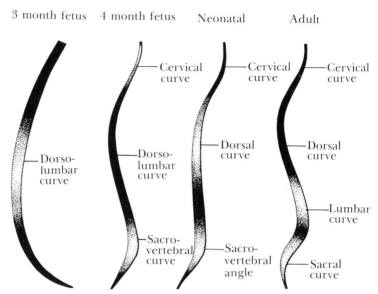

3 month fetus   4 month fetus   Neonatal   Adult

Cervical curve
Cervical curve
Cervical curve

Dorso-lumbar curve
Dorso-lumbar curve

Dorsal curve
Dorsal curve

Lumbar curve

Sacro-vertebral curve
Sacro-vertebral angle
Sacral curve

Figure 1-5   This diagram illustrates the evolution of the spinal curves from the earliest simple C-shaped curve to the mature configuration with a cervical lordosis, thoracic kyphosis and lumbar lordosis.

foramina. The foramina are longer in their vertical dimension than in their horizontal one. Through these intervertebral foramina pass the spinal nerves which usually occupy the uppermost portion of the foramina.

Cervical Vertebrae

The osseous elements of the cervical spine comprise seven vertebrae. Between each vertebral body below the level of the second vertebra is interposed an intervertebral disc. From cephalad to caudad the massiveness of each subsequent vertebra increases progressively. Four of these vertebrae, namely the third, fourth, fifth and sixth, exhibit identical anatomic features and are therefore designated typical vertebrae (Fig. 1-6). The first, second and seventh vertebrae possess distinct anatomic features not encountered elsewhere and are therefore known as atypical vertebrae. It is interesting to note in the examination of a typical vertebra that the height of the body anteriorly is usually less than posteriorly, so that the cervical curve is due to the configuration of the discs rather than the bodies.

The body of a typical cervical vertebra is elongated transversely so that its width is approximately 50 per cent greater than its anteroposterior dimension. The upper surface is concave from side to side. This concavity is deepened by an uncinate process which is a bony prominence projecting upward from the posterolateral aspect of the rim of the body. The upper surface is also convex in the anteroposterior direction. The lower surface of the vertebral body is convex from side to side and concave in

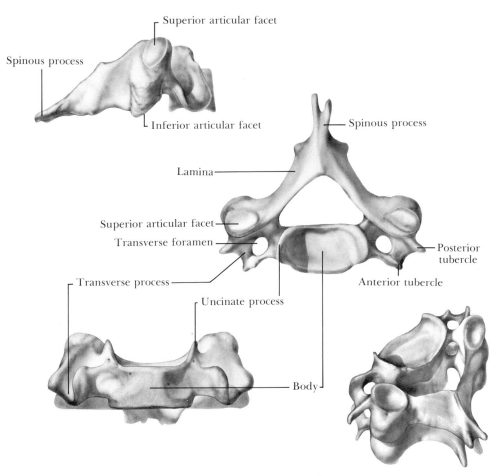

Figure 1-6 Typical cervical vertebra.

the anteroposterior direction. A prominent inferior overhanging lip is noted on the anteroinferior surface of the vertebral body. The inferior and slightly posterolateral aspects of the first vertebral body are beveled and lie in apposition to the uncinate process of the body, below which they form the bony components of the so-called joints of Luschka.

The pedicles are short and bear superior and inferior articular processes. The articular surfaces of the superior facet face upward and posteriorly, whereas those of the inferior articular facet face downward and anteriorly. On either side of the body are situated the transverse processes. These are short at development and developmentally evolve from separate anterior and posterior components. The anterior portion of the transverse process is developmentally a rib, whereas the posterior portion is a true transverse process. These portions fuse, but between them persists the transverse foramen which allows for passage of the vertebral artery. The transverse processes contain a gutter running obliquely from back to front for the spinal nerves. Posteriorly the laminae terminate in a short, slender spinous process which is bifid.

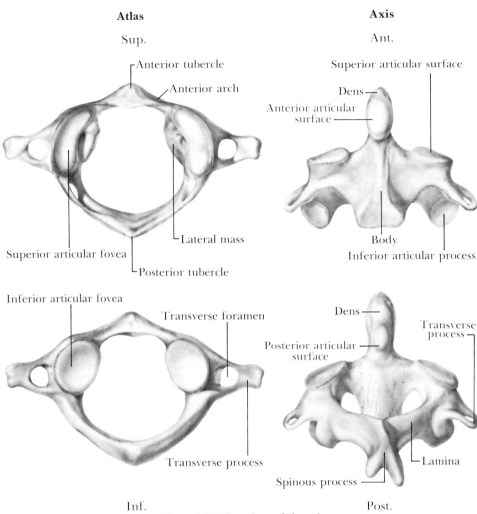

Atlas

Sup.

Anterior tubercle

Anterior arch

Lateral mass

Superior articular fovea

Posterior tubercle

Inferior articular fovea

Transverse foramen

Transverse process

Inf.

Axis

Ant.

Superior articular surface

Dens

Anterior articular surface

Body

Inferior articular process

Dens

Posterior articular surface

Transverse process

Lamina

Spinous process

Post.

Figure 1-7   The atlas and the axis.

The atlas, or first cervical vertebra, possesses no vertebral body (Fig. 1-7). Its body is joined to that of the second cervical vertebra, the axis, to form the odontoid process, or dens. The atlas consists of an anterior and posterior arch and heavy lateral masses which bear the superior and inferior articular surfaces. The superior facets articulate with the occiput and the inferior with the axis. Spanning the lateral masses anteriorly is the slender anterior arch lying in front of the dens. It has on its internal surface a facet for articulation with the dens and on its anterior surface an anterior tubercle for muscular attachments. The posterior arch is longer and bears a small posterior tubercle in place of a spinous process. On its upper surface are found sulci for the vertebral arteries.

The second cervical vertebra, also known as the axis, is identified by the projection of the odontoid process or dens which was developmentally the body of the first vertebra. The dens is continuous with the body of the second vertebra. Its spinous process is massive, elongated and bifid. The superior articular surfaces are large and face upward, posteriorly and laterally. They are placed on heavy masses arising from the body and pedicles. It should be noted parenthetically that the second spinal nerves pass dorsal to the joints between the atlas and axis instead of anterior to the synovial joints as do the remaining spinal nerves.

The seventh cervical vertebra is considered atypical because of its particularly long and unbifurcated spinous process. This is known as the vertebra prominens. The seventh cervical vertebra also has a small transverse foramen since it does not usually transmit the vertebral artery.

Thoracic Vertebrae

The thoracic vertebrae are 12 in number and progress in size as examined from a cranial to caudal direction (Fig. 1-8). They are unique in that they present on each side of the body facets for articulation with the heads of the ribs. Their anterior height is 1 to 2 mm. less than their posterior height; this difference accounts primarily for the thoracic kyphosis. The body surfaces above and below are essentially flat. As noted previously the vertebral notches on the pedicles are deeper on the inferior surface than the superior one and together form the intervertebral foramina.

The laminae are long and overlap the laminae of the succeeding vertebrae. The spinous processes are long and slender and also tend to overlap the succeeding spinous process. The superior articular facets face posterior upward and laterally; the inferior articular facets face anteriorly, inferiorly and medially. The long heavy transverse processes bear facets on their lateral anterior surfaces for articulation with the tubercles of the ribs. These vary somewhat in the first, eleventh and twelfth thoracic vertebrae. The body of a thoracic vertebra may exhibit half of a facet at both its upper and lower borders for articulation with the head of the rib. The arrangement of these facets also varies somewhat at the cranial and caudal extremes of the thoracic spine.

Lumbar Vertebrae

The lumbar vertebrae are easily identified by their large heavy configuration (Fig. 1-9). The bodies are wider transversely than in the anteroposterior direction. The last three lumbar vertebrae tend to have less height anteriorly than posteriorly and are therefore slightly wedge-shaped, as viewed from the side. The pedicles are massive and exhibit a shallow superior vertebral notch and a deep inferior vertebral notch. The transverse processes are long and delicate, being flattened in their anteroposterior direction. On the dorsal surface of the base of each transverse process is an accessory process.

The laminae are directed in a caudal direction from their attachment to the pedicle, forming a V shape. The spinous processes are broad and

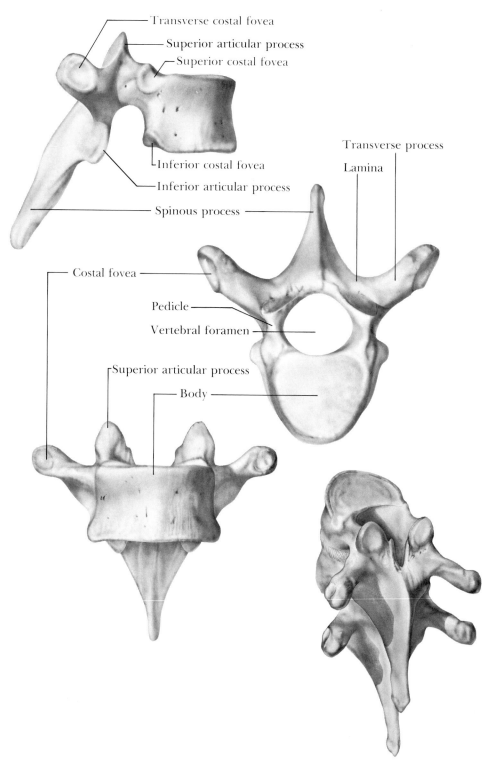

Figure 1-8   Typical thoracic vertebra.

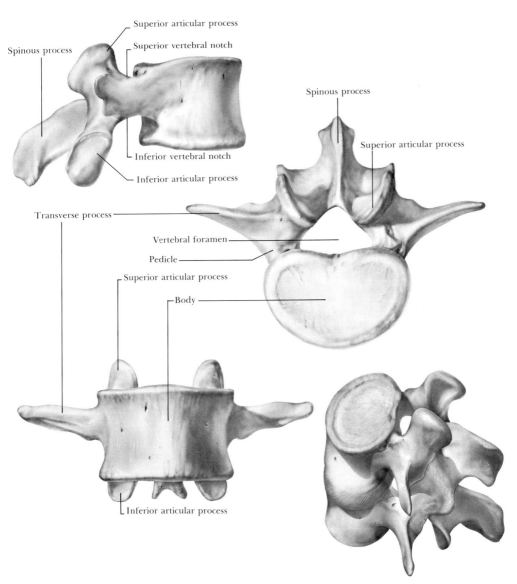

Figure 1-9 Typical lumbar vertebra.

massive with a prominent thickening of the tip. The superior articular processes arise at the junction of the laminae and pedicle and have on their posterior borders a mammillary process. The articular surfaces of the superior articular process face medially and backward. In succeeding vertebrae they tend to face more posteriorly and less medially. The inferior articular process is essentially a mirror image of the superior articular process in regard to its direction.

The Sacrum

The sacrum is composed of five fused sacral vertebrae. The central portion of the sacrum consists of the fused bodies of the five sacral vertebrae. On its dorsal surface a series of tubercles are noted in the midline to form a mean sacral crest. On each side of this crest a series of tubercles are noted forming an intermediate crest, representing the vestigial articular processes. There is a dorsally located sacral hiatus at the lower portion of the sacral canal. The sacral foramina are typically located opposite each other forming a communicating canal from the pelvic to the dorsal surface of the sacrum, which also communicates medially with the sacral portion of the vertebral canal. These allow for the exit of the dorsal and ventral branches of the spinal nerves.

The superior articular processes arise from the dorsal aspect of the sacrum and face posteriorly for articulation with the inferior articular process of the fifth lumbar vertebra. Laterally the sacrum articulates with the ilium. The articular surface which forms the actual articulation resembles an external ear. These represent the small part of the sacroiliac articulation and show a synovial cavity. Dorsal to this articular surface are roughened areas or tuberosities which receive the strong sacroiliac ligaments.

The Coccyx

Four vertebral bodies fuse to form the coccyx. Projecting upward from its dorsal surface are paired cornua, which represent pedicle superior articular processes. The first segment of the coccyx may also exhibit short transverse processes. There may be a vestigial fibrocartilaginous disc between the first and second coccygeal segments. If this is present the coccyx then presents as two bony segments.

The Intervertebral Discs

The intervertebral discs together form approximately 25 per cent of the length of the vertebral column above the sacrum. This percentage varies in the different parts of the spinal column. In the cervical region the disc contributes 22 per cent of the length of the column, in the thoracic region 20 per cent, and in the lumbar area 33 per cent. The discs

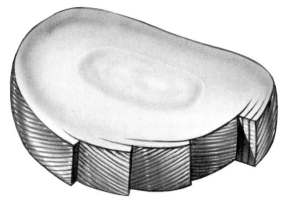

Figure 1-10 Diagram illustrating the alternating layers of the annulus fibrosus, in which the fibers run in alternating oblique directions.

form the chief structural units between adjacent vertebral bodies. They serve to allow greater motion between the vertebral bodies than if they were in direct apposition. More important, they distribute weight over a large surface of the vertebral body during bending motions, weight that would otherwise be concentrated on the edge toward which the spine is bent. They also serve a shock-absorbing function during direct vertical loading.

The annulus fibrosus forms the outer boundary of the disc and is composed of fibrocartilaginous tissue in which fibrous tissue predominates. These fibers are arranged in concentric lamellae from which the fibers run obliquely from one vertebra to the next. In successive layers the fibers slant in alternate directions, so that the fibers of each ring cross those of the two adjacent rings at an angle (Fig. 1-10). The peripheral fibers pass over the edge of the cartilaginous endplates to unite with the bone of the vertebral body as Sharpey's fibers. The deeper fibers insert into the hyaline cartilage at each end of the disc. The most superficial anterior fibers blend with the anterior longitudinal ligament as the posterior fibers blend with the posterior longitudinal ligament.

The annulus tends to be thicker anteriorly than posteriorly, which may be one of the factors responsible for the predominance of posterior protrusion of the nucleus pulposus. In addition, the anterior longitudinal ligament is stronger, and in the lumbar region broader. The annulus fibrosus is basophilic, a property which increases towards the nucleus. Superficially the layers stain acidophilic as do the longitudinal ligaments.

The nucleus pulposus is centrally situated and consists of collagen fibrils enmeshed in a mucoprotein gel. It occupies approximately 40 per cent of the disc's cross-sectional area. The nucleus pulposus has a high water content which decreases with age. The line of delineation between the nucleus pulposus and annulus is rather clear in young specimens and becomes less so in adults. The nucleus is usually located between the middle and posterior thirds of the disc. Microscopically, cells of a notochordal type are found at birth but with aging become less prominent as the nucleus becomes more fibrous and dense. In adulthood the cells of the nucleus resemble chondrocytes and fibroblasts in a gelatinous matrix.

The cartilaginous plates limit the upper and lower borders of the disc and are composed of hyaline cartilage. They are at the zone of junction between the bone and the vertebra and the fibrous portion of the disc. This cartilage covers the perforated bony endplate but does not cover the compact peripheral epiphysis. Much of the collagen fibers which lead to the annulus fibrosus take origin from these cartilaginous plates. Whether this cartilaginous plate is a portion of the disc or of the vertebral body is merely a question of terminology.

The discs in the cervical region are thicker anteriorly than posteriorly and are entirely responsible for the normal cervical lordosis. They do not conform completely to the surface of the vertebral bodies with which they are connected, being slightly smaller in width than the vertebral bodies. The discs bulge anteriorly beyond the adjacent vertebrae. The nucleus pulposus in the cervical spine is located more anteriorly than in other portions of the spine.

The relationship of the lateral portion of the disc to the so-called joints of Luschka is very controversial. Our studies support the findings of those workers who are of the opinion that there exists an uncinate portion of the annulus fibrosus which extends laterally between the beveled inferior portion of the superior vertebrae and the uncinate portion of the inferior vertebrae. We feel this precludes the opinion that the joints of Luschka are true synovial joints. Because of the relatively free range of motion between cervical vertebrae, the annulus fibrosus in this region, with time, laminates layers of fibers and eventually forms actual spaces, which may be erroneously interpreted as synovial cavities, between them. This region is of clinical importance because it forms one of the boundaries of the intervertebral foramina and lies in close relationship to the cervical nerve root as it traverses the foramen.

The discs in the thoracic region are of equal height anteriorly and posteriorly, and thus the thoracic kyphosis is due primarily to the shape of the body of the vertebra rather than to that of the disc. The thoracic discs are thinner than those in the cervical or lumbar area. One might then expect the mobility of the thoracic vertebral column to be somewhat restricted as compared to that of the cervical and lumbar spine.

The lumbar intervertebral discs tend to be of greater height anteriorly than posteriorly and this tendency is most marked in the fifth lumbar disc. In the upper portion of the lumbar spine, the lordosis is due almost entirely to the shape of the disc, but in the lower lumbar area the shape of the vertebral body is also a contributory factor.

Ligaments of the Vertebral Column

The anterior longitudinal ligament is a broad, strong ligament placed on the anterior and anterolateral aspects of the vertebral bodies from the atlas to the sacrum. Its deepest fibers blend with the intervertebral disc and extend from the body of one vertebra, to the disc, to that of the adjacent vertebra. These deep fibers bind the discs and the margins of the vertebrae. More superficial fibers extend over several vertebrae, oc-

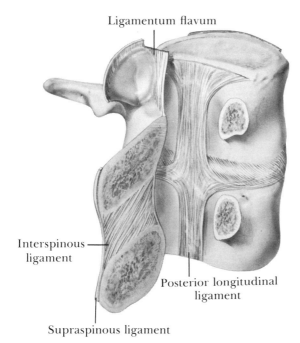

Ligamentum flavum

Interspinous ligament

Posterior longitudinal ligament

Supraspinous ligament

Figure 1-11   Ligamentous structure of the spine in the lumbar region.

casionally spanning as many as five. This ligament is most firmly bound to the vertebral bodies at their periphery. The edges of the ligament are thinner than the centermost portion (Fig. 1-11).

The posterior longitudinal ligament lies on the posterior surface of the bodies of the vertebrae from the axis to the sacrum. The tectorial membrane is continuous, and the ligament passes to the occiput. This ligament is attached most firmly to the ends of the vertebrae and most deeply to the intervening discs. A midportion of the body is only loosely attached to this ligament. As previously noted, the deepest fibers in the anterior ligament run only to adjacent vertebrae, whereas the more superficial fibers span several vertebrae. In the thoracic and lumbar regions the ligament becomes narrow as it passes over the vertebral bodies and then expands over the discs. It thus takes on the configuration of an hourglass. The lateral expansions over the intervertebral discs are rather weak and form a vulnerable point for disc herniations compared to the strong central band.

Capsular ligaments are present surrounding the synovial joints between the superior and inferior articular processes of adjacent vertebrae. Of necessity these ligaments are lax to allow the necessary gliding motion between these joints and they add little stability. Best developed in the lumbar region, the intertransverse ligaments join the transverse processes of adjacent vertebrae.

Posteriorly between adjacent laminae are found the ligamenta flava. These yellow ligaments, which have been studied extensively,[32] extend from the roots of the articular process on one side to those on the opposite, and, contrary to earlier statements found in the literature, there is no gross cleavage in the midline. These ligaments extend laterally into the intervertebral foramen forming a portion of the roof of the foramen and in certain areas, such as the thoracic spine, actually turn dorsally out of the foramen and fuse with the capsule of the apophyseal joint. The ligamenta flava are attached inferiorly to the superior edge and the posterosuperior surfaces of the laminae. Superiorly they are attached to the inferior and antero-inferior surfaces of the laminae. This unique attachment, combined with the anterior tilting of the laminae, has the effect of creating an extremely smooth postero-inferior wall of the spinal canal. This wall remains smooth in the various postural positions and serves to protect the neural elements. Most investigators have come to discard the concept of "hypertrophy" of the ligamenta flava as a clinical entity.

The supraspinous and interspinous ligaments are found between adjacent spinous processes. The supraspinous ligament is a thin ligament, composed of a high percentage of elastic tissue, running over the tips of the spinous processes. In the cervical region it is continuous with the ligamenta nuchae. The interspinous ligaments are thin and relatively weak, passing from one spinous process to the adjacent one. They are best developed in the lumbar area.

ATLANTO-OCCIPITAL AND ATLANTOAXIAL JOINTS AND LIGAMENTS

There are two large articulations between the occiput and the atlas. Each joint is formed by the deeply concave, oval, superior articular surface of the lateral mass of the atlas and the corresponding convex condyle of the occiput. The joints are condyloid in configuration, and the articular surfaces are reciprocally curved. In spite of the massiveness of this joint, strong accessory ligaments are necessary to provide stability in this area. The anterior atlanto-occipital membrane is a strong, dense band composed of interweaving fibers which stretch the anterior margin of the foramen magnum above to the upper border of the anterior arch of the atlas below. In the midline there is a round, tough band of fibers connecting the anterior tubercle of the atlas with the occiput. This can be considered a continuation of the anterior longitudinal ligament. The posterior atlanto-occipital membrane is thinner than its anterior counterpart and connects the posterior margin of the foramen magnum with the upper border of the posterior arch of the atlas. Inferiorly and laterally, there is an arched defect which permits the passage of the vertebral artery and the first cervical nerve. The articular capsules of the atlanto-occipital joints are loose, thin structures connecting the condyles of the occiput with the superior articular process of the axis (Fig. 1-12).

In addition to the ligaments between the occiput and the atlas, stability of the cranium on the vertebral column is further insured by a group of ligaments between the occiput and the axis.

The alar ligaments are short, strong bundles of fibrous tissue directed

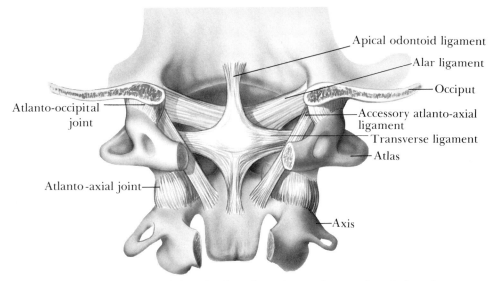

Apical odontoid ligament

Alar ligament

Occiput

Accessory atlanto-axial ligament

Transverse ligament

Atlas

Atlanto-occipital joint

Atlanto-axial joint

Axis

Figure 1-12   Ligaments of the spine from the occiput to the second cervical vertebra.

obliquely upward and laterally from either side of the upper part of the odontoid process to the medial aspect of the condyles of the occiput. Because these ligaments restrict rotation of the head on the atlas they are often referred to as check ligaments.

The apical odontoid ligament is a tough, fibrous cord arising from the apex of the odontoid process between the alar ligaments. It inserts into the anterior margin of the foramen magnum.

The tectorial membrane or occipito-axial ligament is a broad, strong band lying in the vertebral column and immediately behind the body of the axis and its ligaments. Below, it is anchored to the posterior surface of the body of the axis and, above, to the basilar groove of the occiput. The structure, essentially, is a continuation upward of the posterior longitudinal ligament.

There are three true synovial articulations between the atlas and the axis, the two lateral atlantoaxial joints and the median atlantoaxial joint. The lateral joints are formed by the inferior articular surfaces of the atlas and the superior articular surfaces of the axis. They are a large mass of arthrodial or gliding joints, second in size only to the atlanto-occipital joints. Their broad surfaces are directed slightly downward and laterally. The median atlantoaxial joint is essentially a pivot joint with two synovial cavities, one anteriorly between the dens and the posterior surface of the anterior arch of the atlas, and the other between the posterior aspect of the dens and front of the transverse ligament of the atlas.

As in the atlanto-occipital region, important ligaments are found which add stability to the atlas and axis. These are the articular capsules and their accessory ligaments. The capsular tissues are loose, but they are reinforced posteriorly and medially by stout fibrous bands termed accessory ligaments. These are anchored below to the body of the axis on

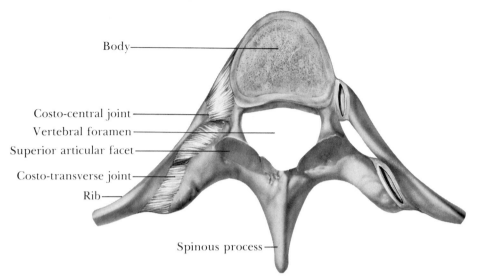

Body

Costo-central joint

Vertebral foramen

Superior articular facet

Costo-transverse joint

Rib

Spinous process

Figure 1-13   Ligamentous structures in the thoracic spine.

either side of the odontoid process and above to the lateral mass of the atlas in relation to the transverse ligament. The anterior atlantoaxial ligament is a broad, dense membrane extending from the interior border of the anterior arch of the atlas to the anterior aspect of the body of the axis. Anteriorly and in the midline, it is reinforced by a round cord which is a continuation of the anterior longitudinal ligament. It is attached above to the tubercle of the anterior arch of the atlas and below to the body of the axis.

The posterior atlantoaxial ligament is also a broad, fibrous band, but thinner than its anterior counterpart. It stretches from the lower border of the posterior arch of the atlas to the upper margin of the laminae of the axis. Essentially it corresponds to the ligamenta flava of the lower vertebrae.

The transverse ligament of the atlas is undoubtedly the most important component of the system of ligaments of this region. It is a broad, strong, triangular ligament arching across the ring of the atlas and firmly anchored on each side to a tubercle in the medial surfaces of the lateral masses of the atlas. Note that it is concave in front and convex behind. It divides the ring into two compartments, a small anterior and a large posterior one. In the anterior compartment lies the odontoid process, which is held firmly against the anterior arch of the atlas by the transverse ligament. There are two synovial cavities, one between the arch of the atlas and the dens anteriorly, and the other between the transverse ligament and the dens posteriorly. The posterior compartment is occupied by the medulla spinalis and its membranes. The transverse ligament gives off two strong fasciculi. The superior fasciculus is prolonged upward to the basal part of the occiput; the inferior is attached to the posterior surface of the body of the axis. This arrangement gives the transverse ligament a cruciate configuration (Fig. 1-13).

NERVE SUPPLY

The problem of the source of pain in degenerative disease of the spine has not yet been answered. Two general approaches have been used, in an attempt to solve this problem. The first method of approach has been the gross and histologic study of the nerve supply in the osseous and soft tissue elements of the spine. If nerve endings associated by physiologists with the sensation of pain are found in a particular structure, it might be presumed that the structure is one of the sources of back pain. The second approach is the introduction of certain noxious stimuli, such as the injection of hypertonic saline or the mechanical pinching of a structure, in order to reproduce pain.

Both of these approaches provide incomplete answers. It is obvious that the noxious stimuli utilized by investigators for the most part are artifactual and not comparable to the actual degenerative processes which occur. The fact that a ligament, when injected with hypertonic saline reproduces a back pain syndrome, does not provide conclusive evidence that this ligament is the source of difficulty when this syndrome is found in a patient. It is also readily evident to the student of physiology or microscopic anatomy that there is a very poor correlation between the anatomic location of various nerve endings and the various sensory modalities perceived from this area.

It is generally assumed that the sinuvertebral nerve carries many of the important sensory fibers from the organs concerned with the production of low back pain. The sinuvertebral nerve arises from its spinal nerve near the ramus communicans.[30] The nerve enters the spinal canal by way of the intervertebral foramen and curves upwards around the base of the pedicle proceeding toward the midline on the posterior longitudinal ligament. It supplies the posterior longitudinal ligament, the blood vessels of the epidural space, the dura mater and the periosteum. Pedersen further studied the posterior rami of the spinal nerves and found that they supply branches to skin, muscle, intertransverse ligaments and apophyseal joints. He concluded that both a sympathetic and spinal component were present in both of these nerves.

In histochemical studies utilizing the methylene blue immersion technique[21] and silver nitrate and Gomori cholinesterase techniques,[26] soft tissue, bone and articular structures were studied for the presence of nerve endings. The lumbodorsal fascia, supraspinous ligaments and interspinous ligaments exhibited both fine free fibers and complex unencapsulated nerve endings. In the ligamenta flava, fine free fibers were found in the outermost layers but no nerve structures were found in the deeper substances of these structures.

Hirsch demonstrated fine free fiber and complex unencapsulated endings in the anterior and posterior longitudinal ligaments.[21] The outermost layers of the annulus fibrosus demonstrated free fiber endings although the deeper layers of the annulus and the nucleus are apparently free of all nerve fibers. The intervertebral joint capsules exhibited the usual triad of nerve endings found in all other synovial joint capsules, that is, fine free fibers, complex unencapsulated and small encapsulated nerve endings. The vertebral periosteum exhibited both fine free fibers and complex unencapsulated nerve endings. Again, it must be stressed that there is no definitive correlation between the structure and function of these sensory elements.

When injected with a noxious substance (hypertonic saline — 11%),[21] many anatomic locations gave rise to back pain. The disc proper, the apophyseal joints, the ligamenta flava and interspinous ligaments produced various patterns of back pain. Cloward and Compere have demonstrated that pain can be caused by pinching the annulus fibrosus or the anterior longitudinal ligament.[9]

In studies specifically of the cervical spine, it has been shown that nerve fibers were found in the anterior and posterior longitudinal ligaments and in the superficial layers of the annulus fibrosus.[14]

The Blood Supply of the Disc

There is general agreement that the nucleus pulposus and the annulus fibrosus are completely without vessels during the adult phase of life.[10, 19] Up to the age of eight years, there are small blood vessels supplying the disc through the cartilaginous endplates. There is a central axial vessel running a vertical course from the osseous vertebrae to the plate and two additional ventral dorsal vessels, termed the marginal vessels. During the first three decades of life these vessels are gradually obliterated leaving scars in the cartilaginous plate. By the time growth has ceased, these vessels are completely obliterated leaving the nucleus pulposus and annulus fibrosus without a blood supply.

RELATIONAL ANATOMY

Relations of the Spinal Cord

The upper end of the spinal cord may be defined by the beginnings of the first rootlets of the first cervical nerve or the foramen magnum. The average length of the spinal cord is found to be 45 cm. in the male and 42 cm. in the female. The termination of the cord is usually located between the upper border of the first and the upper border of the second lumbar vertebrae.[23]

There is a marked variation in the cross-sectional configuration of the cord. For the most part its lateral dimension is greater than its anteroposterior one. The average width of the cord in the cervical prominence is 13.2 mm., in the thoracic region 8 mm., and in the lumbar area 9.6 mm. The average depth in the cervical area is 7.7 mm., 6.5 mm. in the thoracic region and 8.0 mm. in the lumbar area.

It is significant to compare these dimensions with those of the vertebral canal as reported by Aeby. In the cervical region the width was 24.5 mm., the anteroposterior depth 14.7 mm.; in the thoracic spine 17.2 mm.

and 16.8 mm. respectively; and in the lumbar spine 23.4 and 17.4 mm. It is obvious that in the lumbar area, these dimensions are not critical as the cord self-terminates before it drops below the level of L2.

In the cervical spine the relationship between the cord and vertebral canal is more critical. In certain individuals the cervical cord fills a substantially larger percentage of the anteroposterior diameter of the canal than others. In these persons, should spondylosis develop, a significant myelopathy could occur. The shape of the spinal cord is oval, whereas that of the canal in the cervical spine is triangular. This lack of uniformity between the canal and the cord allows the formation of a gutter anterolaterally between the cord and the walls of the canal. This recess permits some narrowing of the canal anterolaterally without compression of the spinal cord. The effect of disc herniations in relationship to the above noted dimensions will determine the clinical significance of the herniation.

Relations of the Spinal Nerves

The dorsal roots arise through a series of rootlets which attach to the spinal cord from the posterolateral sulcus. The ventral rootlets arise in an anterolateral position with no sulcus. The rootlets run separately through the subarachnoid space with a caudal inclination (below the level of C3) with increasing obliquity in a caudal direction to reach their respective foramina. At the level of the intervertebral foramina, the roots, still separate, turn laterally (in sheaths represented by both dura and arachnoid) to unite with each other just distal to the dorsal nerve root ganglia. These ganglia are found at the level of the intervertebral foramina. The average length of these nerve rootlets varies from 3 mm. in the cervical area to 266 mm. in the coccygeal area.[23]

At and below the level of the fifth cervical nerve, the obliquity of these nerve rootlets is such that the zone of exit of the respective roots is opposite a disc that is one level higher than the foramen transversed by the roots. For example, the cord segment of the sixth cervical nerve lies opposite the C4-5 intervertebral disc, but the sixth radicular nerve, as it approaches its foramen, lies opposite the C5-6 disc. In a similar fashion the posterior roots at and below the fifth cervical area enter the cord at a higher level than their respective foramina.

It should be noted that the dorsal root of any one nerve is considerably larger than its ventral root. The dural sleeve that surrounds the nerve roots becomes continuous with the epineurium of the spinal nerve as it exits the intervertebral foramen. In the lumbar area the major portion of the nerve roots lie in the lumbar cistern of the cauda equina. In this cistern the nerve roots are loose and follow a sinuous course.

Although the rootlets of the lumbar and sacral nerves are normally lax, in ventro-flexion there is a marked increase in tension due to a lengthening of the spinal canal with a subsequent stretching of the cord. Since this cord is anchored at its extremities, a marked increase in the tension of the nerve rootlets results.[6] The clinical significance of this is evident when one considers the stress-strain phenomena which have been demonstrated in human spinal nerve roots.[34] Sunderland has shown that these nerve roots fail at low values which may be created by the various pathologic entities such as a degenerated lumbar disc.

Relations of the Intervertebral Foramina

In the cervical spine the intervertebral foramina are of special significance (Fig. 1-14). They are essentially small canals approximately four mm. in length directed anterolaterally and inferiorly. They are ovoid in shape with vertical diameters of approximately ten mm. in height. The anteroposterior diameter is approximately half of this. The roofs and floors of the foramina comprise the grooves in the bases of the adjacent vertebral arches. The posterolateral wall of each foramen is formed by the adjacent posterolateral articular processes. The superior process of the caudad vertebra contributes more to the formation of this boundary than the inferior process of the cephalad vertebra. The anterolateral wall of each foramen is formed by the lateral portion of the adjacent bodies, the uncovertebral joints and the inferior portion of the superior vertebra.

All of the cervical spinal nerves except the first and second are contained in the intervertebral foramina. The first cervical nerve lies in close relation to the superior articulation of the atlas and the vertebral artery, and the second in close proximity to the atlanto-axial articulation of the vertebral artery.

The nerve roots and mixed spinal nerve completely fill the anteroposterior diameter of the intervertebral foramina. The upper one-quarter of the canal is filled with areolar tissue and small veins. In addition to these structures, small arteries arising from the vertebral

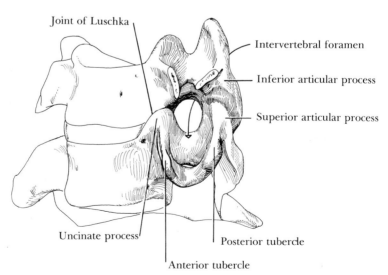

Joint of Luschka

Intervertebral foramen

Inferior articular process

Superior articular process

Uncinate process

Posterior tubercle

Anterior tubercle

Figure 1-14 The osseous structures which contribute to the cervical intervertebral foramen. Note the relationships of the joints of Luschka and the apophyseal joint to this foramen. Hypertrophy of these structures can readily lead to constriction in this area.

arteries and the sinuvertebral nerves traverse the canals. Any space-taking lesion which pinches on the anteroposterior diameter of the intervertebral foramen might be expected to cause compression of the nervous tissue elements traversing this limited space. The close proximity of the contents of the intervertebral foramen to the uncovertebral joints anteromedially and to the apophyseal joints posterolaterally should be noted, since these are potential sites of hyperplastic processes which may constrict the canal. Flexion of the cervical spine will increase the vertical diameter of the foramen while extension decreases it.

In the lumbar area, the intervertebral foramen is limited in front by a portion of the adjacent vertebral bodies and the disc. The pedicles of the adjacent vertebrae above and below form the superior and inferior boundaries of the foramen. Posteriorly, the superior and inferior articular processes together with the ligamenta flava form the remainder of the border of the canal.

The lumbar intervertebral foramen is normally five to six times the diameter of the spinal nerve which traverses it, permitting it relatively great freedom from constriction.[17] Extension and lateral flexion may decrease the diameter of this foramen significantly. In the lumbar area the foramina are sufficiently elongated that the spinal nerve exits at a level across the vertebral body above the disc space rather than across from the disc proper. Thus, a protruding lumbar disc will narrow the foramen below the level of the exit of the nerve. A disc will then produce its clinical effect by compressing through the dura the most laterally situated nerve of the cauda equina at that level, that is, the nerve that makes its exit at the foramen below the level of the disc. Hence, a degenerated disc at the L5 level will produce an S1 radiculitis.

Nerve-Disc Relationship

All spinal nerves below the cervical level emerge from the intervertebral foramina below the corresponding numbered vertebrae. Thus, the L5 spinal nerve exits in the intervertebral foramen between L5 and the sacrum. In the cervical spine however, the cervical nerves emerge above the similarly numbered vertebrae. The fifth cervical nerve, for instance, emerges between the fourth and fifth cervical vertebrae.

In attempting to localize a disc lesion by the affected nerve root, several factors should be recalled. As noted earlier, the lumbar nerves are nestled sufficiently high in the intervertebral foramina that they will not be affected by a degenerated disc at the same level unless the disc fragment migrates cranialward. The fifth lumbar nerve root, therefore, will be compressed not by a degenerated L5-S1 disc but more often by a degenerated L4-5 disc. In the cervical spine a disc protrusion will usually affect the nerve root exiting at the same level as the disc, but the numbering system is different. It should also be noted that the rootlets in the cervical spine may arise from a rather wide area from one segment above or below the level of exit of the nerve and thus a disc one segment above or below may cause compression of a particular nerve root.

Relations of the Sympathetic Nervous System

Many of the cervical syndromes present bizarre manifestations related to the sympathetic nervous system. No sympathetic fibers are found in the cervical nerve roots which comprise sensory and motor roots only. This is in contradistinction to the segmental nerves from T1 to L2 as the anterior roots contain preganglionic fibers arising from cells in the lateral horn of the spinal segments.

The cervical nerves are connected to the sympathetic system by way of the preganglionic fibers, which arise in the lateral horn cells of spinal segments T3 to T6. These issue from the spinal cord to the corresponding anterior roots and pass through the proximal portion of the anterior primary rami. Here they split off in a mass to form the white rami communicantes joining the sympathetic chain. They continue upward, and the chain can reach the stellate and middle cervical ganglion where they synapse with the postganglionic fibers. These fibers proceed to the anterior primary rami of the cervical nerves and pass through the peripheral nerves to blood vessels, sweat glands and pyeloerector muscles.

Other postganglionic fibers proceed directly from the stellate and upper thoracic sympathetic ganglion to the subclavian artery to reach the blood vessels of the upper arm. Of great importance is the relation of the sympathetic fibers extending to the orbital structures. The preganglionic fibers concerned with ocular functions arise in the lateral horn cells of spinal segments T1 and T2, traverse the anterior roots' mixed nerves, and anterior primary rami. They then join as white rami communicantes the sympathetic chain proceeding upward to reach the superior cervical ganglion where they end and synapse with the postganglionic fibers. The latter fibers proceed directly to the internal carotid and ophthalmic arteries and with these reach the orbit. Here they supply the back of the eye, the dilator muscle of the pupil and the smooth muscles of the upper lid.

Interruption of these fibers produces Horner's syndrome, whereas the irritation of these fibers results in manifestations which are directly opposite. Other postganglionic fibers proceed to many of the cranial nerves, either directly or indirectly, and are distributed to the larynx, pharynx and heart; still others, reaching the vertebral artery and its branches, are distributed to the vestibular portion of the ear.

The Vertebral Artery

The vertebral artery ascends in the foramina of the transverse processes of the cervical vertebrae, in most instances beginning at the level of the sixth cervical vertebra. It lies anterior to the anterior primary rami of the third to sixth cervical nerves inclusive. The second cervical nerve, as previously noted, has no foramen and lies posterior to the vertebral artery. The first cervical nerve, after emerging from the dura, lies on the posterior arch of the atlas immediately beneath the vertebral artery. It has been demonstrated that flexion, extension and rotation of the cervical spine may alter the blood flow in one or both vertebral arteries.[8] It is also felt that muscle spasm in the posterior and superior cervical region might produce vascular impairment in a vertebral artery.

KINESIOLOGY OF THE SPINE

Normal Motions of the Spine

Cineroentgenography of the spine has added much to our knowledge of the normal and pathologic motion of the spine.[15] In the atlanto-occipital articulation only flexion and extension are possible. Approximately ten degrees of flexion and 25 degrees of extension are possible.

The atlantoepistrophic articulation allows rotation, flexion, extension and vertical approximation. In the early stages of rotation, the skull and first cervical vertebra move together on the second cervical vertebra. Subsequent to this the remaining portions of the cervical spine partake in rotation. The total range of rotary motion is 142 degrees.[13] With lateral flexion of the head there is associated rotation of the second cervical vertebra.[15] Ten degrees of extension and five degrees of flexion are permitted at this level. During rotation C1 rides upwards in relationship to C2 as the neutral position is approached. The vertical approximation which occurs during rotation is responsible for obliteration of the joint space noted on x-ray when rotation is present.[22]

At those levels below the second cervical vertebra, flexion, extension, lateral inclination and rotation occur. During forward flexion the superior vertebra will shift anteriorly over the inferior one. While this is occurring, there is anterior narrowing of the disc space and posterior widening. The reverse is true during extension. As this disc deformation occurs, facet gliding in the apophyseal joints will also occur. During flexion, the superior facets will glide forward and upward as the vertebral body shifts forward. It has been noted that greater flexion will occur at the level of the fifth cervical vertebra in apparently normal individuals.[15] Rotation in the cervical region is always accompanied by some flexion. This is due to the fact that during lateral flexion the configuration of the apophyseal joints is such that the inferior articular process on the side toward which the neck is bent will glide downward and backward, while on the opposite side the inferior articular process glides upward and forward resulting in rotation.[23] The total range of motion in the cervical spine is 127 degrees for flexion and extension, 73 degrees total inclination, 142 degrees total rotation.[13] Individuals with thick, short, muscular necks showed less motion than those with long, thin ones. A progressively decreased range of motion was noted with aging.

The small size of the thoracic intervertebral discs limits the motion in the thoracic spine. This limitation is further enhanced by the rib cage. The frontal direction of the apophyseal joints serves to limit flexion and extension. Rotation might be expected to be relatively free due to the configuration of the facets, but this motion is also limited by the sternum and ribs. The rib cage also limits lateral bending.

Flexion and extension are free in the lumbar spine. There is a gradual transition in the relationship of the articular processes of the apophyseal joints from the upper to the lower lumbar spine, so that the upper areas of the superior articular processes face more medially and, as they descend, gradually face more posteriorly. The inferior articular processes gradually face more anteriorly and less laterally. There is a large variation in this tendency, but for the most part there is a greater amount of rotation present in the lower lumbar area than in the upper lumbar area. In young women the mean total motion between the first lumbar vertebra and the sacrum for maximal flexion to maximal extension was 92 degrees.[7] The greatest motion was present between the fifth lumbar vertebra and the sacrum, a progressive decline in motion being present with each successive vertebra in a cranial direction. The studies tend to support the earlier work of Allbrook.[1]

The Mechanical Response of the Disc

There is general agreement in the literature today that the intervertebral disc has the ability to convert a vertical pressure to a horizontal thrust, extending its energy on the annulus fibrosus. The fluid behavior of the nucleus pulposus is essential in distributing this vertical thrust. In some way, the annulus must behave as an elastic mechanism to provide for increase in the radius of the disc.[25] As the radius of the disc increases, the distance between the cartilaginous endplates decreases. It is possible that such an increase in radius can be achieved by the relative movement of adjacent uniaxial sheets of collagen fibers as are present in the annulus. Measurements of the anterior and posterior expansions of the nucleus fibrosus when compressing intervertebral discs have revealed figures of 0.5 mm. expansion with 50 kg. loads and 0.75 mm. for 100 kg. loads.[20] With degeneration this expansion increases. It has also been shown that with aging, greater stiffness and decreased residual deformation is present.[35]

When the tensile properties of the annulus fibrosus were studied in detail, it was noted that the response of the annulus varied according to the direction in which the samples were cut.[16] The annulus appeared stiffest and exhibited lowest deformation and energy dissipation in the horizontal axis. As the samples were cut in a more vertical direction, they became more extensible and had poorer recovery properties. It was also noted, as sections were sampled from the midline to the periphery of a disc across the horizontal axis, that stiffness increased and recovery properties improved. These findings are in keeping with our conceptual model of the disc as a mechanism to convert vertical thrust into horizontal thrust, which is absorbed by the elastic mechanism of the annulus. The annulus extends with ease along the vertical axis allowing motion, while its resistance against horizontal displacement provides stability.

During vertical loading there is a much greater amount of energy absorbed by the disc than during flexion or lateral bending.[12] As would be expected, the load-deflection curves during vertical loading are steeper.

This factor is of importance in evaluating injuries arising from a suddenly applied external force such as the high-speed ejection seats found in modern aircraft.

Function of the Spine

Many complex models have been constructed over the past century in an effort to understand the function of the erect human spine. The most useful and perhaps the most accurate is that of Asmussen and Klausen[3] in which the spine is considered to be a segmented pole joined to the parts lying caudal to it. This segmented pole is stabilized by guy-wires represented by the muscles of a trunk; the abdominal muscles in the front and side and the erector spinae in the back and side.

Because of the constant changing position of the spine, even during so-called quiet standing, it would seem that the spine must be kept in position by active forces primarily, rather than a balanced equilibrium. Electromyographic studies have demonstrated that only one set of these muscles is generally active during quiet standing.[3] In the majority of cases the erector spinae muscles were found to be active in counteracting gravity. It could then be assumed that, in these individuals, the center of gravity for that part of the body above the lumbar lordosis would lie ventral to the axis of movement. The earlier models constructed by Steindler[33] are at variance with these findings. X-ray studies of normal adults revealed that on the average the center of gravity passed 1 cm. ventral to the fourth lumbar vertebral body and therefore ventral to the axis of movement of the lumbar spine.[2]

When, in addition to the weight of the body, a load is added anteriorly, an entirely new situation exists. As the spine bends forward and picks up this heavy weight, it then acts as a crane for the creation of tremendous forces. Geometric calculations indicated that a disc pressure of 1600 lbs. will result when the hands lift a weight of 100 lbs.[5] These theoretical calculations are not in keeping with what is known about the yield points of the annulus fibrosus,[4, 35] which are known to have a mean of 710 lbs. Discs have been demonstrated to break down completely with a pressure of 750 lbs., and thus they would not be able to withstand the theoretical pressures calculated by Bradford and Spurling.[5] It is therefore necessary to theorize additional support for the spine under the stress of weight lifting.

It has been demonstrated that intra-abdominal pressure can act as a force in the body to aid the erector spinae and act against compression of the disc. The intra-abdominal pressure will tend to strengthen and elongate the spine by creating a moment of force in front of the disc.[4, 11] The intra-abdominal pressure can reach 140 mm. Hg. which, although it is a relatively small force, acts on a lever arm of considerable length. Under extreme circumstances increasing the intrathoracic pressure against the closed glottis will provide further support (Fig. 1-15).

It has already been implied that the theoretical approaches to the stresses on the lumbar discs may well be in error. Recently it has been

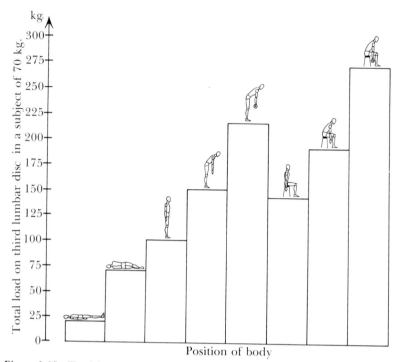

Figure 1-15 Total load on the third lumbar disc in different positions. Note that the minimum load is found in the supine horizontal position and the marked increase in load with standing in forward flexion and sitting in forward flexion. (Modified from Nachemson, A.: Acta Orthop. Scand. 36:426, 1965.)

possible to study directly, through a pressure transducer placed in the intervertebral disc, the stress that is created in various postural positions.[28] In the sitting position, the load on the disc is directly proportional to the body weight above the level of the disc. In the standing position, it was demonstrated that there is a decrease in the pressure of 30 per cent as compared to the sitting position. In the reclining position, the decrease in the load of 50 per cent was noted as compared with the sitting position. Forward leaning significantly increased the load in the sitting position as compared with erect sitting. It was demonstrated that if a 70 kg. man in a standing position lifts a 50 kg. weight and leans forward at an angle of 40 degrees, the stress in his lower lumbar disc will be about 660 lbs. The marked difference between this direct measurement in a theoretical calculation could be explained by the stress relieving effect of intra-abdominal pressure.

REFERENCES

1. Allbrook, D.: Movements of the lumbar spinal column. J. Bone Joint Surg. 39-B:339-345, 1957.
2. Asmussen, E.: The weight-carrying function of the human spine. Acta Orthop. Scand. 29:276-290, 1960.
3. Asmussen, E. et al.: Form and function of the erect human spine. Clin. Orthop. 25:55-63, 1962.

4. Bartelink, D. L.: The role of abdominal pressure in relieving the pressure on the lumbar intervertebral discs. J. Bone Joint Surg. 39-B:718-725, 1957.
5. Bradford, F. K. and Spurling, R. G.: The Intervertebral Disc. Springfield, Illinois, Charles C Thomas, 1945.
6. Breig, A. et al.: Biomechanics of the lumbo-sacral nerve roots. Acta Radiol. (Diag.) (Stockholm) 1:1141-1160, 1963.
7. Clayson, S. J. et al.: Evaluation of mobility of hip and lumbar vertebrae of normal young women. Arch. Phys. Med. 43:1-8, 1962.
8. Coburn, D.: Vertebral artery involvement in cervical trauma. Clin. Orthop. 24:61-63, 1962.
9. Compere, E. L.: Origin, anatomy, physiology, and pathology of the intervertebral disc. Instruc. Lect. Amer. Acad. Orthop. Surg. 18:15-20, 1961.
10. Coventry, M. B. et al.: The intervertebral disc: Its microscopic anatomy and pathology. Part I: Anatomy, development and physiology. J. Bone Joint Surg. 27:105-112, 1945.
11. Eie, N. et al.: Measurements of the intra-abdominal pressure in relation to weight bearing of the lumbrosacral spine. J. Oslo City Hosp. 12:205-217, 1962.
12. Evans, F. G. et al.: Biomechanical studies on the lumbar spine and pelvis. J. Bone Joint Surg. 41-A:278-290, 1959.
13. Ferlic, D.: The range of motion of the "normal" cervical spine. Bull. Johns Hopkins Hosp. 110:59-65, 1962.
14. Ferlic, D. C.: The nerve supply of the cervical intervertebral disc in man. Bull. Johns Hopkins Hosp. 113:347-351, 1963.
15. Fielding, J. W.: Cineroentgenography of the normal cervical spine. J. Bone Joint Surg. 39-A:1280-1288, 1957.
16. Galante, J. O.: Tensile properties of the human lumbar annulus fibrosus. Acta Orthop. Scand. Suppl. 100: 1-91, 1967.
17. Hadley, L. A.: Constriction of the intervertebral foramen: A cause of nerve root pressure. J.A.M.A. 140:473-476, 1949.
18. Hamilton, W. J., Boyd, J. D., and Mossman, H. W.: Human Embryology. Baltimore, Williams & Wilkins, 1962.
19. Hirsch, C. et al.: Studies on structural changes in the lumbar annulus fibrosis. Acta Orthop. Scand. 22:184-231, 1952.
20. Hirsch, C. et al.: New observations on the mechanical behavior of lumbar discs. Acta Orthop. Scand. 23:254-283, 1954.
21. Hirsch, C. et al.: The anatomical basis for low back pain. Studies on the presence of sensory nerve endings in ligamentous, capsular and intervertebral disc structures in the human lumbar spine. Acta Orthop. Scand. 33:1-17, 1963.
22. Hohl, M.: Normal motions in the upper portion of the cervical spine. J. Bone Joint Surg. 46-A:1777-1779, 1964.
23. Hollinshead, W. H.: Anatomy for Surgeons. Vol. 3: The Back and Limbs. New York, Paul B. Hoeber, Inc., 1958.
24. Hollinshead, W. H.: Anatomy of the spine: Points of interest to orthopedic surgeons. J. Bone Joint Surg. 47-A:209-215, 1965.
25. Horton, W. G.: Further observations on the elastic mechanism of the intervertebral disc. J. Bone Joint Surg. 40-B:552-557, 1958.
26. Jackson, H. C. et al.: Nerve endings in the human lumbar spinal column and related structures. J. Bone Joint Surg. 48-A:1272-1281, 1966.
27. Keyes, D. C. et al.: The normal and pathological physiology of the nucleus pulposus of the intervertebral disc. J. Bone Joint Surg. 14:897, 1932.
28. Nachemson, A.: The load on lumbar disks in different positions of the body. Clin. Orthop. 45:107-122, 1966.
29. Peacock, A.: Observations on the prenatal development of the intervertebral disc in man. J. Anat. 85:260, 1951.
30. Pedersen, H. E.: The anatomy of lumbosacral posterior rami and meningeal branches of spinal nerves (sinuvertebral nerves), with an experimental study of their functions. J. Bone Joint Surg. 38-A:377-391, 1956.
31a. Prader, A.: Die frühembryonal Entwicklung der menschlichen Zwischenwirbelscheibe. Acta Anat., 3:68-83, 1947a.
31b. Prader, A.: Die Entwicklung der Zwischenwirbelscheibe beim menschlichen Keimling. Acta Anat. 3:115-152, 1947b.
32. Ramsey, R. H.: The anatomy of the ligamenta flava, Clin. Orthop. 44:129-40, 1966.
33. Steindler, A.: Kinesiology of the Human Body, 2nd ed. Springfield, Illinois, Charles C Thomas, 1955.
34. Sunderland, S. et al.: Stress-strain phenomena in human spinal nerve roots. Brain 84:120-24, 1961.
35. Virgin, W. J.: Experimental investigations into the physical properties of the intervertebral disc. J. Bone Joint Surg. 33-B:607-611, 1951.

Chapter 2

PATHOLOGY

The understanding of the process of aging in man is the greatest challenge facing medical science today. There has been a great resurgence of interest in the cellular biology of the aging process. This heightened interest stems from agreement that comprehension of the basic mechanisms in the aging process is a necessary prerequisite to the effective treatment and prevention of diseases of senescence. Also, our basic fund of knowledge of cellular function in biochemical and biophysical terms has progressed to the point that reasonable and testable mechanisms can now be proposed and evaluated.

Biologic changes associated with aging and pathologic processes are not identical, and whenever possible these processes should be differentiated. The term "pathology" implies a deviation from normal, associated with a disease process. The concept of aging is not that simply defined. A reasonable definition is that proposed by Comfort: "Senescence is a deteriorative process. What is being measured when we measure it is a decrease in viability and an increase in vulnerability."[5] The individual is rendered progressively more likely to die from accidental causes, "Accidental" is used in its broadest sense, implying that no death is completely natural and that no one dies from the burden of years alone.

Four criteria of aging have been outlined by Strehler.[31] These are universality, progressiveness, intrinsicality and deleteriousness. The concept of universality would place a particular phenomenon as part of the aging process if it would eventually occur in all older members of a particular species. It should be recognized that certain basic universal age changes may or may not express themselves depending on the environmental situation. A predisposition to cancer, which is closely associated with basic aging processes, may not be expressed simply because the individuals have not been exposed to the appropriate tumor-inducing external agent.

A second factor is intrinsicality, which would eliminate the changes which are age correlated but due to extrinsic factors. External radiation would meet the criteria of universality but it is basically extrinsic to the system and would not be considered a basic aging process.

Progressiveness is a third factor that is used in the definition of an aging process. Most aging processes occur gradually because they are due to cellular or subcellular changes which may not become evident until they have reached the level of an organ system or the organism as a whole. Thus an individual event at a molecular level may occur suddenly and in a very short time, but large numbers of these events may be necessary to produce a gross change that will be readily apparent.

The fourth and final criterion is implied in our original definition of aging, and that is deleteriousness. The aging process should, by definition, lead to a decline in the functional capacity of the individual. This definition and criterion for the processes involved in aging is difficult to evolve and often difficult to apply to particular incidents. However, it will become apparent, as the pathology of age changes of the intervertebral disc are considered, that we must constantly appraise what is a normal aging process and what is a disease process.

It should be pointed out that in the broad biologic realm aging and natural death are not universal. Natural death as such does not occur until the metazoan species of development is reached. The unicellular organism has the potential, like the gods of ancient Greece, to live forever. Numerous examples of species can be mentioned in which there is only a minimally increased mortality as a function of age. The family of birds, particularly the parrot, the fish, with the sturgeon as an example, and certain reptiles, such as the box turtle, give good evidence that certain species are free from the ravages of senescence. It is of course the hope of investigators concerned with gerontology that by a more complete understanding other processes of aging can be controlled and eventually prevented.

Aging can be thought of in terms of tissues, cells and subcellular components. Recently much work has been directed towards the understanding of the age changes of connective tissues. This will be discussed in some detail in subsequent sections. The angry housewife who has purchased a piece of old beefsteak is readily aware of the consequences of the increased amount of collagen found in aged connective tissue.

There is a decreased regularity of the arrangement of cells and a greater variability in nuclear size with the passage of time. There is a concomitant accumulation of pigment in certain cell lines. Recent evidence suggests that there is not only a decrease in the number of functioning cells but a decrease in functional activity per cell with the passage of time. The rate of regeneration of various tissues in young animals is greater than in the old. Changes in the subcellular components such as the endoplasmic reticulum, nuclei, and mitochondria have been described with aging but require a more detailed analysis than is possible here.

It is necessary to briefly consider the three basic theories evolving today regarding the causation of age-related changes. The developmental theory of aging has as its basic concept a failure in the basic mechanisms of embryonic tissue and cellular development. A second theory is based on intercellular relationships, with particular emphasis on immunologic competition between cells. Finally, a third theory is based on the instability of certain cellular structures, due to failure of the genetic coding and read-out machinery, which results in a failure of steady-state energy maintenance.

BIOCHEMICAL CHANGES IN AGING AND DISEASE

CHANGES IN HYDRATION

The efficient functioning of the intervertebral disc depends largely on the physical properties of the nucleus pulposus which in turn are closely related to its water-binding capacity. It has been repeatedly demonstrated that there is a progressive lowering of the degree of hydration of the intervertebral disc from early life, where it has been demonstrated that the water content approaches 88 per cent, to a level of 69 per cent in the eighth decade of life.[25]

A basic question which must be posed is the mechanism whereby water is retained by the disc. Two possibilities exist, either osmotic pressure exerted by the individual molecules or imbibition pressure exerted by the protein-polysaccharide gel. There are many theoretical difficulties which prevent the acceptance of osmosis as the source of hydrophilia of the nucleus. These are outlined in detail by Hendry.[16] It is more likely that hydration of the nucleus is predominantly due to the imbibition pressure of the gel. The imbibition characteristics of normal and pathologic specimens have been found to be markedly different. The imbibition index, which is a measure of the water-binding capacity of the disc, was markedly depressed in degenerated discs. Not only were they less hydrophilic than the normal discs but they showed a greater than normal susceptibility to changes in pressure.

Several results may occur from this reduction in the imbibition pressure of the nucleus. Mainly, a greater percentage of the total strain will be transmitted to the annulus; the normal pattern of alternating tension and compression on the annulus will be modified to continual compression; and finally, a pathologic disc which has imbibed fluid may be unable to retain it when stressed. The former factors could lead directly to injury to the annulus; the latter might lead to a herniation.

COLLAGEN INCREASE

Aging is accompanied by a gradual increase in the collagen content of the human intervertebral disc.[14] This may be more marked in the pathologic than in the normal disc.[22] Naylor has pointed out that as aging progresses in the human intervertebral disc there is increasing loss of gel structure by the nucleus due to an increase in the collagen.[23] This is associated with precipitation and fibrillation of the collagen. There is an associated reduction in the elastic properties of the annulus. Coincident with the increase in collagen content is a reduction of polysaccharides. A second noncollagenous protein, termed beta-protein, appears in the discs of elderly subjects.

LIPID CHANGES

Little attention has been paid in the literature to the relationship of function and quantitative and qualitative changes of lipids of the intervertebral disc with aging. Franklin and Hoe have made a thorough analysis of the methodologies involved in lipid extraction from connective tissues and have found that the average lipid content of intervertebral disc material was 0.6 and 1.8 per cent of the tissue wet weight, for dry and wet extractions.[10]

MUCOPOLYSACCHARIDE CHANGES

Studies of degenerated intervertebral discs reveal a rather constant pattern of biochemical change. There is an increase in insoluble collagen which is poorly oriented, a general reduction in polysaccharide content, a reduction in hydration and a decrease in chondroitin sulfate without a comparable decrease in keratosulfate.[7] These findings suggest that disc herniations have as their basis a biochemical abnormality. Depolymerization of the mucopolysaccharides may be the initiating factor in the disordered gel function which occurs early in disorders of the intervertebral disc.

A basic requirement for normal disc function is perfect gel characteristics of the nucleus pulposus. With loss of chondroitin sulfate and increase in the collagen content which is fibrillated and disoriented, the nucleus is no longer capable of normal absorption and redistribution of the stresses placed upon it.[23] The work of Mitchell suggests that the biochemical differences in regard to polysaccharides are much more striking when normal and pathologic discs, rather than only young and aged discs, are compared.[22] It is his feeling that the breakdown of the protein polysaccharide linkage is the underlying aging process in the nucleus pulposus, and that in a prolapsing disc this process, which is normally seen with aging, occurs much more rapidly. Such a breakdown could lead to altered imbibition characteristics which have been demonstrated in prolapsed discs.

In summary, a series of biochemical events might be postulated in which there is a rapid breakdown of the protein polysaccharide linkages in the intervertebral disc. During this rapid breakdown of mucopolysaccharides there is a disproportionate loss of chondroitin sulfate as compared to keratosulfate. As this process is occurring there is a simultaneous rise in the collagen content and the "unmasking of a beta-protein." These changes in the macromolecular structure of the disc result in altered fluid behavior of the disc and in a reduction in the imbibition index of the disc.

If we will recall, normal function of the disc requires the presence of a perfect gel in the nucleus to evenly distribute pressure, together with high tensile strength in the annulus with associated elastic properties. These changes lead to a loss of the gel behavior in the nucleus and the desired mechanical properties of the annulus. Pressure then placed upon the nucleus will be unevenly distributed to a weakened and inelastic annulus, and a rupture or herniation may occur. This proposed model is of course simplified and, to a certain degree, hypothetical but appears reasonable in the light of today's knowledge.

GENETIC FACTORS IN INTERVERTEBRAL DISC DEGENERATION

Extensive investigation of the genetic factors in human intervertebral disc degeneration has not been performed. Berry has demonstrated that in certain genetic mutations in mice, the intervertebral discs will show greatly accelerated age changes.[3] He demonstrated that the effect of this abnormal change was a reduction in the mitotic rate of the notochord early in gestation. It was his feeling that the greatly accelerated age changes in the abnormal discs of the mice were a direct consequence of their reduced size.

AUTO-IMMUNE PHENOMENON

An auto-immune etiology for the degeneration of the intervertebral disc has been proposed by Bobechko.[4] The totally avascular nature of the mucoprotein in the nucleus pulposus makes an auto-immune phenomenon plausible. When this avascular protein becomes exposed to the general circulation it is possible that this protein serves as an antigen, which will subsequently be rejected by the host lymphocyte by an auto-immune reaction. If this is so, it might be expected that the regional lymph nodes would exhibit changes consistent with an auto-antibody response. Evidence of this process has not been conclusive and rests on the demonstration of a pyronine staining reaction within the cytoplasm of lymphoid cells in the regional lymph nodes. Certain nonspecific fluorescence indicators have also been demonstrated in these lymphoid cells. Hyperplasia and enlargement of regional para-aortic lymph nodes have been noted during the operation for anterior exploration of degenerated intervertebral discs.[4] This area, that today remains highly speculative, deserves intensive investigation in the future.

POSTURE AND PATHOLOGY

Erectness of the trunk can be regarded as an essential primate characteristic. Along with this truncal erectness, there is a marked tendency for the forelimbs to assume a dominant role. Many of the primates engage in standing, walking and running; however, man alone stands with knee extended and indulges in prolonged standing.[30] Fossil evidence suggests that this erect bipedal type of posture had its beginnings approximately 12 million years ago in the early Pliocene era. It is evident that modern man has imperfectly adapted to this upright posture, as shown not only by degenerated intervertebral discs but also by varicose veins, hemorrhoids, and hernia. The structural shortcomings of the quadruped skeleton were transformed into an erect bipedal posture, the evolution of which has been beautifully demonstrated by Yamada.[35] He amputated the forelegs and tails of rats in the first postnatal week. Subsequently, those rats that survived assumed an upright bipedal posture. Histologic examination of the intervertebral discs revealed changes typical of intervertebral disc degeneration in man.

GROSS AND MICROSCOPIC PATHOLOGY OF THE INTERVERTEBRAL DISC

One must explain herniation of the nucleus pulposus on the basis of either an extraordinarily high pressure in the nucleus, or a weakening of the annulus or both. It is the authors' feeling that the most realistic explanation for disc protrusion lies in a series of biochemical changes through which the nucleus pulposus loses its gel behavior and its ability to evenly distribute stresses transmitted to it.[23] Thus, the nucleus will transmit high pressures to certain areas of the annulus. It has been demonstrated that certain pathologic biochemical changes also occur in the annulus, with structural changes that allow herniation of the nucleus. The relationship between biochemical changes and structural stresses is not entirely clear. It is possible that the stresses placed upon the intervertebral disc by the upright posture may lead to the previously described sequence of biochemical abnormalities. It is also possible that the biochemical abnormalities occur as an independent process to weaken the structure of the disc, which will ultimately decompensate when subjected to mechanical stresses. At present these questions lack a definitive answer.

Before a detailed description of the pathologic changes in the intervertebral disc is presented, we must recall that the changes associated with aging and pathologic discs are not necessarily synonymous. Closely aligned with this problem is the question constantly posed by the thoughtful clinician, "Which of the pathologic changes described are actually producing the patients' symptoms?" This question is deceivingly simple, yet difficult to answer.

To come to a definitive answer as to which specific pathologic entities give rise to symptoms, one would ideally like to examine two large groups of spines throughout the various decades of life, one group asymptomatic and the other with symptoms of spine disease. An investigator would then be able to say with some certainty which of the findings are associated with symptoms and which are incidental. Few studies of this type are to be found in the literature.

HISTOCHEMICAL CHANGES IN THE INTERVERTEBRAL DISC

In a sequential histologic and histochemical examination of the annulus fibrosus from childhood to old age,[33] it has been found that histochemical changes make their first appearance in the third decade of life. The innermost lamellae of the annulus fibrosus show an irregular distribution of the P.A.S.-positive and Alcian blue-positive polysaccharides. There is a loss of homogeneity and enrichment of the polysaccharides in the pericellular areas, and a loss of the regularity of the fibrous pattern, with tears and holes in certain areas. The appearance of groups of typical cartilage cells can also be noted. In later age groups, the distinction between the nucleus pulposus and annulus fibrosus becomes increasingly obscure. Whether these changes are due to accumulative mechanical stresses or to a metabolic disease is as yet unclear.

The nucleus pulposus shows considerable structural changes with aging. At birth the nucleus is a well-defined structure, clearly demarcated from the annulus. It consists of a loose network of primitive mesenchymal cells. By the second and third decades of life the border between the nucleus and the annulus becomes less well-defined, the cellular content becomes sparser and the fibrous components more prominent. In the fourth and fifth decades evidence of cavitation and desiccation in the center of the nucleus may be noted, and nests of cartilage cells scattered throughout the nucleus pulposus. As yet it is not possible to say which of these changes may be classified as characteristic of aging and which as definitely pathologic.

DESCRIPTIVE PATHOLOGY OF THE CERVICAL SPINE

In discussing disc lesions and degeneration in the cervical spine, one must be precise in his terminology. There is an acute type of pathology of the intervertebral disc comprised of nuclear herniations, and there is a more diffuse, annular protrusion. In nuclear herniation, a circumscribed mass is formed by the extrusion of nuclear material through a tear in the annulus. This is a lesion found in young people and frequently associated with trauma.[34] Middle-aged and elderly people are more prone to annular protrusion. When using these terms we are speaking primarily of a problem of the intervertebral disc itself. Both of these lesions may with time develop into a diffuse degeneration of the disc and its associated, ligamentous and osseous structures, termed "cervical spondylosis." The term "degenerative arthritis" refers to synovial joints and therefore should be applied only to degeneration of the apophyseal joints.

The acute disc protrusions may be classified as dorsal, intraforaminal, lateral or ventral. Most investigators today agree that there is an intimate relationship between intervertebral disc degenerations and cervical spondylosis. Narrowing of the intervertebral discs allows close proximation of the bodies of the adjacent vertebrae, which in turn leads to the deformation of the uncus and to the formation of osteophytes along the superior margins of the distal vertebrae and the inferior margins of the proximal vertebrae. Ridge formation also develops on the anterior wall of the spinal canal with varying degrees of occlusion of the intervertebral foramen.

The authors have studied in detail 70 cervical spines, ranging in age from 38 to 95 years, obtained from the anatomic laboratory. The spines were studied grossly, microscopically and radiographically. Degeneration of the cervical intervertebral discs was not seen as an isolated process but as one which affected the entire structure of the cervical spine. Degeneration of the cervical discs was found to be closely associated with aging. The majority of spines after the fourth decade showed implication of one or more discs and, after the fifth decade, a sharp rise in the severity of the degenerative process. Of the specimens over the age of 70, 72 per cent had severe abnormalities.

Those discs that were most frequently implicated also showed the most severe alterations. In general, the discs below the C3-4 level exhibited a higher incidence of involvement and more severe changes. The C5-6 level was most frequently involved; the next most frequently altered disc was at the C6-7 level. The disc at the C2-3 level was least often affected (Table 2-1).

When several discs are involved, changes in their configuration and decrease in their height produce alterations in the adjacent vertebral bodies and in the normal alignment of the cervical column. The anterior superior surface of the bodies may become rounded and the bodies elongated. The height of the cervical column is reduced and the normal lordotic curve may be decreased, straightened or even reversed (Fig. 2-1).

Fissures in the central portion of the discs extended frequently in a lateral direction and became continuous with fissures in the joints of Luschka. Nuclear material was found to be extruded under the longitudinal ligament, laterally into the joints of Luschka and superiorly or inferiorly through the cartilaginous plates into the adjacent vertebral bodies (Fig. 2-2). Extrusions of nuclear material under the longitudinal ligament were thought to be of particular significance because they are capable of exerting pressure on the anterior surface of the spinal cord and the adjacent nerve rootlets. This was particularly true when the

Table 2-1 *Incidence of Disc Degeneration (in per cent)*

Level	Severity of change	
	≥ 1	≥ 3
C2-C3	40	16
C3-C4	70	22
C4-C5	70	38
C5-C6	86	48
C6-C7	75	38
C7-T1	66	14

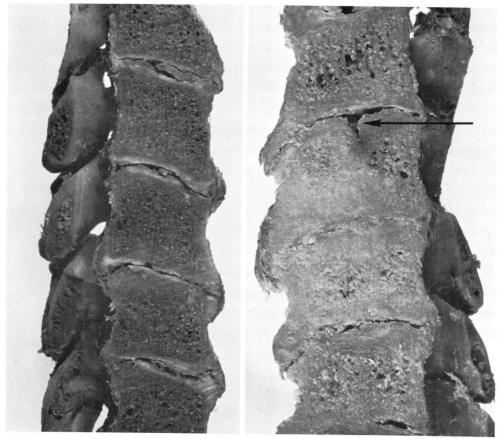

Figure 2-1   Figure 2-2

Figure 2-1   Marked multilevel disc degeneration in the cervical spine with drying and loss of substance of the intervertebral disc, collapse of the disc space, and osteophyte formation.

Figure 2-2   Herniation of the nucleus into the body of the adjacent cervical vertebra as indicated by the arrow. Note also the marked disc degeneration at other levels in the cervical spine.

protrusions were associated with large, marginal osteophytes arising from the posterior surface of the vertebral body (Fig. 2-3).

Disc degeneration results in close approximation of adjacent vertebral bodies. This in turn is followed by a reactive process producing osteophytes at the superior and inferior peripheral attachments of the discs to the vertebral bodies. A high statistical correlation was noted between disc degeneration and posterior osteophyte formation. The level most frequently involved in posterior osteophyte formation was the C6-7 level (Table 2-2). These posterior osteophytes were capable of decreasing the anteroposterior diameter of the spinal canal and of exerting pressure on the spinal cord and nerve roots. They also narrowed the intervertebral foramina (Fig. 2-4).

Anterior osteophyte formation differed from posterior osteophyte formation in that it was not as closely related to disc degenerations. It was felt that ligamentous stress played a greater role in initiating the reactive process involved in anterior osteophyte formation. The anterior osteo-

Table 2-2   *Incidence of Posterior Osteophytes
(in per cent)*

Level	Severity of change	
	≥ 1	≥ 3
C2-C3	35	0
C3-C4	65	4
C4-C5	80	4
C5-C6	86	4
C6-C7	88	10
C7-T1	84	4

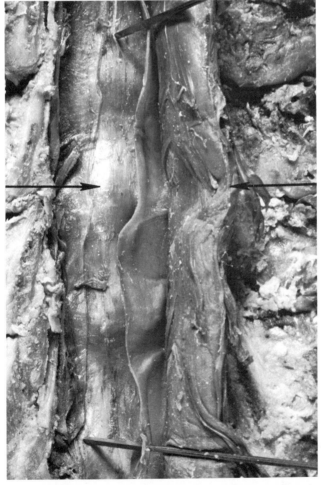

Figure 2-3 Photograph illustrating pressure of posterior osteophyte (arrow on left) which has indented the cervical cord (arrow on right). This type of cervical disc pathology is a frequent cause of myelopathy.

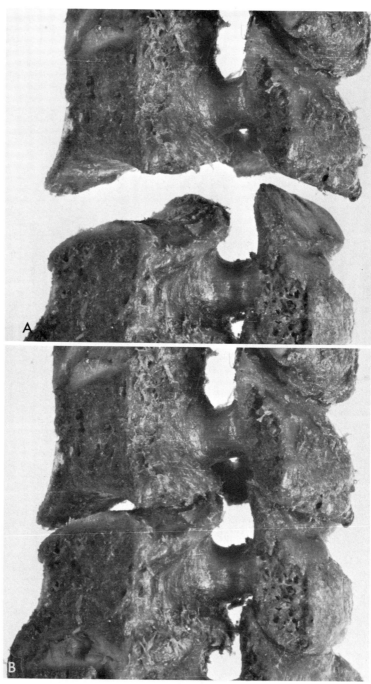

Figure 2-4 These photographs illustrate marked posterior osteophyte formation in the cervical spine. Viewed with vertebrae separated, *A*, and vertebrae opposed, *B*. Note encroachment of the intervertebral foramen by these posterior osteophytes.

Table 2-3   *Incidence of Anterior Osteophytes*
(in per cent)

Level	Severity of change	
	≥1	≥3
C2-C3	60	0
C3-C4	98	26
C4-C5	100	50
C5-C6	100	50
C6-C7	100	58
C7-T1	98	44

phytes were noted to be more prominent than their posterior counterparts and to be most frequent below the fourth cervical vertebra (Figs. 2-5 and 2-6) (Table 2-3).

Reactive changes in the region of the joints of Luschka also appeared to be closely related to disc degeneration. Severe alterations in the joints of Luschka were most often encountered in the lower three levels of the cervical spine, the highest incidence being at the C5-6 level (Table 2-4).

The frequency of severity of changes in the apophyseal joints showed a progression commensurate with aging. However, these articulations are not frequently involved and the changes are rarely severe (Table 2-5). Subluxation of the facets of the apophyseal joint was noted frequently with advanced disc degeneration. This is of significance because it may cause constriction of the adjacent intervertebral foramina, particularly when associated with osteophyte formation about the facets (Figs. 2-7 and 2-8).

Changes in the various components of the cervical spine are of particular significance if they decrease the lumina of the intervertebral foramina and thereby compress their contents. When compromised intervertebral foramina were evaluated, it was found that the joints of Luschka were involved in 79 per cent, the discs in 78 per cent, and the apophyseal joints in 79 per cent. It is thus apparent that all three areas can play a major role in producing narrowing of the intervertebral foramina. The most frequently involved foramina were at the C3-4, C4-5 and C5-6 levels.

Table 2-4   *Incidence of Degenerative Changes*
in Joints of Luschka (in per cent)

Level	Severity of change	
	≥1	≥3
C2-C3	49	1
C3-C4	86	15
C4-C5	88	17
C5-C6	88	24
C6-C7	77	4
C7-T1	58	0

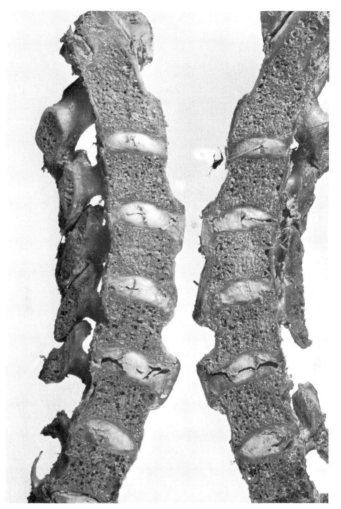

Figure 2-5 Photograph of sagittal section of a cervical spine illustrating multilevel disc degeneration with marked anterior osteophyte formation. These osteophytes may produce symptoms by encroaching on the soft tissues in the neck.

Table 2-5 *Incidence of Degenerative Changes in Apophyseal Joints (in per cent)*

Level	Severity of change	
	≥ 1	≥ 3
C2-C3	56	3
C3-C4	67	10
C4-C5	76	10
C5-C6	85	11
C6-C7	87	9
C7-T1	78	1

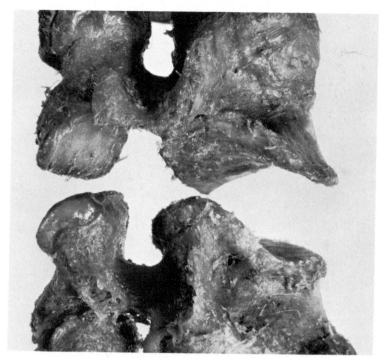

Figure 2-6 Photograph of the osseous changes in cervical spondylosis with osteophyte formation circumferentially about the entire vertebra. In routine x-rays we would describe these as anterior and posterior osteophytes, although in actuality they are frequently present about the entire circumference of the vertebral body.

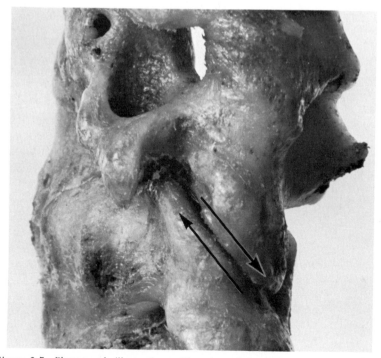

Figure 2-7 Photograph illustrating subluxation of the articular facets comprising an apophyseal joint. Note how the subluxation can compromise the size of the intervertebral foramen producing nerve root compression.

43

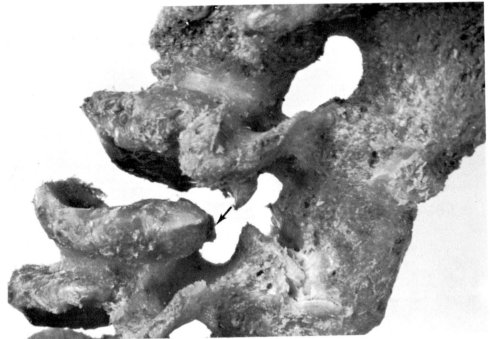

Figure 2-8 Illustration of apophyseal joint degenerative changes in which hypertrophic facets have intruded upon the intervertebral foramen.

Bony ankylosis between two adjacent vertebrae is invariably associated with resorption of the osteophytes surrounding the foramina (Table 2-6).

The correlation between the gross anatomic and roentgenographic findings when applied to the discs and intervertebral foramina was found to be extremely high. The findings just reported agree in general terms with other pathologic descriptions noted in the literature.[12, 24, 29]

The prominent anterior osteophytes have been reported to cause pressure symptoms not only on the esophagus but also on the trachea.[9] Their occurrence to this degree is not common but should be considered in obscure causes of esophageal tracheal compromise.

From C3 through C7 the average measurement of the cervical canal is 17 mm.[24] It is generally agreed that spinal cord compression will occur only if this figure is reduced to 10 mm. or less.[34] In cervical spondylosis some reduction will usually take place in the anteroposterior diameter of the spinal canal and, when associated with a canal which was initially

Table 2-6 *Contribution to Foraminal Narrowing by Component (in per cent)*

Component	Incidence
Apophyseal joint	79
Joints of Luschka	79
Disc	78

small, myelopathy can occur. It should be noted that the cervical cord is oval, whereas the canal is roughly triangular in shape, producing the recess to the anterolateral direction. Because of the presence of this canal, some reduction of canal size can occur in a lateral direction without resultant cord compression, and, secondly, when the cord is compressed in the midline this recess may remain open to serve as a pathway for cerebrospinal fluid.

The work of Friedenberg and Miller is helpful in attempting to correlate changes seen on x-ray with patient symptomatology.[13] They evaluated two large groups of patients, one symptomatic and the other asymptomatic in regard to the cervical spine. They were evaluated radiographically with roentgenograms of the cervical columns of the anteroposterior, lateral and oblique projections. It was striking to note that in the asymptomatic group, 25 per cent of patients in the fifth decade of life exhibited degenerative changes and, by the seventh decade, 75 per cent showed degenerative changes. In both the symptomatic and asymptomatic groups the highest incidence of abnormalities was noted between the fifth and sixth and sixth and seventh vertebral bodies. It was significant to note that the incidence of narrowing of the interspaces between the fifth and sixth and the sixth and seventh cervical vertebrae was higher in the symptomatic than in the asymptomatic group. No differences were noted between these two groups in incidence of changes at the joints of Luschka, the intervertebral foramina or the posterior articular processes. These studies should give the clinician some cause for hesitation before deciding that the changes noted on routine x-rays of the cervical spine are causing a particular patient's clinical syndrome. It is felt that over-reliance on routine x-ray as a guide to operative intervention has often resulted in the incorrect disc being removed with a resultant surgical failure.

It has been pointed out by Robinson that after surgical fusion osteophyte resorption can take place.[28] It is thought that this may explain the mechanism of relief of radicular pain in cervical spondylosis after interbody fusion even when the osteophytes are not removed. In addition to the common type of chronic disc degeneration previously described, there is a group of cervical intervertebral disc lesions associated with major trauma to the cervical spine with or without fractures and dislocations. Disc injury can be indirectly surmised radiographically in fractures and dislocations when there is either a decreased height of the intervertebral disc space or an abnormal increased width of the intervertebral disc space when the neck is subjected to traction.[2]

In flexion-type fracture dislocations there is frequently an avulsion of the disc from its attachment to the superior vertebra and less frequently from its inferior vertebra. The line of disruption is most frequently at the junction of the disc with the cartilaginous plate. In hyperextension injuries where there is a teardrop type of fracture, the nucleus may herniate into the fracture site itself.[2]

It has been the authors' experience that in certain patients with extensive laminectomy, particularly when the articular facets have been implicated, a degree of instability may result, which will subsequently lead to intervertebral disc degeneration. This is particularly true in individuals with weak cervical musculature who cannot compensate for loss of the posterior stabilizing structures. Relief in these individuals can only be obtained by cervical fusion preferably through the anterior route.

PATHOLOGY OF THE LUMBAR INTERVERTEBRAL DISC

The lumbar intervertebral disc undergoes a pattern of degeneration which in many respects is different from the pattern found in the cervical spine. Although spondylosis is the chief cause of neck pain associated with radiculitis, disc degeneration per se is the most common cause for low-back pain with radiculitis. In both the cervical and lumbar areas, disc degeneration is not usually due to one major traumatic insult but rather to the combined ravages of the biochemical and metabolic changes of aging, associated with long-standing chronic mechanical stress. A history of injury which may have precipitated a low-back syndrome may often be elicited, but this injury has played an incidental role in what is truly a chronic degenerative process. The sequential pathology of the lumbar intervertebral disc has been well described by many authors.[1, 6, 11, 15, 17, 18, 20, 27, 29]

Ballooned Discs

Ballooning of the intervertebral disc is characteristically found in association with diseases which weaken the vertebral body. Classically, osteoporosis, more accurately termed osteopenia, will sufficiently weaken the vertebral body to allow expansion of the intervertebral disc into the upper and lower plates of the body. For this to occur the disc must still have its elastic gelatinous nucleus.[6] If the disc has lost its integrity, collapse and wedging of the vertebral body will occur rather than ballooning of the disc. Malignant processes such as multiple myeloma will produce sufficient weakness of the vertebral body to allow this ballooning to take place (Fig. 2-9).

Intraspongy Nuclear Herniations

It has been noted for over one hundred years that the intervertebral disc can herniate through the cartilaginous endplate into the cancellous bone of the vertebral body. This herniation of disc material takes place through a defect in the cartilaginous plate which may represent the point of passage of blood vessels from the vertebral body to the disc during early life. These herniations are irregular in size and shape and tend to be surrounded eventually by a rim of bony sclerosis. These defects are found in the younger age groups as well as the older.[29] The adjacent disc frequently exhibits thinning.

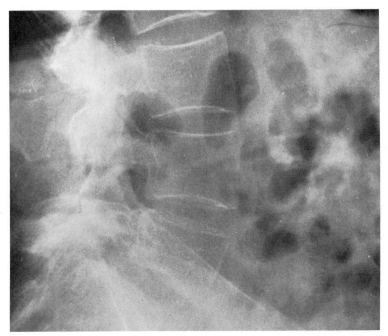

Figure 2-9 Ballooning of the intervertebral disc space in the lumbar spine secondary to osteoporosis.

Osteophyte Formation

Peripheral osteophyte formations, anteriorly and laterally and to a lesser extent posteriorly, were often found in the bodies of lumbar vertebrae associated with disc degeneration. These osteophytes represent pathologic stimulation of new bone formation at the attachment of the longitudinal ligaments to the bodies or the attachment of the annulus to the bodies. This stimulation may be due to hypermobility of the vertebral bodies or abnormal distribution of stresses on the annulus and ligaments associated with degeneration of the intervertebral disc.

The decreased incidence of posterior osteophytes as compared to those in the anterior and lateral position may be explained by the absence of a strong attachment of the posterior longitudinal ligament to bone. This osteophyte formation in association with disc degeneration may be termed lumbar spondylosis, which has its counterpart in cervical spondylosis. In certain instances the intervertebral foramina may be compromised by prominent osteophytes sufficiently to cause clinical radiculitis. This is particularly true when thinning of the disc space has progressed to the point where the facets of the apophyseal joints have "settled" and narrowed the diameters of the intervertebral foramina (Fig. 2-11).

Thinned Discs

Three distinct situations are present which may be associated with thinning of the disc space. The first situation occurs in the presence of a

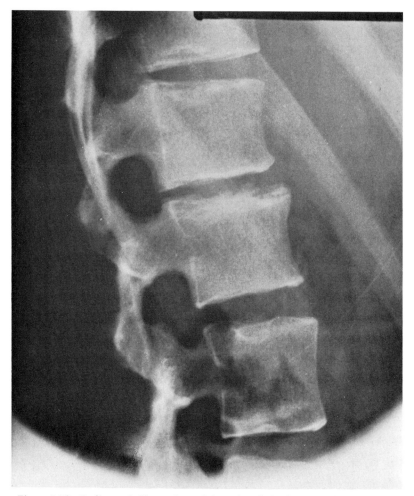

Figure 2-10 Radiograph illustrating a Schmorl node in the upper lumbar spine.

transitional fifth lumbar vertebra (Fig. 2-12). Between the transitional vertebra and the sacrum a vestigial disc is often found which is devoid of nucleus pulposus and not a product of degenerative changes.[15] When the transverse process of this transitional vertebra is incompletely sacralized on one side and normal on the other it is possible that the caudal intervertebral disc may be degenerated. More often there is a broad sacralization of the transverse processes, either unilaterally or bilaterally, and a vestigial nondegenerated disc. In these situations one should look for disc degeneration above this transitional vertebra rather than below it.

A second group of thinned intervertebral discs are associated with the rupture of the annulus and loss of nuclear material or herniation of the nuclear material into the adjacent vertebra (Fig. 2-13). This mechanical loss of disc material is often associated with invasion of granulation tissue through the rents in the annulus. Subsequent to the loss of disc material, dehydration of the disc and eventually fibrosis can occur.

A third group of thinned intervertebral discs consists of those in

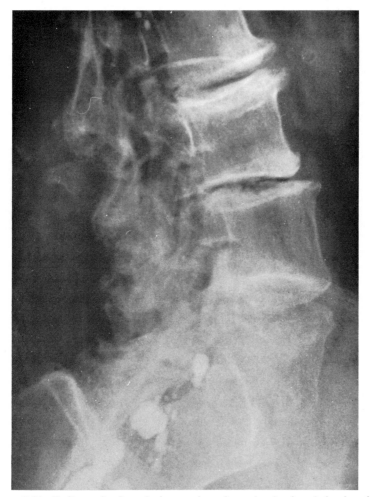

Figure 2-11 Radiograph of marked osteophyte formation in chronic lumbar disc degeneration. Note also the marked sclerosis and loss of height of the disc space.

which there has been a marked dehydration of the disc with desiccation and necrosis of the nucleus pulposus. This is not associated with a rent in the annulus or with a herniation through the cartilaginous endplate.

Disc thinning may also occur with disc space infections but this will be discussed separately in a later section.

Disc Protrusions

The process of nuclear herniation and annular protrusion is caused by a combination of biochemical factors previously discussed, chronic degenerative structural changes and superimposed mechanical stresses. The pathologic cycle has been well described by Armstrong.[1] Before there is actual displacement of disc material, the nucleus and annulus undergo certain structural changes. Radiating cracks in the annulus fibrosus

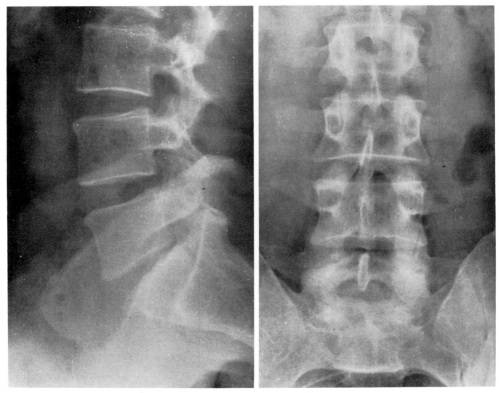

Figure 2-12 Radiographs of a transitional vertebra with an associated thin disc. This is not to be confused with loss of height of a disc space due to disc degeneration.

develop in the most centrally situated lamellae and extend outward toward the periphery.[17] These radiating cliffs in the annulus progressively weaken its resistance to nuclear herniation. They may heal by fibrosis and scar formation or, if subject to persistent mechanical pressures, may permit herniation of the nucleus pulposus. In younger individuals from the age of 30 to 50, having good turgor in the nucleus, it is more likely that persistent pressure which may lead to herniation will be present. In the elderly individual, in whom the nucleus is desiccated and fibrotic, these fissures will more often progress to fibrosis and healing so that a degenerated thin disc may develop without any of the signs and symptoms of an acute disc syndrome. This may be the explanation for the predominance of acute disc syndromes of the middle-aged population and its rarity in the elderly.

Posterior displacement of the nucleus pulposus may occur in a variety of fashions (Fig. 2-14). On the one extreme, there may be a massive nuclear retropulsion, in which a large volume of disc material is suddenly thrust into the spinal canal, producing a profound neurologic catastrophe. More commonly the extrusion is a gradual and intermittent process. The nucleus progressively bulges through a defect in the annulus, being retained in position by the posterior longitudinal ligament. This ligament may be stretched and detached by the herniating nuclear

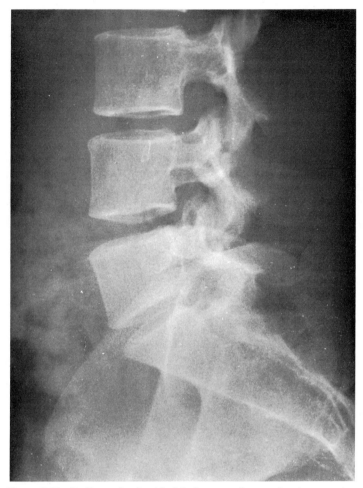

Figure 2-13   Radiograph of a thin L5 disc secondary to disc degeneration.

material as it projects backward into the spinal canal. This ligament may rupture with the formation of free sequestra into the spinal canal which may migrate encephalad-caudad or into the intervertebral foramina. It is not only the size of the nuclear herniation which determines its clinical significance but the direction in which this herniation takes place. In addition, the shape of the spinal canal has been shown to be of great importance.[15] Failure to recognize the variety of types of disc pathology having significant spatial relationships will lead to inadequate surgical treatment of these problems. It should also be pointed out that posterior protrusion of disc material may often occur at some site other than that of an obviously thin disc.[6]

Subsequent to loss of integrity of the annulus fibrosus there may be invasion of the disc by granulation tissue, either through rents in the annulus or through cracks in the cartilaginous endplate. The role of this granulation tissue and the production of pain is as yet unclear.

It has been demonstrated that a high degree of correlation exists

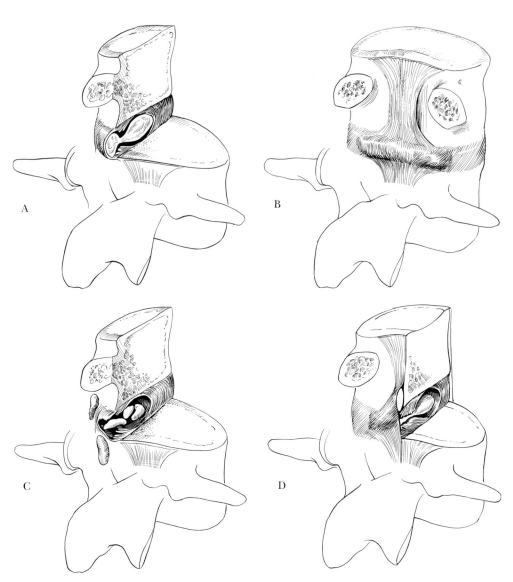

Figure 2-14 *A*, Herniation of a lumbar disc beneath the posterior longitudinal ligament in the common lateral position. *B*, Herniation of a lumbar disc in the less frequent central position beneath the strong portion of the posterior longitudinal ligament. *C*, Complete herniation of a lumbar through a rupture in the annulus and the posterior longitudinal ligament, with free fragments in the neural canal. These fragments may migrate cranially, caudally, or into the intervertebral foramen. *D*, Herniation of a lumbar disc, with upward migration of the disc fragments, beneath the posterior longitudinal ligaments. These fragments may go unnoticed unless specific exploration in these areas is undertaken.

between degenerative processes in the interspinous ligament and degeneration of the lumbar intervertebral discs. These two areas of degeneration appear to be concurrent and not consecutive.[27]

Calcification of the Intervertebral Disc

Two distinct processes should be delineated when discussing calcification of the intervertebral disc. In adults, calcification of the intervertebral disc is a manifestation of a degenerative process in the disc and is itself of only minor clinical significance (Fig. 2-15). The calcific deposits may be found beneath the cartilaginous plate, in the annulus or in the nucleus itself. The exact metabolic pathways involved in this type of pathologic calcification are not clear.[6] X-ray diffraction and electron microscopic studies of these pathologic calcium deposits reveal the predominant mineral constituent to be hydroxyapatite.[32]

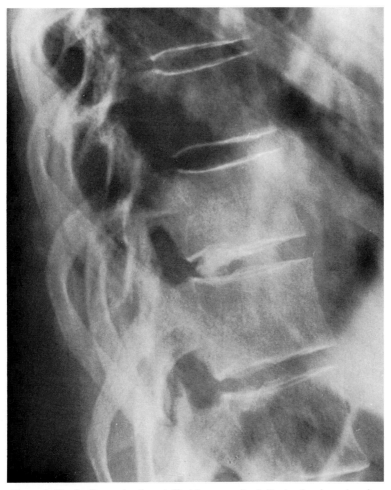

Figure 2-15   Radiograph of a calcified intervertebral disc in the thoracic spine.

Calcification of the intervertebral discs in children represents a different and distinct pathologic entity. This calcification has been subdivided into three types: disappearing, dormant and silent.[26] The disappearing form of disc calcification is a clinical syndrome associated with a calcific deposit in the nucleus pulposus. Most often the cervical discs are involved; less frequently the thoracic and lumbar areas. The nuclear site of calcification is in contrast with the adult type of calcification which is more often found in the annulus or in the region of the endplates. This form is associated with acute symptoms of pain, tenderness and systemic evidence of inflammation. Usually the clinical signs and symptoms spontaneously abate with eventual disappearance of the calcification in the disc.[21, 26] The involved discs may prolapse and require surgical intervention.

In the dormant form the calcific deposit may be noted incidentally on roentgenograms of the spine, and at some later date acute symptomatology will develop. Subsequent disappearance of the calcific deposit is the usual course.

Silent disc calcification refers to those individuals in whom it was incidentally noted that disc space calcification was present with no associated signs or symptoms.

Intervertebral Disc Space Infections

Intervertebral disc space infections are classified as either pyogenic or tuberculous. Pyogenic infections of the intervertebral disc are of two types. The first is that found in childhood in which the infecting organism is carried to the disc by the blood stream or lymphatics. As has been previously noted, the blood supply to the disc becomes obliterated by the end of the second decade so it is not surprising that hematogenous disc space infections are limited to the first and second decades of life.

Characteristically, these infections are manifested by episodes of acute back pain, but these may be associated with meningeal symptoms of abdominal or hip pain. A low-grade fever may or may not be present. Within two to three weeks of the onset of the infection, narrowing of the disc space occurs as the disc is progressively destroyed by the acute inflammatory process. Over a period of several months the pathologic process will resolve with sclerosis of the adjacent vertebral bodies. Occasionally spontaneous interbody fusion may occur.[19] The organism most often involved is *Staphylococcus aureus*.

A second group of pyogenic disc space infections is found in individuals exposed to intervertebral disc surgery. It is presumed that the organism is introduced at the time of surgery. As the infection progresses in the disc space, back pain will become predominant, with or without signs of systemic reaction. It is not unusual for a disc space infection to be associated with no abnormalities of temperature. Usually an elevated sedimentation rate and leukocytosis will be present. Radiographic evaluation of the spine at the site of the disc space infection will reveal irregularity of the adjacent vertebral borders with rapid loss of height of the disc space and a varying amount of sclerotic bone reaction.

Tuberculous disc space infections are usually secondary to tuberculous infection of the adjacent vertebral body. The negative tuberculin skin test will usually but not always preclude the diagnosis of tuberculous spondylitis. In occasional cases the disc space will be the primary site of the infection. If this is the case, vascularity must be present in the disc, and thus it will occur in the younger age groups. Roentgenographically, narrowing of the disc space will occur before bony destruction when the disc is primarily involved. The characteristic osseous changes of osteolysis and collapse will be present before disc thinning if the infection was primarily in the bone.

Ochronosis

Ochronosis is an inborn error of metabolism in which the enzyme homogentisic acid oxidase is quantitatively deficient. Because of the inability of the body to metabolize homogentisic acid, it is excreted in the urine, producing alkaptonuria. Ochronosis refers to the pigmentation of cartilage tendon and ligament by homogentisic acid which grossly appears grey or blue-black but under the microscope yellow, leading to the nomenclature of ochronosis. The intervertebral discs appear as elliptical, opaque wafers particularly in the lumbar area. This opacity may be due to secondary calcification which follows the deposition of homogentisic acid. Alkaptonuria and ochronosis have been reported in association with acute rupture of a lumbar intervertebral disc[8] (Fig. 2-16).

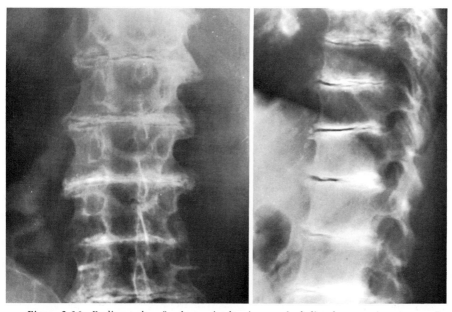

Figure 2-16 Radiographs of ochronosis showing marked disc degeneration at several levels in the lumbar spine. Note deposition of radiopaque material in the substance of the intervertebral disc and the extensive changes present at all levels in the spine.

REFERENCES

1. Armstrong, J. R.: Lumbar Disc Lesions. Baltimore, Williams & Wilkins, 1965.
2. Bailey, R.W.: Observations of cervical intervertebral disc lesions in fracture and dislocations. J. Bone Joint Surg. 45-A:461-470, 1963.
3. Berry, R. J.: Genetically controlled degeneration of the nucleus pulposus in the mouse. J. Bone Joint Surg. 43-B:387-393, 1961.
4. Bobechko, W. P. et al.: Auto immune response to nucleus pulposus in the rabbit. J. Bone Joint Surg. 47-B:574-580, 1965.
5. Comfort, A.: The Biology of Senescence. New York, Rinehart, 1956.
6. Coventry, M. B. et al.: The intervertebral disc: Its microscopic anatomy and pathology. Part III: Pathologic changes in the intervertebral disc. J. Bone Joint Surg. 27:460-474, 1945.
7. Davidson, E. A. et al.: Biochemical alterations in herniated intervertebral discs. J. Biol. Chem. 234:2951-2954, 1959.
8. Eisenberg, H.: Alkaptonuria, ochronosis, arthritis and ruptured intervertebral disc, complicated by homologous serum reaction. Arch. Int. Med. 86:79-86, 1950.
9. el-Sallab, R. A. et al.: Oesophageal and tracheal pseudo-tumors due to anterior cervical osteophytes. Brit. J. Radiol. 38:682-684, 1965.
10. Franklin, L. et al.: Lipid content of the intervertebral disc. Clin. Chem. 12:253-257, 1966.
11. Friberg, S. et al.: Anatomical and clinical studies in lumbar disc degeneration, Acta Orthop. Scand. 19:222-242, 1949.
12. Friedenberg, Z. B. et al.: Degenerative changes in the cervical spine, Anat. Study, J. Bone Joint Surg. 41-A:61-70, 1959.
13. Friedenberg, Z. B. et al.: Degenerative disc disease of the cervical spine, J. Bone Joint Surg. 45-A:1171-1178, 1963.
14. Hallen, A.: The collagen and ground substance of human intervertebral disc at different ages. Acta Chem. Scand. 16:705, 1962.
15. Harmon, P. H.: Congenital and acquired anatomic variations, including degenerative changes of the lower lumbar spine; role in production of painful back and lower extremity syndromes. Clin. Orthop. 44:171-186, 1966.
16. Hendry, N. G. C.: The hydration of the nucleus pulposus and its relation to intervertebral disc derangement. J. Bone Joint Surg. 40-B:132-144, 1968.
17. Hirsch, C. et al.: Studies on structural changes in the lumbar annulus fibrosis. Acta Orthop. Scand. 22:184-231, 1952.
18. Joplin, R. J.: The intervertebral disc: Embryology, anatomy, physiology and pathology. Surg., Gynec. and Obstet. 61:591-599, 1935.
19. Keiser, M. D. et al.: Intervertebral disc space infections in children. Clin. Orthop. 30:163-66, 1963.
20. Keyes, D. C. et al.: The normal and pathological physiology of the nucleus pulposus of the intervertebral disc. J. Bone Joint Surg. 14:897, 1932.
21. Lindberg, T.: Intervertebral calcinosis in childhood. Ann. Paediat. (Basel) 201:172-184, 1963.
22. Mitchell, P. E. et al.: The chemical background of intervertebral disc prolapse. J. Bone Joint Surg. 43-B:141-51, 1961.
23. Naylor, A.: The biophysical and biochemical aspects of intervertebral disc herniation and degeneration. Ann. Roy. Coll. Surg. Eng. 31:91-114, 1962.
24. Payne, E. E. et al.: The cervical spine, an anatomicopathological study of 70 specimens (using a special technic) with particular reference to the problem of cervical spondylosis. Brain 80:571-596, 1957.
25. Puschel, J.: Der wasserergehalt normaler und degenerierter zwischenwirbelscheiben. Beitr. Path. Anat. 84:123-130, 1930.
26. Rechtman, A. M. et al.: Calcification of the intervertebral disc—disappearing, dormant and silent. Clin. Orthop. 7:218-225, 1956.
27. Rissanen, P. M.: Comparison of pathologic changes in intervertebral discs and interspinous ligaments of the lower part of the lumbar spine in the light of autopsy findings. Acta Orthop. Scand. 34:54-65, 1964.
28. Robinson, R. A.: The results of anterior interbody fusion of the cervical spine. J. Bone Joint Surg. 44A:1569-1586, 1962.
29. Saunders, J. B. de C. B. and Inman, V. T.: Pathology of the intervertebral disk. A.M.A. Arch. Surg. 40:389-416, 1940.
30. Straus, W. Jr.: Fossil evidence of the evolution of the erect, bipedal posture. Clin. Orthop. 25:9-19, 1962.
31. Strehler, B. L.: Time, Cells, and Aging. New York, Academic Press, 1962.

32. Taylor, T. K. et al.: Calcification in the intervertebral disc. Nature (London) 199:612-13, 1963.
33. van den Hooff, A.: Histological age changes in the annulus fibrosis of the human intervertebral disc; With a discussion of the problem of disc herniation. Gerontologia (Basel) 9:136-49, 1964.
34. Wilkinson, M.: The anatomy and pathology of cervical spondylosis. Proc. Roy. Soc. Med. 57:159-62, 1964.
35. Yamada, K.: The dynamics of experimental posture. Experimental study of intervertebral disc herniation in bipedal animals. Clin. Orthop. 25:20-31, 1962.

Chapter 3

LUMBAR DISC LESIONS: ANATOMIC AND PATHOLOGIC FEATURES AND THE CLINICAL SYNDROME

The manifestations of the clinical syndrome of the lumbar disc are many and varied. They are related to the different phases of the pathologic process in the lumbar disc and to secondary changes occurring in the surrounding tissues. In order to arrive at the correct diagnosis it is most essential to be able to correlate both the subjective and objective clinical features with these changes.

Invariably the patient seeks medical aid because of pain in the lower back, with or without pain in one or both legs. The nature of the pain is governed by the components of the nerve root involved and by stimulation of the sensory nerve endings in the surrounding soft tissues. It will be shown subsequently that many of the typical features of the lumbar disc syndrome, such as posture, restriction of motion, muscle spasm, sensory, motor and reflex abnormalities, are directly or indirectly related to the neural elements affected by the pathologic process in the disc.

Therefore, at this point it is important to recapitulate briefly the pertinent anatomic relationships of the lumbar spinal column and its contents and to again emphasize the different phases of the processes which affect both the normal and the pathologic intervertebral disc.

MOTOR SEGMENT UNIT

The intervertebral disc is considered by some observers as one of the amphiarthroses of the body.[11, 13] In order to fit the intervertebral disc into this category, the nucleus pulposus must be considered as a joint cavity, the annulus fibrosus as the investing ligamentous apparatus, and the articular plates of the superior and inferior surfaces of the vertebral bodies as the articular cartilages.[11, 25] However, in considering movements between two vertebrae, structures that permit and others that limit motion must be included. These comprise the posterior articular joints and their capsular and ligamentous apparatuses, the anterior and posterior longitudinal ligaments, the ligamentum flavum, the interspinous ligament and the extensor muscles of the back crossing the level of the intervertebral disc. All these structures function as a unit, are closely interrelated and comprise a motor segment unit, of which there are 23 or 24.[11] To this segment of the spine must be added the spinal canal and the intervertebral foramina and their contents (Fig. 3-1). It should be understood that the elements comprising the motor unit are not the only structures providing spinal mobility and sustaining the mechanical stresses to which the spine is habitually exposed during normal function. It has already been recorded that the body muscles, especially the muscles of the abdomen and thorax, by raising the intra-abdominal and intrathoracic pressures, afford additional support to the spine and sustain forces which would otherwise fall on the spine.[2, 16, 17]

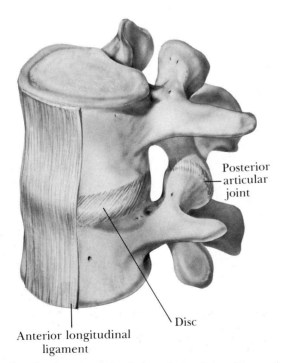

Posterior articular joint

Disc

Anterior longitudinal ligament

Figure 3-1 Functional motor unit of the spinal column; it comprises two vertebral bodies and the disc between them, the two posterior joints and the ligamentous structures binding the two vertebrae to one another.

SINUVERTEBRAL NERVE AND THE POSTERIOR PRIMARY DIVISION OF THE LUMBAR NERVE ROOT

The nerve supply of the soft tissue elements of the motor units and the relation of the nerve roots in their extrathecal course to the intervertebral discs readily explain the location and pattern of pain observed in the lumbar disc complex.[4, 14, 21, 23] In general, the soft tissue components of the motor units are innervated by the sinuvertebral nerves and the posterior primary divisions of the lumbar nerve roots. Both these nerves contain sympathetic and sensory fibers. Many of the fibers are myelinated, of which the smaller fibers are, in all probability, pain fibers, whereas the larger ones are proprioceptive fibers. The sinuvertebral nerve takes origin near the spinal ganglion; one or two segments above the foramen it enters to regain access to the spinal canal. In the canal it breaks up into ascending and descending branches, which proceed toward the disc above and the disc below and supply the peripheral layers of the annulus fibrosus. Other branches innervate the dura mater, the vascular elements, the posterior longitudinal ligament and the periosteum. In the spinal canal, filaments of the adjacent nerves anastomose with each other, and some fibers even cross the midline (Fig. 3-2).

The posterior rami amply supply the skin and muscles of the lumbar region and, in addition, distribute sensory fibers to fasciae, ligaments, the periosteum and the intervertebral joints. The areas of distribution of

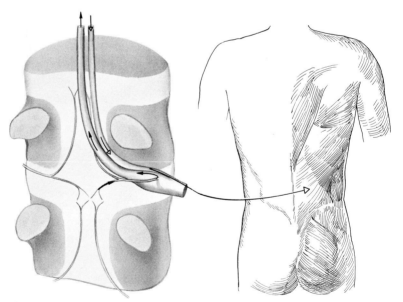

Figure 3-2 Origin and course of the sinuvertebral nerve. Note the wide distribution of the fibers within the spinal canal; it sends fibers to the peripheral layers of the annulus, the dura mater, vascular elements in this region, the posterior longitudinal ligament and the periosteum. Filaments of adjacent nerves anastomose with each other; some fibers cross the midline. Reflex phenomena (deep pain and muscle spasm) may occur in the posterior structures following stimulation of the endings of the sinuvertebral nerve; the impulses produced take the pathways shown diagrammatically in this illustration.

adjacent posterior rami overlap considerably. Each synovial joint is innervated by two nerves. The posterior rami supply the ligamenta flava and the supraspinous and interspinous ligaments; like the posterior synovial joints, the spinal ligaments receive innervation from two spinal nerves.

The endings of the sinuvertebral nerve, when stimulated by noxious agents, such as occurs in tearing of the posterior annulus and extrusion of disc material, not only evoke deep local pain but also produce reflex muscle spasm, the severity of which depends upon the intensity of the stimulus. If the stimulus is of great intensity, pain may radiate into the hip, the region of the sacroiliac joint and the posterior aspect of the thigh. This type of radiating pain is diffuse and deep in nature and is poorly localized by the patient; it may be accompanied by a vasovagal response. It is often referred to as discogenic pain in contrast to neurogenic pain, which is caused by direct irritation of a nerve root.[5] The reflex muscle spasm associated with stimulation of the nerve endings of the sinuvertebral nerve produces the characteristic clinical changes in the back of a patient with an acute lumbar disc lesion, namely, obliteration or flattening of the normal lumbar lordosis and sciatic scoliosis.

This same pain pattern can be reproduced experimentally by puncturing the outer fibers of the annulus while the patient is under local anesthesia. If a pathologic disc is stimulated, the patient's pain will be reproduced. The same response is attained when, in the process of doing a discogram, the pathologic disc is distended by the opaque solution.

SHAPE AND SIZE OF THE SPINAL CANAL

When nuclear herniations occur, the shape and size of the lumbar spinal canal may determine the character and the intensity of the symptoms. It was previously noted that the average width of the lumbar spinal canal is 23.4 mm. and the anteroposterior depth is 17.4 mm. However, these dimensions vary considerably in different individuals, and in some there may exist an actual stricture of the canal.[24, 28] A small canal existing alone or together with other structural abnormalities, such as spondylolisthesis or a very acute lumbosacral angle, complicates profoundly the nature of the clinical manifestations of disc herniations. The shape of the canal also shows wide variations from one individual to another; it may be round or ovoid, triangular or trefoil.[1] Canals that are trefoil in shape have lateral recesses, a configuration which renders the lumbar roots particularly vulnerable to compression (Fig. 3-3).[24, 25]

RELATION OF THE LUMBAR NERVE ROOTS

The thecal and extrathecal relationships of the lumbar nerve roots are of particular importance in lesions of the lumbar discs. In the great majority of individuals (95 per cent) the spinal cord terminates within the limits of the bodies of the first and second lumbar vertebrae. The lumbar rootlets together with the conus medullaris and its continuation, the filum

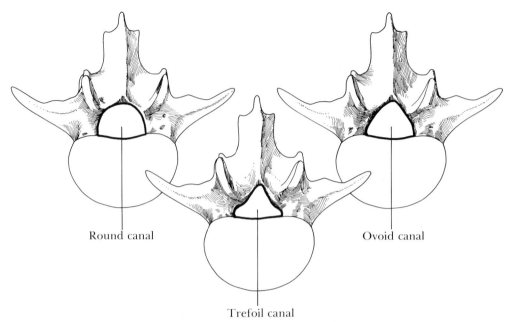

Round canal   Ovoid canal

Trefoil canal

Figure 3-3   The three variations of the spinal canal: round, ovoid and trefoil. The lateral recesses of the trefoil canal render the lumbar roots particularly vulnerable to compression by extruded disc material.

terminale, comprise the cauda equina. In the lumbar spine the intrathecal portions of the roots are extremely loose; also in this region, the posterior portion of the dura mater, which is relatively inelastic, exhibits considerable redundancy. These features permit extreme flexion of the spine without imposing undue tension on the nerve roots or the posterior dura. On the other hand, the anterior portion of the dura lies in close apposition to the anterior surface of the spinal canal formed by the posterior surfaces of the vertebral bodies and intervertebral discs. Additional fixation of the anterior dura is provided by the nerve roots as they become extrathecal and take with them a sheath of the dura. The excursion of motion of the anterior wall of the spinal canal is less than that of the posterior wall. It has been estimated that in full flexion the posterior wall lengthens 11 mm. and the anterior wall 5 mm.[4] A range of 5 mm. is well within the tolerance of the anterior dura and the five extrathecal roots. Of clinical significance is the observation that the lower lumbar roots (fourth and fifth lumbar and first sacral) are capable of a certain range of movement in their respective foramina when the extended leg is raised. There is some variability of the range noted in cadavers by different observers; but most estimates of range fall between 2 and 8 mm. Also, when the extended leg is raised, the lower lumbar roots on the contralateral side advance a little from their foramina and tend to slip toward the opposite side and also toward the anterior wall of the spinal canal.[27] When disc protrusions compress the lower lumbar roots or put great tension on them, straight leg-raising imposes even more tension on the nerve root and thereby produces a painful response. The degree to which

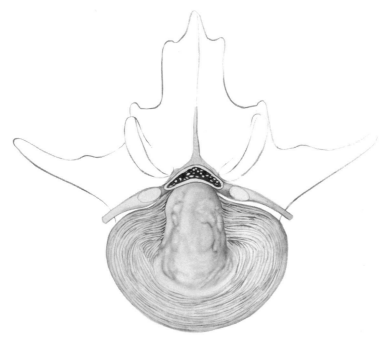

Figure 3-4 A massive extrusion of disc material may obliterate the spinal canal almost completely, especially if the canal is small and trefoil in shape; a complete cauda equina syndrome may result.

the leg can be raised without a painful response is a good index of the irritability of the nerve root.

The relationship of the lumbar roots and the lumbar discs is of major clinical importance. A massive extrusion posteriorly of one of the lumbar discs may severely injure the cauda equina (both the intrathecal and extrathecal roots). Although these lesions are rare, they do occur. In these instances, the size and shape of the spinal canal and the size of the mass extruded are major factors in the severity of the clinical syndrome. Complete paralysis may result if the extruded mass is large and the canal is small, in which case the mass obliterates the spinal canal (Fig. 3-4).

It was previously noted that after the roots emerge from the dura they pursue a course caudalward and laterally within the spinal canal before they enter their respective foramina. They leave the anterior dura opposite to and one vertebral segment above their foramina of exit. In their oblique and downward course they cross the posterolateral aspects of the discs below and opposite the vertebral bodies from which they emerged, then continue across the upper and posterolateral aspect of the bodies below the discs. Finally, they swing laterally beneath the pedicles and enter the intervertebral foramina. Therefore, the first sacral nerve root leaves the dura above the level of the L5-S1 disc and opposite the posterior aspect of the fifth vertebral body; it enters the foramen formed by the first and second sacral segments. This same relationship is true for the fifth and fourth lumbar roots.[7] Knowledge of the relationship of the extrathecal portion of the lumbar nerve roots in the spinal canal is of major clinical and surgical importance. It permits definitive localization

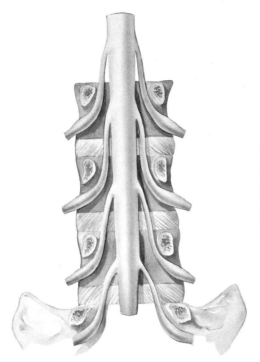

Figure 3-5 Relationship of lumbar nerve root to the vertebral bodies and the intervertebral discs. Note that the roots leave the anterior dura opposite one vertebral body above their foramina of exit; also, the roots cross the posterolateral aspect of the disc below the vertebral body opposite which they emerged.

of the disc affected and the nerve root involved. In addition, it provides an explanation for the varied features that the clinical picture may present (Fig. 3-5).

RELATIONS OF THE INTERVERTEBRAL FORAMINA

The intervertebral foramina of the lumbar spine provide the routes of exit for the lumbar nerve roots. Their relationship to the discs is of clinical significance because their anterior boundaries are formed by the posterior and lateral aspects of the vertebral bodies and the intervertebral discs. It was noted earlier that the downward paths of the roots cross the intervertebral discs. It becomes apparent that herniations of the discs may compress the nerve roots before they enter the foramina. The lumbar foramen is an elongated canal which is five or six times the size of the nerve which passes through it. This spatial difference provides much freedom for the nerve and protects it from constriction. However, large sequestrated disc fragments sometimes migrate into the foramen and occlude it completely; thus, the nerve root becomes severely compressed. In disc lesions, secondary inflammatory changes may occur within the foramen which is compressing the nerve root. Osteophytes may develop on the posterolateral surface of the vertebral bodies and on the posterior articular joints. These structures form part of the anterior and posterior walls of the foramen; osteophytes in these locations severely reduce the diameter of the foramen and compress the lumbar root it contains.

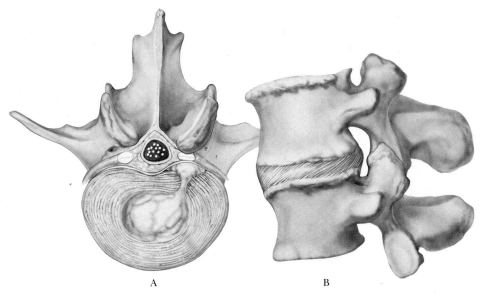

Figure 3-6 *A*, A large sequestrated disc fragment may migrate into the foramen and severely compress the nerve root. *B*, Note the anatomical boundaries of a lumbar intervertebral foramen. With degeneration of the disc secondary changes occur in the posterolateral surfaces of the vertebral bodies and on the posterior articular joints; these osteophytes decrease the diameter of the foramen and may compress the nerve root within the foramen.

Although these degenerative changes are commoner in the cervical spine, they do occur in the lumbar spine more frequently than generally realized (Fig. 3-6).

THE PATHOLOGIC PROCESS IN THE LUMBAR DISC

Armstrong has recorded clearly the progressive nature of the pathologic process that occurs in lumbar disc lesions. This process can be followed step by step, and each phase can logically be correlated with the accompanying symptoms. There is a definite beginning and end; the whole cycle spans many months and even years. Unless the physician has a clear understanding of this pathologic process the clinical picture will be beset by many bizarre and confusing features. However, if one has full comprehension of the cyclic changes of the pathologic process that occurs in the disc and the secondary changes that occur in the surrounding tissues, then all the manifestations of the clinical syndrome, both objective and subjective, fall into their proper places, unfolding a crystal-clear picture.

It should be understood that certain progressive biochemical changes which are associated with aging occur in the discs of man. The etiological factors producing these events are not clear. These physiological changes may never produce symptoms and never reach the end point that the pathologic process responsible for the lumbar disc syndrome reaches.

Nevertheless, in the beginning the biochemical abnormalities are the same but of a different tempo.[9, 10, 15]

The intervertebral disc is a highly specialized organ whose internal biochemical structure is adapted to withstand tremendous stress. Under normal conditions, the nucleus pulposus is a perfect gel with a high imbibition index (or water-binding capacity) confined within and blending with the elastic annulus fibrosus around its circumference and with the articular cartilaginous plates of the adjacent vertebrae. The normal disc, by virtue of its biochemical composition, has the capacity to absorb fluid and, when subjected to compressing vertical forces, converts them to horizontal forces and distributes them equally to all sides of the elastic annulus. By this phenomenon, the extent of hydration of the nucleus and the compressing forces acting upon it are in constant equilibrium.[4, 6, 9, 10, 18, 27] The nucleus is constantly subjected to forces of tension and compression of varying magnitudes resulting from muscular activity and muscle tone.

It was previously noted that the nucleus is composed of a protein-polysaccharide complex imbedding fine fibrils of collagen, and also that the imbibition index of the nucleus is dependent upon the quantitive ratio between the collagen and protein-polysaccharide complex. It is postulated that with aging there is a gradual depolymerization of the mucopolysaccharides resulting in an increase in collagen and a decrease in polysaccharides. When this occurs the gel characteristics of the nucleus are impaired, its lower imbibition index is reduced, it can no longer equalize the forces of compression and tension, nor distribute them to the annulus equally.[8, 18] It will be recalled that in early life the water content of the nucleus is approximately 88 per cent, but in the eighth decade it approaches 69 per cent.[22] In the young, by virtue of the physical characteristics of the nucleus, this structure is elastic and resilient and the annulus is flexible and elastic. The nucleus functions as a perfect gel, distributing forces of compression and tension equally to all parts of the annulus. With aging, because of the biochemical changes that occur in the nucleus, it becomes less elastic and more fibrous as a result of the increase in disorganized collagen and in polysaccharides; its gel characteristics become somewhat impaired, and forces are unevenly distributed to the annulus and the articular plates. The annulus is subjected to abnormal compression and shows evidence of degeneration.[12] The process is progressive with increasing age. The individual reaches old age with discs functioning markedly less effectively than they performed in youth, if the discs are not subjected to some noxious factors. Nevertheless, the discs are still capable of meeting the demands of activity imposed upon them in the late decades of life. These physiological abnormalities of the discs render them vulnerable to abnormal stresses. It is for this reason that the incidence of lumbar disc lesion is so high in the fourth and fifth decades, a time when the process is at its height and the individual is still in a very active stage of life (Fig. 3-7).

In the pathologic disc, the biochemical changes occurring in the nucleus and the deterioration of its gel characteristics pursue a much more rapid course, until the nucleus is totally destroyed and the function

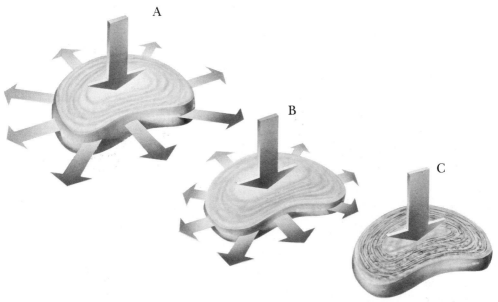

Figure 3-7 Distribution of forces in the normal and abnormal disc. *A*, When the disc functions normally, as in the early decades of life, the nucleus pulposus distributes the forces of compression and tension equally to all parts of annulus. *B*, With degeneration, the nucleus no longer functions as a perfect gel. Now the forces distributed to the annulus are less and not equal. *C*, With advanced degeneration of the nucleus, the distribution of forces to the annulus from within is completely lost; the degenerated annulus can now be compared to a flat tire.

of the motor unit is severely impaired.[9, 10, 15] Let us now consider the primary changes that occur in the pathologic disc and the secondary alterations that occur in the adjacent tissues, and correlate these observations with the symptoms. Essentially the continuing pathologic process can be considered in three phases or stages. (See Armstrong[1] and Hendry.[9, 10])

The Early Phase of the Pathologic Process

It should be remembered that in a normal disc the nucleus and annulus are distinct structures, one blending with the other. The fibrils of the collagen in the nucleus intermingle and fuse with the inner fibers of the annulus and with the articular plates above and below. In the early phase of the pathologic process, the hydrophilic properties of the nucleus are impaired because of the breakdown of its polysaccharides and buildup of its collagen. As the collagen fibers increase in number, they group themselves in a disorganized fashion to form free-floating fragments in a semifluid matrix.

Concurrently with these changes the annulus begins to show evidence of early degeneration. Its texture becomes less elastic; its posterior inner fibers fibrillate and tear apart, producing irregular perforations. The

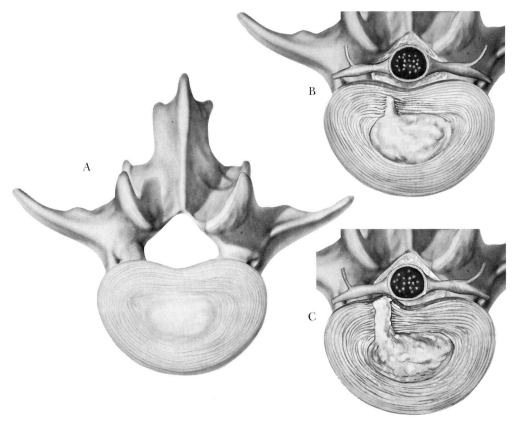

Figure 3-8   Phases of degeneration of the intervertebral disc. *A*, This represents a normal disc. The nucleus and annulus are distinct structures, one blending with the other. *B*, Early phase of degeneration. Increasing numbers of free-floating bodies are seen in the nucleus caused by an increase in the collagen content. Also note the fenestrations occurring in the annulus especially in the posterior fibers. Nuclear material is beginning to push out into the defects in the annulus. This is the end of the early phase. The posterior longitudinal ligament is intact. *C*, Intermediate phase. Nuclear material extrudes through the annulus and even may perforate the posterior longitudinal ligament.

process is more pronounced at varying distances from the midline of the posterior annulus. At this point, the nuclear material is confined to the intervertebral space only by the posterior longitudinal ligament, and here the early phase terminates.

Because the imbibition index of the nucleus is lowered, its gel characteristics are seriously impaired; therefore, the annulus, particularly its posterior portion, is subjected to constant ever-increasing forces that cause further degeneration of the annular fibers. At this stage the disc is indeed vulnerable; if it should be exposed to excessive stresses incident to normal activity or to other forms of trauma, the nucleus may break through the annulus or even through the posterior longitudinal ligament, which is the last barrier between it and the spinal canal. With the termination of the early phase, the nucleus and the annulus lose their distinctive features and the nucleus assumes characteristics of the fibrous annulus (Fig. 3-8 *A* and *B*).

The Intermediate Phase of the Pathologic Process

During this phase, extrusions of sequestrated nuclear material occur; they vary in size from very small, shredded particles to the entire nucleus. Extrusion of the complete nucleus is rare. Several factors govern the mechanism of escape of nuclear fragments. Clinical experience reveals that, generally, most nuclear extrusions occur gradually and intermittently and only a few occur suddenly. In those whose clinical manifestations suggest sudden displacement resulting from injury, it must be assumed that the herniation was already present and that the injury was responsible only for further retropulsion of the fragment and perhaps perforation of a defective posterior longitudinal ligament. It was previously noted that gravity, muscular activity and muscle tone maintain the nucleus under varying degrees of positive pressure at all times, and that the annulus which confines the nucleus is constantly slightly distended.[4] Even when the normal dynamics of the nucleus is impaired, the nucleus keeps the annulus in a state of slight tension. When the annulus perforates, an intact nucleus tends to bulge into the defect; however, if the nucleus is broken down into free sequestrae, some of these fragments herniate into the annular fenestrations. They are now contained only by the posterior longitudinal ligament (Fig. 3-8 C).

Loss of nuclear mass brings about a reduction in the positive pressure within the annulus; extrusions continue to occur until the internal pressure equals the external pressure, at which point a state of balanced pressures is reached and further extrusion of nuclear fragments ceases. This state of equilibrium may be disturbed by subjecting the motor unit to excessive compression forces; should this occur, more nuclear tissue may be forced out of the intervertebral space. Also, with loss of the gel characteristics of the nucleus, the forces of compression, which are acting constantly, force the vertebral bodies closer together. The annulus then becomes the only structure separating the vertebral bodies and is the recipient of constant, compressive insults. This repeated trauma, sustained by the annulus, not only initiates further degenerative changes within it but also sets the stage for the development of secondary changes in the surrounding tissues.[12]

TYPES OF PROTRUSIONS

Only the surgeon who has explored many hundreds of disc spaces can fully appreciate the great variability in size and shape of nuclear protrusions and can correlate the accompanying symptoms or lack of them with the different types of lesions. A classification based on the site of the protrusions and their relationship to the neural elements in the affected region is helpful in the clarification of the clinical picture.

Most nuclear protrusions associated with lumbar disc lesions can be grouped into three categories: lateral protrusions, intraforaminal protrusions and dorsal protrusions.

LATERAL PROTRUSIONS

The weakest portion of the posterior annulus is to either side of the midline where it lacks reinforcement by the strong central fibers of the posterior longitudinal ligament. This is also the commonest site of nuclear protrusions in the lumbar spine. Having penetrated the annulus, the protrusion lodges under the posterior longitudinal ligament, which is stretched commensurate with the size of the fragment and the degree of internal pressure within the disc. In this position it appears as a firm, smooth mound. To accommodate the sequestrated fragment the posterior ligament is lifted off the vertebral bodies. As the nuclear mass increases in size, further stripping of the ligament occurs; now the mass may migrate in any direction—cephalad, caudad, medially or laterally. Generally, it moves in a lateral direction close to and parallel to a nerve root and may even extend into the intervertebral foramen. Under the ligament, the mass lies tightly compressed and folded upon itself; it may be completely

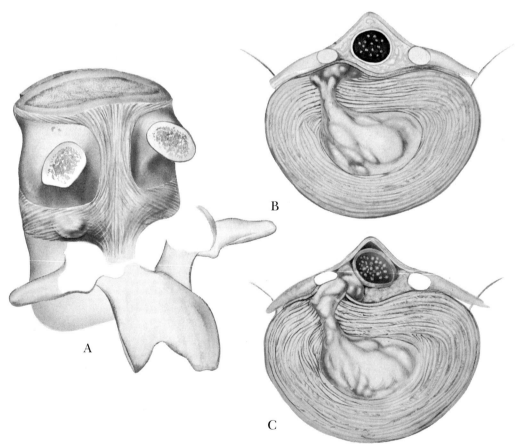

Figure 3-9 *A*, Lateral protrusion. The protrusion lies lateral to the midline and lateral to the strong central fibers of the posterior longitudinal ligament. This is the weakest portion of the annulus. *B*, The nuclear material is still confined by the posterior longitudinal ligament. *C*, The nuclear material has penetrated the posterior longitudinal ligament and now lies in the spinal canal.

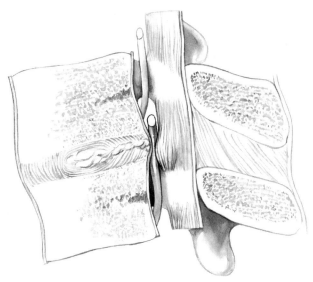

Figure 3-10 Large protrusions of nuclear material may compress the nerve root against the bony laminae or a hypertrophied ligamentum flavum.

free or it may still be attached to material in the nucleus by strands of irregular, stringy, fibrous tissue. This type of protrusion is by far the commonest lesion encountered (Fig. 3-9).

Occasionally, a dissecting protrusion may erode through the posterior ligament at a distance from its site of exit from the annulus. More commonly, the fragment is retropulsed through the annulus and the ligament at the same time. These free sequestrae, regardless of their mode of origin, may move in any direction in the spinal canal. The usual course is along one of the extrathecal nerve roots and they may lodge in the intervertebral foramen (Fig. 3-9).

It becomes apparent that both the dissecting and the extruded nuclear materials may make contact with one of the nerve roots anywhere from the point of exit at the dura to the intervertebral foramen. In most instances, the nuclear material lodges directly under or slightly to either side of the root, putting it in great tension. Because of the lack of elasticity of the roots outside the dura, even a small protrusion is capable of putting the root in tension. In this position, local secondary inflammatory changes bind the root tightly to the underlying nuclear mound so that the root can be displaced to one side or the other of the mass only with great difficulty. In cases of long standing, the root may actually become embedded in the heap of local fibrous tissue formed. The root also responds to the abnormal situation; it becomes injected, edematous and cordlike. Within the nerve sheath, granulation tissue appears which, with maturation, is converted to dense fibrous tissue binding the nerve fasciculi together and in some instances actually destroying the fibers. The neurologic deficits resulting from this process may be permanent.

Large protrusions, in addition to creating tension in a nerve root, may also compress the nerve root against the bony laminae or a hypertrophied ligamentum flavum (Fig. 3-10). If by chance, the spinal canal is narrowed, either by congenital or acquired abnormalities, compression of the root becomes even more likely. Hypertrophy of the ligamentum flavum is not recognized as a cause of compression by some observers; however, in the authors' opinion this is a very likely causative factor, particularly in unstable vertebral motor units. Also, in lumbar spines with an exaggerated lumbar angle and an almost horizontal sacrum, the laminae of the fifth lumbar vertebra may actually dig into the dural sac like a tight collar around a thick neck. When compression rather than tension of a nerve root is predominant, sensory and motor deficits are the chief complaints, and pain is assigned an insignificant role in the clinical picture.

INTRAFORAMINAL PROTRUSIONS

As stated previously, a posterior protrusion may be retropulsed into the spinal canal, rupturing through the posterior annulus and the posterior ligament instantaneously and finally coming to lodge in one of the intervertebral foramina. Also, a dissecting protrusion may eventually break through the posterior ligament, gaining access to the spinal canal and eventually migrating into a foramen. Once in the foramen, the nuclear mass is more apt to compress a nerve root than to put it in tension. On the other hand, the local reactive changes that occur in the bony canal often bind the root firmly in the canal so that the slightest tension, such as produced by straight leg-raising, causes severe pain (Fig. 3-11).

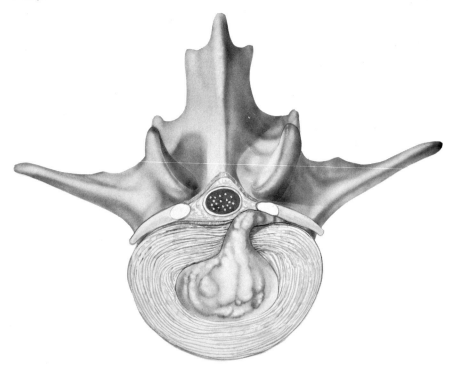

Figure 3-11 Intraforaminal protrusion. The sequestrum may migrate into the foramen and cause severe compression of the nerve root.

Dorsal protrusions

A true dorsal protrusion occurs when the nuclear material is extruded through the central portion of the annulus but contained by the posterior longitudinal ligament. At this site the central fibers of the posterior longitudinal ligament add considerable reinforcement to the posterior annulus; therefore, complete ruptures at this point are extremely rare. However, the ligament may rupture, particularly when the spine is subjected to violent flexion forces. The nuclear material is retropulsed through the posterior ligament into the spinal canal. From this point, its behavior is similar to that of lateral extrusions and it is capable of causing tension and compression of the extrathecal roots. When the nuclear material is contained by the posterior ligament, no involvement of the roots occurs, but the posterior ligament may be severely stretched, producing back pain without radicular pain. The protrusion may not retain this position; subsequent stress may force the mass to a lateral position (Fig. 3-12).

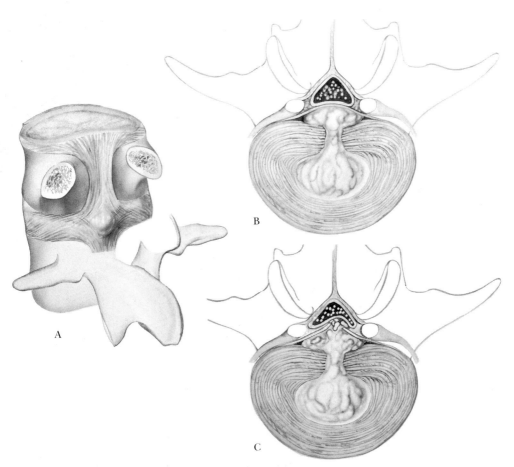

Figure 3-12 *A*, Dorsal protrusion. The nuclear material migrates directly backward, opposite the strong central fibers of the posterior longitudinal ligament. Rupture of the posterior ligament is rare. *B*, The nuclear material is confined by the posterior longitudinal ligament. *C*, The nuclear material has extruded through the posterior ligament and now lies in the spinal canal.

VARIATIONS OF THE USUAL TYPES OF DISC LESIONS

So far the usual types of disc lesions encountered have been considered. There are variations of these which may produce a bizarre and confusing clinical picture; yet, if one understands the nature of these lesions the symptom complex becomes clear.

MASSIVE EXTRUSION

From time to time a massive herniation may occur as the result of severe flexion forces applied to the lumbar spine. The extruded nuclear fragment may be a large portion of the nucleus pulposus or the entire nucleus. It may be retained by the posterior ligament or it may extrude through it. Often portions of the annulus of varying size accompany the nuclear material. The clinical picture resulting from sudden compression of the dural sac and the cauda equina is very characteristic (Fig. 3-13). A rapid onset of paraplegia with loss of sphincter control follows. Unless this lesion is recognized and treatment instituted immediately, irreversible changes in the cauda equina set in; even when adequate decompression of the cauda equina is promptly performed, recovery is slow and more often than not incomplete.

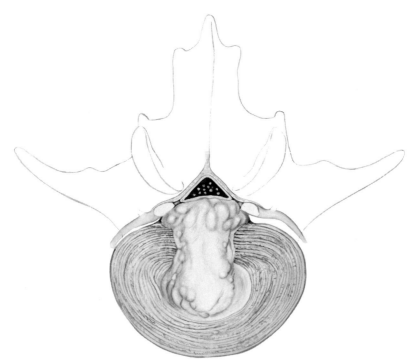

Figure 3-13   Massive extrusion of nuclear material which has penetrated the posterior longitudinal ligament and is compressing the cauda equina.

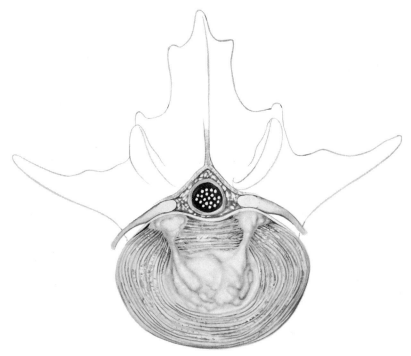

Figure 3-14   Bilateral disc lesion. The nuclear material has penetrated the defective annulus on both sides of the midline producing two lateral protrusions at the same level.

BILATERAL DISC LESIONS

The posterior annulus may degenerate sufficiently on both sides of the midline to allow fragments of nuclear material to extrude on both sides simultaneously or at different times. Patients with such lesions may have pain in both extremities or the pain may appear first on one side and then on the opposite side. Another variation is a single lesion on one side which gradually becomes larger and migrates medially under the central portion of the posterior ligament and appears finally on the opposite side of the midline (Fig. 3-14).

DISC LESIONS AT DIFFERENT LEVELS

It has been pointed out that the pathologic process affecting discs may occur simultaneously at several or all levels of the lumbar spine. There may be a difference in the speed of the process at different levels and herniations may occur at one level and not at another. However, not infrequently (10 to 20 per cent of all lumbar disc lesions), extrusion of nuclear material occurs at two levels, usually but not necessarily in contiguous discs and on the same side. Only one lesion may be responsible for the clinical syndrome presented, but the other is surely a potential source of future trouble. The possibility of multiple lesions should be kept in mind when surgical treatment is instituted.

TRAPPED NUCLEAR MATERIAL

Nuclear material extruding through the annulus may be trapped between the rims of the contiguous vertebral bodies, producing a sudden onset of pain of varying intensity in the lumbar region. Generally the pain is severe and is aggravated by all spinal movements. It may disappear as suddenly as it appears or after a few days may be accompanied by severe sciatica. Armstrong's explanation of this phenomenon is the most logical one of all the mechanisms offered so far.[1] The displaced material may either recede into the disc space or be extruded beyond the rims of the vertebral bodies. This "unlocking" of the joint explains the sudden relief of pain. If the extruded sequestrum migrates laterally and comes into contact with the nerve root, radicular pain will be produced. Unlocking of the joint may also follow shrinkage of the nuclear material. When this occurs, the symptoms recede slowly and finally disappear.

The Final Phase of the Pathologic Process

This phase is characterized by complete disintegration of the nucleus and the annulus, followed by an active reparative process which terminates in replacement of the disc by dense fibrous tissue that firmly binds the vertebral bodies one to the other. This is a continuous process with no definitive line of cleavage separating it from the intermediate phase; indeed, there is considerable overlap between the two. It was previously pointed out that, concurrent with degeneration of the gel of the nucleus, changes are also discernible in the inner layers of the annulus. Here, radiating clefts and fenestrations appear; also, fibrillation of and defects in the articular cartilage of the adjacent vertebral plates occur. Through these defects, granulation tissue infiltrates the disc space and eventually replaces the entire disc. It is obvious that nuclear extrusions can and do occur during the phase of fibrous tissue formation; when this process is the predominant feature, the final stage is in full progress.

It should be understood that not all the nuclear material is sequestrated and extruded in the intermediate stage. Much of the degenerated nuclear material remains in the disc space; some remains attached to the annulus and the vertebral plates and some lies free. In this portion of the nucleus the breaking-down process of the mucopolysaccharides and the increase of irregularly formed collagen continues until the nuclear tissue has lost all its hydrophilic properties and assumes the characteristics of the degenerated annulus fibrosus. On the other hand, it should not be assumed that nuclear extrusions do not occur in the final stage. From time to time, an elderly individual presents the classic picture of a lumbar disc lesion with nerve root irritation. The authors have seen many elderly patients in whom the dominating feature of the syndrome was sciatica with little or no back pain. The motor unit in these individuals is firmly fixed by fibrosis, but the reparative process is still not completed. This accounts for the absence of back pain and the extrusion of small fragments of free nuclear material.

This phase terminates when the reparative process is complete; at this point all nuclear tissue and the entire annulus are converted into mature fibrous tissue; the motor unit becomes completely stable. The fate of extruded nuclear material is the same as that within the disc space. It too undergoes fibrosis and finally even bone formation, appearing as small osteophytes attached to the vertebral rims. The entire process may take many years. Slight narrowing of the disc, seen on radiographs, may be noted relatively early, but advanced collapse of the disc space with secondary changes in the vertebral bodies and the posterior articulations may not be discernible for many years (Fig. 3-15).

The secondary alterations that occur in the wake of degeneration of the nucleus pulposus implicate all the elements comprising the motor unit. In addition to destruction of the nucleus and the annulus, the articular plates degenerate. Because the hydrostatic mechanism between the vertebrae is lost, the anterior portions of the vertebral bodies come closer together and become directly subjected to compressive forces. This results in condensation of the subchondral bone of the bodies and, in some instances, diffuse sclerosis of one or both vertebrae. The annulus and the surrounding ligaments are also subjected to the ravages of compressive forces, resulting in the formation of osteophytes, often beak-shaped, along the rims of the vertebral bodies. Finally, with approximation of the vertebrae, there is telescoping of the articular facets of the

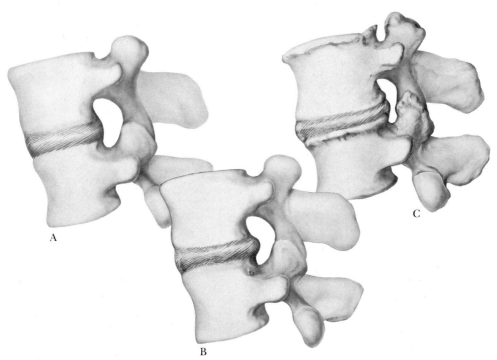

Figure 3-15 Progressive degeneration of a lumbar disc. *A*, The disc is intact and shows no evidence of collapse. *B*, As the degenerative process advances the height of the disc decreases and the annulus fibrosis begins to collapse. *C*, In the final stage, there is complete collapse of the disc with secondary changes in the posterior joints and along the adjacent rims of the vertebral bodies of the motor unit. Observe that these hypertrophic bony changes decrease the width of the intervertebral foramen.

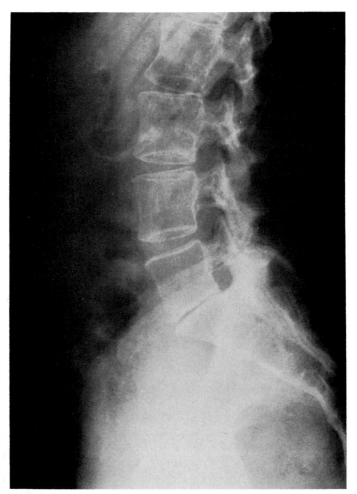

Figure 3-16   The final phase of lumbar disc disease. Note the almost complete obliteration of the L5-S1 disc space and the condensation of subchondral bone of the vertebral bodies adjacent to the disc. There is also considerable sclerosis in the region of the posterior articular joints. In this instance the amount of hypertrophic formation along the rims of the L5 and S1 vertebrae adjacent to the disc is minimal. This patient (female, 45 years old) complained of only occasional minimal discomfort in her lower back. She never had pain in her legs.

posterior joints and stretching of their capsules. All the posterior ligaments of the motor unit (the supraspinous ligament, the interspinous ligament and the ligamenta flava) are placed in a state of constant tension, which eventually results in pronounced thickening of these structures. The resulting incongruity of the articular surface causes degeneration of the articular cartilage, subchondral sclerosis of the facets and some spurring at the joint margins. It should be remembered that the posterior articular joints form the posteromedial boundaries of the intervertebral foramina and that the discs and posterior surfaces of the vertebral bodies form the anterior boundaries. Bony spurs formed at these sites may project into the foramina and even compress the nerve roots. We have

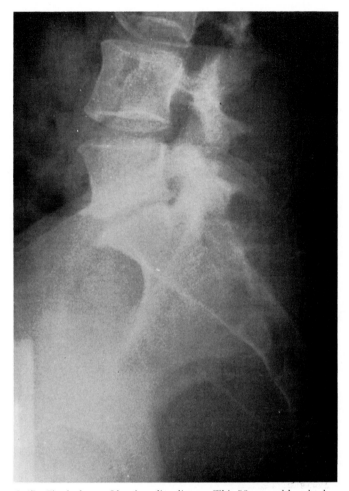

Figure 3-17   Final phase of lumbar disc disease. This 52-year-old male shows advanced degeneration of the L5-S1 disc. Observe the marked hypertrophic bone formation along the rims of the vertebrae; also note the increased density of the bone of both vertebrae adjacent to the disc. A large posterior spur on the posterior inferior rim of the fifth lumbar vertebra projects directly backward into the foramen. This patient had little or no back pain but did have persistent sciatica in the left leg. The symptoms were relieved by decompressing the left S1 nerve root by a foramenotomy.

demonstrated this pathologic process many times at the operating table. Root irritation caused in this manner can only be relieved by a foramenotomy (Figs. 3-16, 3-17, and 3-18).

In some instances, individuals are spared the painful phase of extrusion of nuclear fragments. For some reason not clear, the degenerated nuclear material is retained at all times within the disc space, and the pathologic process progresses from the phase of degeneration of the gel of the nucleus directly to the reparative phase, which culminates in total replacement of the disc by fibrous tissue. This is not a rare occurrence and is frequently demonstrable by radiographs of elderly individuals who have never had serious back disabilities.

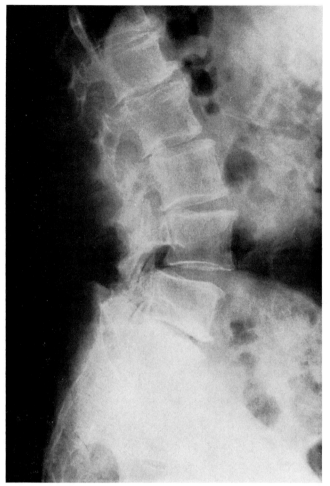

Figure 3-18 Degeneration of multiple discs. All the lumbar discs show varying degrees of degeneration. The discs more severely involved are the T12-L1, L1-L2 and the L5-S1 discs. This 62-year-old male had repeated episodes of back pain for many years and only one severe attack of sciatica in the right leg which did not respond to conservative measures. At operation, extruded disc material was found at the L4-L5 level; the right L5 nerve root was implicated.

FURTHER CONSIDERATION OF ROOT-PROTRUSION RELATIONSHIP

It was pointed out that in the lower lumbar spine the nerve root leaves the dura one vertebral segment above its foramen of exit. Therefore, in order to reach the foramen, the root must cross the posterolateral aspect of the disc below the vertebral body opposite which it emerged. A dissecting disc which migrates directly laterally may implicate the nerve root traversing the foramen. More specifically, the fourth lumbar nerve root emerges at the interspace between the fourth and fifth lumbar vertebrae. However, because the inferior vertebral notch is so far distal, the root leaves the canal posterior to the lower end of the fourth lumbar

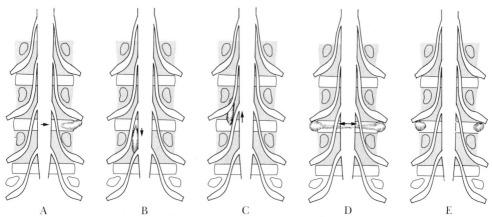

A   B   C   D   E

Figure 3-19 Different pathways extruded disc material may take. *A*, If a protrusion arises from the L4-L5 disc and migrates directly laterally, it may implicate the fourth lumbar root. This is a rare situation. *B*, Generally the protrusion migrates downward and laterally and involves the fifth root before it reaches the foramen at the L5-S1 level or it may proceed into the foramen. *C*, The protrusion may travel upward and involve the fourth root before it enters the L4-L5 foramen. *D*, Posterolateral protrusions usually involve the root crossing the disc from which the protrusion originated. *E*, Large or double protrusions may involve both roots at this level.

vertebra and, therefore, passes above rather than across the disc at this interspace (Fig. 3-5). Because of this anatomic peculiarity, extruded nuclear material from the L4-L5 disc does not affect the fourth root, but rather involves the fifth root, which is the most lateral root and which crosses the L4-L5 disc as it proceeds downward and laterally. The fourth root may be involved by extrusions from the L4-L5 disc if the nuclear mass is sufficiently large to push the root against the pedicle of the fourth lumbar vertebra or against the ligamentum flavum.

Stated in another way, if the protrusion arises from the L4-L5 disc and occupies the foramen between the L4-L5 vertebral bodies, the fourth lumbar root is affected. However, the protrusion may migrate downward and laterally and involve the fifth root before it reaches the foramen at the L5-S1 level, or it may proceed into the L5-S1 foramen and there trap the fifth root. The protrusion may also travel upward and involve the fourth root before it reaches its foramen of exit. Posterolateral protrusion usually involves the nerve root crossing the disc from which the protrusion originated; large or double posterolateral protrusions may implicate both roots at this level (Fig. 3-19).

The relationship of the disc to the nerve root frequently determines the posture the patient presents. Generally, during an acute episode, the individual assumes one of two postures: (1) the normal lumbar curve is flattened or even reversed without scoliosis of the trunk, or, (2) the lumbar curve is flattened and associated with scoliosis to one or the other side. Occasionally the scoliosis may shift from one side to the other. Invariably individuals exhibiting these postures also have pronounced spasm of the paravertebral muscles. Clinically, it is obvious that the different postures and the muscle spasm are protective measures to attain relief of pain. Scoliosis is an involuntary attempt on the part of the

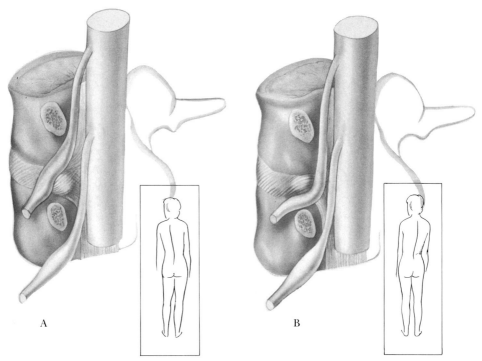

A   B

Figure 3-20   Relation of the disc protrusion to the nerve root when the patient presents sciatic scoliosis. *A*, When the lesion is lateral to the root and displaces it medially, tension on the root is reduced by bending the trunk away from the lesion. *B*, When the lesion is medial to the nerve root and displaces it laterally, tension on the root is reduced by bending the spine toward the lesion.

individual to reduce nerve root irritation by reducing the forces of compression and tension acting on it; therefore, if the protrusion lies to the medial side of the nerve root and displaces it laterally, the effect of these forces is lessened by bending the spine toward the side of the lesion. On the other hand, if the protrusion is on the lateral side of the nerve root, displacing the root medially, tension is reduced by bending the spine away from the side of the lesion (Fig. 3-20). Frequently, these individuals complain of radiating pain in one leg without associated back pain, indicating that nerve root irritation is the predominant cause of the presenting symptom complex. Simple flattening or even reversal of the lumbar curve is frequently not associated with radicular pain; the pain is localized in the lower lumbar spine and any movement of the spine accentuates the pain. It appears that, in these instances, the prime pathologic feature is disruption of an intervertebral joint rather than root irritation. The postures and associated muscle spasm are methods to prevent all motion at the affected joint. It is not uncommon to observe patients with severe spasm of the lumbar muscles, complete obliteration of the normal lumbar lordosis and no back pain.

In summation the features deserving special emphasis are as follows.

1. From beginning to end, the pathologic process affecting the lumbar discs is continuous.

2. Three phases are discernible, but these overlap.

3. The early phase is typified by disintegration of the nucleus pulposus, which, under normal conditions, functions as a perfect gel. The essential biochemical change is a breaking down of the mucopolysaccharides, resulting in an increase in collagen and a decrease in polysaccharides.

4. There is a gradual loss of the hydrophilic properties of the nucleus until it is hydrostatically inert.

5. Concurrently with changes in the nucleus, degenerative changes occur in the annulus, beginning with its inner fibers.

6. The intermediate phase is characterized by extrusion of fragments of degenerated nuclear material. This phase goes on intermittently for many years.

7. The site of extrusion from the posterior annulus can be used as a basis for the classification of the different forms of extrusions.

8. The presenting clinical picture can be closely correlated with the stage of development of the pathologic process and with the nature and behavior of displaced nuclear fragments.

9. The end point of the process is fibrous ankylosis of the contiguous vertebral bodies, at which time symptoms disappear.

10. Characteristic secondary changes occur in all the parts of the motor unit and these changes, in some instances, may produce symptoms.

11. Finally, the process spans a period of many months and even years.

REFERENCES

1. Armstrong, J. R.: Lumbar Disc Lesions. Baltimore, Williams & Wilkins, 1965.
2. Bartelink, D. L.: Role of abdominal pressure in relieving pressure on the lumbar intervertebral discs. J. Bone Joint Surg. 38-B:718-725, 1957.
3. Charnley, J.: Orthopaedic signs in diagnosis of disc protrusion, with special reference to straight-leg-raising test. Lancet 1:186-192, 1951.
4. Charnley, J.: Imbibition of fluid as cause of herniation of nucleus pulposus. Lancet 1:124-127, 1952.
5. Cloward, R. B.: The clinical significance of the sinuvertebral nerve of the cervical spine in relation to the cervical disc syndrome. J. Neurol. Neurosurg. Psychiat. 23:321-6, 1960.
6. Davidson, E. A. et al.: Biochemical alterations in herniated intervertebral discs. J. Biol. Chem. 234:2951, 1959.
7. Falconer, M. A. et al: Observations on cause and mechanism of symptom-production in sciatica and low back pain. J. Neurol. Neurosurg. and Psychiat. 11:13-26, 1948.
8. Hall, D. A. et al.: Mucopolysaccharides of human nuclei pulposi. Nature (Lond.) 179:1078, 1957.
9. Hendry, N. G. C.: The hydration of the nucleus pulposus and its relation to intervertebral disc derangement. J. Bone Joint Surg. 40-B:132-144, 1958.
10. Hendry, N. G. C.: Physical changes in the prolapsed disc. Lancet 2:158, 1958.
11. Junghanns, H.: Der lumbosakralwinkel. Dtsch. Zschr. Chir. 213-322, 1929.
12. Lindblom, K.: Intervertebral disc degeneration considered as a pressure atrophy. J. Bone Joint Surg. 39-A:933-945, 1957.
13. Luschka, H.: Die halbgelenke des menschlicken. Kärpess, Berlin, 1858.
14. Luschka, H.: Die nerven des menschlicken wirbelkanals. Tubingen, 1850.
15. Mitchell, P. E. et al.: The chemical background of intervertebral disc prolapse. J.Bone Joint Surg. (B), 43-B:141-151, 1961.

16. Morris, J. H., Lucas, D. B., and Bresler, B.: Role of the trunk in stability of the spine. J. Bone Joint Surg. 43-A:327-351.

17. Nachemson, A. and Morris, J. M.: In vivo measurements of interdiscal pressure. J. Bone Joint Surg. 46-A:1077-1092, 1964.

18. Naylor, A. and Smare, D. L.: Fluid content of the nucleus pulposus as a factor in the disc syndrome. Preliminary report. Brit. Med. J. 2:975, 1953.

19. Naylor, A. et al.: Collagenous changes in intervertebral disc with age and their effect on its elasticity: X-ray crystallographic study. Brit. Med. J. 2:570-573, 1954.

20. Naylor, A.: The biophysical and biochemical aspects of intervertebral disc herniation and degeneration. Ann. Roy. Coll. Surg. Eng. 31:91-114, 1962.

21. Pedersen, H. E., Blunck, C. F. V., and Gardner, E.: The anatomy of the lumbosacral posterior rami and meningeal branches of spinal nerves (sinu-vertebral nerves). J. Bone Joint Surg. 38-A:377-391, 1956.

22. Puschel, J.: Der Wasserergehalt normaler und degenerierter Zwischenwirbelscheiben. Beitr. Path. Anat. 84:123-130, 1930.

23. Roofe, P. G.: Innervation of annulus fibrosus and posterior longitudinal ligament. Arch. Path. 27:201-211, 1939.

24. Sarpyener, M. A.: Congenital stricture of the spinal canal. J. Bone Joint Surg. 27:70-90, 1945.

25. Schlesinger, P. T.: Incarceration of the first sacral nerve in a lateral bony recess of the spinal canal as a cause of sciatica: Anatomy — two case reports. J. Bone Joint Surg. 37-A:115-124, 1955.

26. Schmorl, G.: and Junghanns, H.: The Human Spine in Health and Disease. Grune & Stratton, New York, 1959.

27. Woodhall, B. et al.: The well leg-raising test of Fajerstajn in the diagnosis of ruptured lumbar intervertebral disc. J. Bone Joint Surg. 32-A786-792, 1950.

28. Verbiest, H.: Radicular syndrome from developmental narrowing of the lumbar vertebral canal. J. Bone Joint Surg. 36-B:230-237, 1954.

Chapter 4

THE CLINICAL SYNDROME OF CERVICAL DISC DISEASE

In attempting to delineate the clinical picture of a patient with degenerative disc disease of the cervical spine, one must be fully cognizant of the pathologic processes in this area. In contradistinction to the acute nuclear herniation or annular protrusion of the lumbar spine, chronic disc degeneration with an acute inflammatory process superimposed is more often found in the cervical area. In the chapter on the pathology of the intervertebral disc, detailed descriptions of the pathologic changes found in the cervical spine are presented and will not be reiterated here, except to stress once again that an acute herniation of soft disc material is but one stage of a larger process of disc degeneration having many biochemical and physical changes.

HISTORY

The onset of pain in cervical disc disease may be either insidious or acute. If the onset is related to trauma the patient will usually describe his discomfort as beginning within several hours of the injury, but pain may be delayed for as much as 24 to 48 hours. In those individuals with an atraumatic onset of neck pain, discomfort will usually be noted on awakening in the morning. The character of the pain is usually described as aching, but frequently it is closely associated with a feeling of stiffness.

The majority of patients with a cervical syndrome secondary to degenerative disc disease will at some time develop associated pain in the shoulder girdles, upper extremities and head. The associated symptomatology in cervical spine disorders is best understood if one recalls the various methods of pain production. One might simplify this problem by categorizing associated pain as radicular, referred, myelopathy or pressure phenomena on associated soft tissue.

The pain produced by compression or irritation of nerve roots is the most easily understood of the symptoms in the cervical spine. Pain and sensory changes such as numbness and paresthesia will usually follow the distribution of one or more dermatomes. These have been well described by Murphy and Simmons in their experience with 250 ruptured cervical discs.[16] In addition to the pain and sensory changes found with root compression, the patient will also note weakness of the various muscle groups in the upper extremities and, frequently, difficulty with coordination. An other characteristic which helps to identify radicular pain is that the pain can be accentuated by maneuvers which stretch the involved roots. In addition, this pain is increased by maneuvers which increase intrathoracic or intra-abdominal pressure, such as coughing, sneezing and straining.

Referred pain is produced by stimulation of sensory nerve endings in the structural soft tissues which support the cervical spine and which are part of the cervical disc complex. This type of pain may be reproduced by the injection of hypertonic saline into the annulus fibrosus of an intervertebral disc, producing not only neck pain but pain referred to the muscles of the shoulder girdle and occiput. In attempting to differentiate this type of pain from radicular pain, the physician is helped by the fact that referred pain will usually not localize itself to a clearly defined dermatome. It is often vague, aching in character and without the lancinating quality found in root compression pain. It is usually not accentuated by coughing or sneezing but, like radicular pain, is mechanical in nature, that is, made worse with stress and relieved by rest.

The pain of cervical myelopathy is unique.[3] It is not intensified by motion of the neck or straining; it is frequently poorly localized and seldom radiates; it is usually referred to the anterior aspect of the thighs, the buttocks or the subcostal areas. The pain has been described as having a bursting nature with a thermal quality. It is dull and aching rather than lancinating. In addition to pain, weakness in the lower extremities is often noted together with a sense of instability. Bowel and bladder symptoms may also be prominent.

Chronic cervical disc degeneration, particularly when associated with prominent osteophytes may produce symptomatology by pressure on surrounding soft tissues. Many of the symptoms are rather bizarre in nature and have often led to patients being erroneously classified as psychoneurotic. Dysphagia due to hypertrophic changes in the cervical spine has been described by many investigators.[2, 7, 8, 17] In extreme cases, tracheal compression symptoms may also be present. It is well known that these spurs may present a real danger during endoscopy and lead to an increased risk of esophageal perforation.

In addition to pressure on the esophagus and trachea, it has been well demonstrated that vertebral artery insufficiency may result from changes in the cervical spine.[14] It has been previously noted that the cervical sympathetic chain is in close relationship to the intervertebral disc and many bizarre visual and auditory symptoms will occassionally be noted in a patient with cervical disc disease due to irritation of these anatomic structures.

It has been pointed out by Ruth Jackson that headaches are frequently a pain in the neck and many pains in the neck are headaches.[12] Compression and irritation of cervical nerve roots may give rise to headache by direct nerve root compression. Usually the upper three or four nerve roots are involved in this process. Occipital headaches with occasional radiation to the ear or eye is noted with this type of problem. Irritation of the cervical sympathetic system may also lead to head pain. These headaches are frequently described as burning, pressure-like or throbbing and may be found in association with visual and auditory disturbance. Radicular type headaches in contrast to the described are sharp, shooting or splitting in nature.[4]

Less commonly severe atypical fascial neuralgia[1] or a pain pattern mimicking coronary ischemia may be described[13] in patients with a cervical syndrome.

It is particularly important to note the type of treatment which has been given to a patient with cervical disc disease and his response to this treatment. A prolonged course of unsuccessful conservative treatment will certainly influence the surgeon's position as to whether operative therapy is indicated. One must be aware however of the varying degree of cooperation the patient may have shown in adhering to previous regimens of treatment. If any doubt exists as to the efficacy or adequacy of prior conservative therapy, a repeated course of conservative therapy under the surgeon's personal observation would be indicated. This also offers an opportunity for the surgeon to evaluate the emotional status of the patient and his suitability as a surgical candidate.

PHYSICAL FINDINGS

The physical findings in examination of the cervical spine are of two types. There are in most patients with cervical disc disease certain non-specific findings which do not help to localize the level of the pathological process. There are other findings, particularly the neurologic abnormalities, which help the examiner to accurately localize the level of the lesion.

A decreased range of motion is frequently noted on physical examination. This limitation is due either to pain or, structurally, to abnormal bony and soft tissue elements in the cervical spine. Hyperextension and lateral rotation usually show evidence of less than a complete range of motion. Many patients will complain bitterly when the maneuver of hyperextension is performed. Paravertebral muscle spasm is frequently noted.

Tenderness is an extremely helpful finding in cervical disc disease. Two types of tenderness to palpation can be differentiated. One is diffuse, elicited by compression of the paravertebral muscles and found over a broad area of the posterolateral muscle masses. The second type of tenderness is more specific and, in a lean subject particularly, may help to localize the level of the degenerated disc. This may be elicited by localized pressure over the intervertebral foramina and spinous processes. Compression in these areas will reproduce not only neck pain but occasionally radicular pain of a type usually noted by the patient.

Compression of the vertex of the head will transmit stress to the intervertebral disc and may reproduce the patient's neck pain and radiculitis. This may sometimes be more easily elicited with the neck in lateral flexion or hyperextension.

Stimulation of the cervical sympathetic elements may produce inequality of pupil size or as we have seen on several occasions, a frank Horner's syndrome.

A complete neurologic examination including both the upper and lower extremities is mandatory in cases of cervical disc degeneration. This is necessary not only as a diagnostic measure for radicular compression but also as a baseline for the evaluation of myelopathy should this develop. With degeneration of the fifth cervical disc one usually will find neurologic involvement of the sixth cervical nerve root, although the root above or below may be involved. Examination will reveal numbness in the thumb, weakness of elbow flexion and a decreased biceps reflex (Table 4-1). With involvement of the seventh cervical root by the sixth cervical disc numbness will usually be noted in the index and middle fingers. There will be weakness of elbow extension and a reduced triceps reflex. The less common C8 radiculopathy secondary to a degenerated C7-T1 disc will produce numbness along the ulnar border of the hand on the little finger, moderate intrinsic muscle weakness in the hand and no reflex changes.

Table 4-1   *Nerve Root Patterns*

C5 NERVE ROOT (C4-C5 Disc)
    Pain—neck, tip of shoulder, anterior arm
    Sensory Change—deltoid area
    Motor Change—deltoid, biceps
    Reflex Change—biceps

C6 NERVE ROOT (C5-C6 Disc)
    Pain—neck, shoulder, medial border of scapula, lateral arm, dorsum forearm
    Sensory Change—thumb and index finger
    Motor Change—biceps
    Reflex Change—biceps

C7 NERVE ROOT (C6-C7 Disc)
    Pain—neck, shoulder, medial border of scapula, lateral arm, dorsum forearm
    Sensory Change—index and middle finger
    Motor Change—triceps
    Reflex Change—triceps

C8 NERVE ROOT (C7-T1 Disc)
    Pain—neck, medial border of scapula, medial aspect of arm and forearm
    Sensory Change—ring and little finger
    Motor Change—intrinsic muscles of hand
    Reflex Change—none

RADIOGRAPHIC FINDINGS IN DEGENERATIVE DISC DISEASE

Routine radiographic examination of the cervical spine should include anteroposterior, lateral, oblique and odontoid views of the spine. Flexion-extension views of cineradiography may be helpful in defining abnormalities of mobility. The generally accepted radiographic signs of degenerative disc disease are loss of height of the intervertebral disc space, osteophyte formation, secondary encroachment of the intervertebral foramina and osteoarthritic changes in the apophyseal joints. It has been our observation that in many patients with early disc degeneration, anterior bulging of the disc may be noted as a soft tissue shadow on good quality radiographs. Loss of the normal cervical lordosis may be seen in degenerative disc disease but is of limited significance.[10] This finding has been noted in patients with no evidence of cervical disc degeneration and also may be seen with slight variation in the positioning of the patient.

The difficult problem in regard to radiographic examination of the cervical spine is not the identification of these abnormalities on the roentgenogram but rather how much significance should be attributed to them. The most careful study in this regard was conducted by Friedenberg and Miller in which 92 matched pairs of asymptomatic and symptomatic patients were compared.[11] It was their conclusion that narrowing of the intervertebral space particularly between the fifth and sixth and sixth and seventh cervical vertebra was the most significant of the radiographic findings as related to symptomatology. There was no difference between the two groups in regard to changes at the joint of Luschka, the intervertebral foramina or the posterior articular processes. It has also been shown by Brain that large numbers of asymptomatic patients may show radiographic evidence of advanced degenerative disc disease.[4]

In most instances myelography has not proved helpful in diagnosis of disc degeneration or its localization. It has already been pointed out that most patients with cervical disc degeneration do not have a protrustion of a soft tissue mass into the neural canal as a pathological feature. For this reason myelography will usually be negative in patients with degenerative disc disease. In those instances where an acute soft disc is present in compressing a neural element, the symptoms and physical findings will be such that accurate clinical diagnosis is possible and myelography will be simply confirmatory. It is our feeling that in most instances cervical myelography is superfluous and is indicated only when there is some confusion as to the location or type of pathological process. This opinion is supported by others active in the field of cervical disc surgery.[16]

The injection of a radiopaque solution into the intervertebral disc for diagnostic purposes was first described by Lindbloom. This procedure as a diagnostic aid in cervical disc disease is somewhat controversial. Cloward feels this to be a helpful adjunct in the presurgical evaluation of a patient with cervical disc disease.[6] It is the authors' feeling, supported by the experience of others,[15] that cervical discography falls far short of its goals as a diagnostic tool. That leakage of dye is present by cervical discogram tells us only that certain structural changes are present in this disc. The essential question, that is, which disc is causing the patient's symptomatology, remains unanswered. It is well known that a high percentage of cervical intervertebral discs in middle-aged and elderly patients will show disc degeneration, although the great majority of these do not lead to clinical symptoms.

A cervical disc distention test is now utilized by the authors as a preoperative diagnostic test in most patients who will undergo cervical disc surgery. In this test physiologic saline is injected into the nucleus pulposus of the various cervical intervertebral discs. Usually one of the discs, so distended, will reproduce the patient's symptomatology. This, we feel, is a good index as to which disc is responsible for the patient's problems. This is particularly helpful when routine roentgenography demonstrates multiple levels of cervical disc involvement.

The technique of the cervical disc distention test is not complex. It is performed in the x-ray department with the patient placed on an image intensifier for x-ray guidance. After routine skin preparation with antiseptic solution and sterile draping, a 2-inch, No. 20 needle is inserted into the center of an intervertebral disc. The disc chosen for investigation will usually be that with the most marked degenerative changes by routine roentgenogram. The operator's fingers are placed in a vertical position along the anterior aspect of the sternocleidomastoid muscle. The interval is palpated between the larynx and carotid artery so that the anterior surface of the spine may be felt. When the needle has reached this area it is inserted approximately 1 mm. into the anterior fibers of the annulus. A No. 25, 2½-inch needle is then inserted through the larger needle so that its point will pass to the center of the disc. X-ray control verifies the position of the needle. Subsequently the disc is distended with physiologic saline solution and the patient questioned as to whether this has reproduced his typical pain pattern. If the answer is affirmative it is felt that this disc is contributing to the symptomatology. All discs which are under suspicion are investigated in this manner. No special precautions are taken after the completion of this study, although surgery is usually deferred for 12 to 24 hours.

Cervical vertebral phlebography has as yet not evolved to the point of routine clinical usefulness.

Cineradiography of the cervical spine as described by Fielding[9] and Buonocore[5] may be helpful in evaluating abnormalities of mobility in the cervical spine. These abnormalities may not be evident on static roentgenograms or on physical examination. Cineradiography will be performed in cases of a traumatic cervical syndrome in which routine roentgenograms are negative. A localized area of hypermobility may be demonstrated in this manner and effectively used as a guide of cervical spine stabilization.

Electromyelography has not become a part of the authors' routine diagnostic evaluation of cervical spine disease. It has been their experience that when the physical and neurologic examination is negative the electromyelogram will also be negative. The converse is also true, that is, with an easily demonstrated neurologic abnormality, confirmatory evidence will also be present on the electromyelogram. There is really no information from this examination that can not be demonstrated by other more easily applied modalities.

Once a decision has been reached that conservative therapy has failed and operative intervention is indicated, a second decision must be made as to the level of the proposed surgery. Knowledge of the pertinent anatomy and pathology has shown us that occasionally one may be led astray by strictly following the pattern of the patient's symptoms and his neurologic abnormalities. It is well known that any of three adjacent intervertebral discs may compress a given nerve root. On the other hand, when one combines the clinical picture gained through history and physical examination with routine roentgenographic evaluation and particularly the disc distention test, a reasonably accurate judgment as to which discs in the cervical spine are responsible for the patient's symptoms can be rendered.

REFERENCES

1. Ashkenazy, M.: Severe unilateral face pains as a presenting symptom of cervical spine lesions. Texas J. Med. 58:633-635, 1962.
2. Bettmann, E. H. et al.: Cervical disc pathology resulting in dysphagia in an adolescent boy. New York J. Med. 60:2465-2467, 1960.
3. Bradshaw, P.: Pain caused by cervical spondylosis. Rheumatism 17:2-7, 1961.
4. Brain, L.: Some unsolved problems of cervical spondylosis. Brit. Med. J. 5333:771-777, 1963.
5. Buonocore, E. et al.: Cineradiograms of cervical spine in diagnosis of soft tissue injuries. J.A.M.A. 198:143-147, 1966.
6. Cloward, R. B.: New method of diagnosis and treatment of cervical disc disease. Clin. Neurosurg. 8:93-132, 1962.
7. el-Sallab, R. A. et al.: Oesophageal and tracheal pseudo-tumors due to anterior cervical osteophytes, Brit. J. Radiol. 38:682-684, 1965.
8. Facer, J. C.: Osteophytes of the cervical spine causing dysphagia. Arch. Otolaryng. (Chicago) 86:341-345, 1967.
9. Fielding, J. W.: Cineroentgenography of the normal cervical spine. J.Bone Joint Surg. 39-A:1280-1288, 1957.
10. Fineman, S. et al.: The cervical spine: Transformation of the normal lordotic pattern into a linear pattern in the neutral posture. J. Bone Joint Surg. 45-A:1179-1183, 1963.
11. Friedenberg, Z. B. et al.: Degenerative disc disease of the cervical spine, J. Bone Joint Surg. 45-A:1171-1178, 1963.
12. Jackson, R.: Headaches associated with disorders of the cervical spine, Headache 6:175-179, 1967.
13. Kapoor, S. C. and Tiwary, P. K.: Cervical spondylosis simulating cardiac pain. Indian J. Chest Dis. (Delhi) 8:25-28, 1966.
14. Keggi, K. J. et al.: Vertebral artery insufficiency secondary to trauma and osteoarthritis of the cervical spine. Yale J. Biol. Med. 38:471-478, 1966.
15. Meyer, R. R.: Cervical discography. A help or hindrance in evaluating neck, shoulder, arm pain? Amer. J. Roentgen. 90:1208-1215, 1963.
16. Murphey, R. and Simmons, J.C.: Ruptured cervical disc. Experience with 250 cases. Amer. Surg. 32:83-88, 1966.
17. Perrone, J. A.: Dysphagia due to massive cervical exostoses. Arch. Otolaryng. (Chicago) 86:346-347, 1967.

Chapter 5

CONSERVATIVE TREATMENT OF CERVICAL DISC DISEASE

The majority of patients with cervical disc disease, either acute or chronic, will respond to a conscientious program of conservative therapy. Its efficacy is predicated upon the physician's complete understanding of the pathologic process involved and his ability to translate this knowledge into a rational and pragmatic course of therapy. He must educate the patient to understand the disease process and the reasons for a protracted course of therapy. It is only with a thorough understanding of the problem that the patient can show the necessary patience to persist with what may appear to be a long and burdensome course of therapy.

IMMOBILIZATION

In both acute and chronic disc disease, immobilization of the cervical spine is the cornerstone of therapy. In acute cervical injuries, immobilization serves to allow for healing of torn and attenuated soft tissues such as the anterior longitudinal ligaments and annulus fibrosus. In chronic disc degeneration immobilization is aimed more towards reduction of inflammation in the supporting soft tissues and about the nerve roots in the cervical spine.

Immobilization can be achieved through the use of various types of collars and braces, bedrest and traction. It has been the authors' experience, in the treatment of several thousand cases of cervical disc degeneration, that a soft felt collar is the method of choice. The more rigid and burdensome devices, such as plastic collars and metallic braces, are not only more burdensome for the patient but less effective in the relief of pain. They also lead to more soft tissue atrophy and stiffening than the soft collar.

The construction of this collar is relatively simple, with a felt insert surrounded by stockinette and light-weight stays added anteriorly to prevent collapse of the collar. It is held in place with a narrow elastic bandage. The collar can be made in heights varying from 2 to 4 inches, depending upon the length of the patient's neck. The collar should be placed in such a way that the head is held in a position of slight to moderate flexion (Fig. 5-1). This is far more comfortable than the hyperextended position and allows for maximal opening of the intervertebral foramina.

In an acute cervical injury, the collar is worn on a full-time basis for two to three weeks until the acute pain subsides and the soft tissues have progressed well in regard to healing. If at the end of this time the patient is relatively free of symptoms, he may be started on a course of cervical isometric exercises to strengthen his neck musculature and then gradually weaned from his collar over the next two to three weeks. It should be expected that six weeks will be necessary to recuperate from a significant cervical soft tissue injury.

In the acute phase of a cervical syndrome, occasional patients will fail to get adequate relief with ambulatory treatment and it may be necessary to place these people at bedrest. This will alleviate the cervical spine from the burden of supporting the weight of the head. While at bedrest, these patients should be instructed to continue use of their collar on a full-time basis.

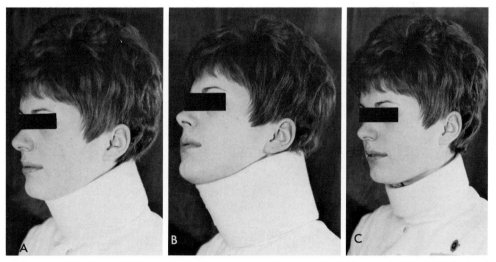

Figure 5-1 *A*, Illustration of the proper height and position of a soft cervical collar. Note the head is in a neutral or slightly flexed position. *B*, Incorrect use of a cervical collar which is excessively high. Note the head is in hyperextension. This is an extremely uncomfortable position for the patient with a cervical syndrome. *C*, Incorrect use of a cervical collar which has insufficient height. Note that the head and neck can be flexed. A low collar such as this gives inadequate support to a patient with a cervical syndrome and does not afford relief.

Cervical traction is rarely indicated in the treatment of soft tissue injuries and disc degeneration in the cervical spine. More often than not, the traction will serve as an irritative phenomenon and may actually increase the patient's discomfort. Its only apparent benefit is that it will enforce a regimen of confinement to bed. When used for this purpose, only minimal amounts of weight (four to six pounds) should be utilized and the direction of pull should be in slight flexion. Traction in the neutral or hyperextended position is contraindicated.

DRUG THERAPY

Acute injuries to the cervical intervertebral discs and the supporting soft tissues of the cervical spine will frequently result in painful muscle spasm. A vicious cycle is established whereby pain leads to muscle spasm, which leads to ischemia and a further increase in pain. Once this cycle is established it tends to be self-perpetuating. An effective muscle relaxant will frequently break this painful cycle and allow for more comfort and an increased range of motion in the cervical spine. An excellent therapeutic effect has been noted with the use of carisoprodol (Soma) 350 mg. every eight hours. A not infrequent side effect of this drug and other skeletal muscle relaxants is drowsiness, which may necessitate reduction in the dosage level.

In addition to muscle relaxants the authors have found it worthwhile to add an anti-inflammatory drug, such as phenylbutazone (Butazolidin), 100 mg. three times daily, to the therapeutic regimen. This drug has been found to be effective in many cases where an inflammatory response is responsible for production of the symptomatology. It should be noted that this drug has several serious side effects of which both the physician and patient should be aware. Among the most common of these is gastrointestinal irritation, which may be prevented by taking this drug with food or an antacid. Blood dyscrasias have been attributed to this drug and periodic complete blood counts are recommended. In those individuals who are unable to tolerate phenylbutazone, a less irritating derivative, oxyphenbutazone (Tandearil), can be used in an equivalent dosage.

Analgesics and sedatives are used as necessary to control discomfort and anxiety associated with these disorders.

CERVICAL ISOMETRIC EXERCISES

Exercises for the cervical spine should be directed at strengthening the paravertebral musculature and not increasing the range of motion. During the acute phase of a cervical injury the patient will be unable to tolerate exercises of any type, and it is not until the acute stage has subsided that an exercise program should be instituted. A typical cervical injury will require two to three weeks for the pain and muscle spasm to subside to the point where an exercise program should be started.

At this time the patient should be instructed in the performance of

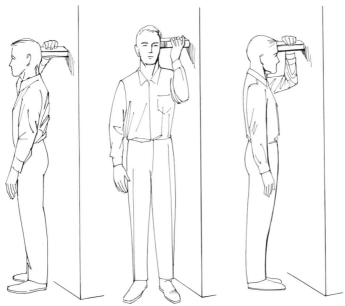

Figure 5-2 Drawing illustrating the correct position for the performance of cervical isometric exercises. A padded book or block of wood is used for support. Note that the cervical spine is maintained in a neutral position during the performance of these exercises. These exercises should be performed twice daily and increased as the patient's tolerance and strength allow.

cervical isometric exercises while he is still in his cervical collar (Fig. 5-2). As he increases strength and stability in his cervical spine, he may gradually be weaned from his cervical collar, at first during the day, and later, at night. In those individuals who are unable to tolerate a program of isometric exercises, muscle strengthening can be achieved by carrying a weight, such as a book or beanbag, balanced on top of the head.

PROCAINE INFILTRATION OF TRIGGER POINTS

Localized tender areas in the paravertebral musculature and the trapezii will be found in many individuals with acute and chronic cervical disc degeneration. Marked relief of symptomatology can often be dramatically achieved by infiltration of the trigger points with 5 to 10 cc. of 1 per cent procaine. The patient should of course be questioned as to sensitivity to procaine and should be lying down or supported during the injection. The more localized the trigger point, the more effective will be this form of therapy. Diffuse tenderness, which cannot be accurately localized, yields disappointing results with this type of approach. It is interesting that although the pharmacological effect of these drugs has worn off in two to three hours, the relief may last for days or even weeks in certain instances. These injections may be repeated at intervals of three days to several weeks.

PHYSICAL THERAPY

If muscle ischemia is one of the mechanisms of pain production in the cervical syndrome, then modalities designed to increase blood flow to muscle might be expected to be beneficial. Hot packs, diathermy and ultrasound will accomplish this goal. It has been our experience that hot turkish towels applied for 10 to 20 minutes, several times a day, are the most effective and least expensive of the modalities mentioned. Light massage combined with the application of this moist heat may also give a measure of temporary relief.

GENERAL MEASURES

There are certain general measures that a patient can take which may hasten his recovery from a cervical syndrome and prevent recurrences. Sleep hygiene is among the most important of these. The patient should be cautioned not to sleep in the prone position which requires his head to be in a forced position of rotation. He may sleep either on his side or back. Extreme flexion, such as that found when the head is propped on three to four pillows, should be avoided. An ideal head support, described by Jackson, is a cylindrical pillow 8 inches in diameter and approximately 18 inches in length and stuffed with a soft filler such as feathers or down.[1] This type of pillow has been demonstrated radiographically to keep the cervical spine in a neutral position whether the patient is sleeping supine or laterally.

The patient should also be cautioned about excessive automobile riding during the acute phase of his syndrome, since the vibration has a deleterious effect on the cervical spine. If travel is necessary, plane is preferred to either automobile or train.

Work areas should be arranged so that during performance of the patient's occupation it is not necessary for him to assume a position of extreme flexion, extension or rotation. This may require rearrangement of desk patterns, typewriters or frequently used equipment. Overhead work in which the patient is forced to hyperextend his spine is particularly difficult for the patient with a cervical spine disorder.

Manipulation is mentioned only to be condemned in the treatment of acute or chronic disc disorders in the cervical spine. Many tragic sequelae have been described in the literature with the use of cervical manipulation, and it is our feeling that manipulation has no place in the armamentarium of the physician treating cervical spine disorders of this type. It is true that certain acute cervical syndromes will enjoy a symptomatic response after manipulation, but we feel the hazards are too serious in nature to warrant its use.

REFERENCES

1. Jackson, R.: The Cervical Syndrome, Springfield, Illinois, Charles C Thomas, 1966.

Chapter 6

OPERATIVE TREATMENT OF CERVICAL DISC DISEASE

SELECTING THE PATIENT FOR OPERATIVE TREATMENT

Planning the operative procedure to be employed in cervical disc disease must take into consideration many factors. The two most important are the nature of the symptom-complex and the objective manifestations of the disease. Being knowledgeable in these areas makes it possible to formulate some conception of the future outlook of the patient. It will be remembered that cervical disc disease expresses itself in many forms, all of which depend on the level of progression of the pathological process involving the disc and on its effect on the neural elements of the cervical spine. For the sake of simplicity, the different patterns of the cervical syndrome, insofar as they relate to the tissues implicated, can be grouped into two major categories: the discogenic and the neurogenic syndromes.[3]

Discogenic Syndrome

In this syndrome the source of pain lies in the structural elements of the motor unit or units affected, particularly the intervertebral disc. Characteristic of the syndrome is the absence of any objective features implicating the nerve roots or the spinal cord; there are no sensory, motor or reflex abnormalities. The clinical manifestations are purely subjective: at first, the patient complains of pain and stiffness in the neck, on the top

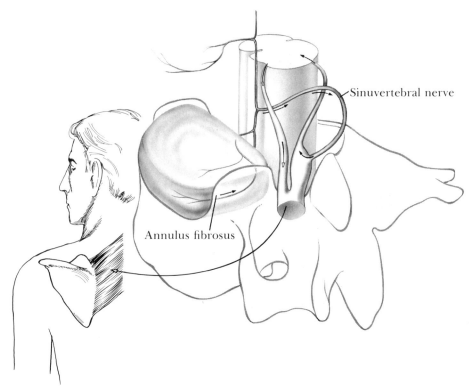

Sinuvertebral nerve

Annulus fibrosus

Figure 6-1   Mechanism of production of discogenic pain. Pain is initiated in the annulus fibrosus and ligaments by stimulation of the sensory receptors of the sinuvertebral nerve.

of the shoulders and in the region of the scapulae; later, the pain descends into the upper arms but rarely goes beyond the elbows. This is not radicular pain but rather it is vague, deep and boring. Usually maximal intensity is in the region of the upper portion of the vertebral border of the scapula, on one or both sides. The pain may be precipitated or, if present, accentuated by certain movements of the neck, particularly hyperextension. Pressure along the upper vertebral borders of the scapulae elicits severe tenderness. In the acute phase, movements may be restricted by local spasm in the trapezius and rhomboid muscles. There are all gradations of this syndrome; the most dramatic clinical picture is seen shortly after flexion and extension injuries of the neck. On the other hand, it may come on slowly and insidiously. In addition, it is episodic, punctuated by remissions and exacerbations.

The mechanism producing the pain in the discogenic syndrome is different than that in the neurogenic syndrome. It is initiated by stimulation of the sensory receptors of the sinuvertebral nerve located in the peripheral fibers of the annulus fibrosus and in the posterior and anterior longitudinal ligaments. The impulses are conveyed by the sinuvertebral nerve to the posterior nerve root and through the spinal cord; they then emerge through the anterior root and motor nerve to the muscles of the scapula (Fig. 6-1). The muscles develop varying gradations of spasm which are responsible for the local pain. Lesions of the discs, produced suddenly or gradually in the form of lacerations, tears and fissures which extend to the periphery of the annulus, are the noxious agents initiating the pain. This type of pain has been produced experimentally by stimulating, under vision, different areas of the annulus.[3] In fact, upon this phenomenon is based the rationale for the disc distention test which we now use routinely to determine the level of the offending disc.

This group comprises the largest segment of patients subjected to surgery (35 to 40 per cent). In the majority of these patients, only one disc is involved, usually the C5-C6 disc, which is implicated in approximately 40 to 50 per cent of all cervical disc lesions. The C4-C5 disc is next frequent, and, in our series, these two constitute 76.9 per cent of all the levels fused. Also, the highest incidence of satisfactory postoperative results are found in this category. It is apparent that patients with a discogenic syndrome have a most favorable outlook. However before operative intervention is considered, conservative methods must be given an adequate trial. If the patient is no longer able or willing to tolerate either the pain or the enforced readjustment of his daily life, operative treatment is justified. Excision of the affected disc through the anterior route and interbody fusion of the involved vertebrae is our treatment of choice.

Localization of the lesion may be difficult in patients with discogenic pain; the subjective symptoms are not particularly significant. Radiological examination is more helpful but again not entirely selective. In young people, radiographs taken during the early phase of the syndrome may be completely normal. However, we have noted not infrequently that one

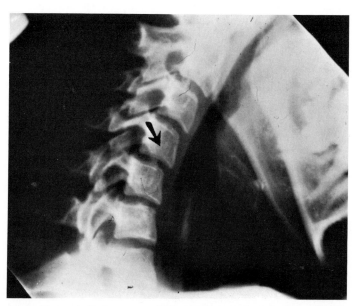

Figure 6-2 Forward displacement of C3 on C4 upon flexion of the spine. This lesion was demonstrable two weeks after a hyperextension injury. Fusion of the C3-C4 level effected complete relief of symptoms.

disc may exhibit considerable anterior bulging compared with the other discs and that invariably it proves to be the site of the trouble. Also, in early cases radiographs taken in extreme flexion and extension may demonstrate pronounced hypermobility of the rostral vertebra of the involved motor unit (Fig. 6-2). Another valuable finding is the gradual narrowing of a disc space seen in serial radiographs taken every four to six weeks over a period of several months.

Lesions of longer duration, in addition to the radiographic findings, will show definite narrowing of an interspace. Still later, the unequivocal signs appear: narrowing of the interspace, anterior and posterior osteophyte formations and possibly narrowing of the intervertebral foramen and changes in the apophyseal joints. However, although these signs are suggestive, they are not conclusive in pinpointing the involved disc. The previously described disc distention test will, in practically all instances, locate the disc or discs responsible for the syndrome. We now perform this examination routinely on all cervical spines in the category of discogenic syndrome.

Neurogenic Syndrome

In this category are patients with objective manifestations of extrinsic compression of the nerve roots or spinal cord or both. There are many patterns of this syndrome that depend upon the location and the size of the extruded nuclear material and on the intensity of the secondary alterations which ensue in a motor unit following degeneration of the disc. Stookey[4] recognized three separate syndromes based on the location of the nuclear lesion: (1) the intraforaminal lesion, (2) ventrolateral lesion and (3) midline lesion.

INTRAFORAMINAL LESION

This syndrome is characterized by compression of a nerve root usually at its site of exit from the spinal canal (Fig. 6-3 *A*). It is the most common of the three types of neurogenic syndromes. The clinical features are pain and stiffness in the neck, pain in the shoulder and radicular pain into the arm and hand, not unlike brachial neuralgia. The sensory distribution is confined to the dermatome of the affected nerve root; the motor deficits are not severe, usually consisting of weakness of the grip and some alterations in the deep reflexes. Some evidence of the root affected is derived from the dermatomal pattern of the pain distribution (Fig. 6-3 *B, C, D*). However, this may be confusing if two roots are involved or if there is a bilateral lesion at the same level. These possibilities are rare but they do occur. Broadly speaking, usually one root is involved and the levels most commonly affected in our series were the C5-C6 and the C4-C5 levels. As with the discogenic syndrome, the clinical picture of lesions compressing a nerve root is episodic, and the accentuation of the symptoms, often associated with recurrences, is mostly due to further extrusion of nuclear material and greater nerve root irritation.

Radiological study should be complete including anteroposterior, lateral and oblique views. It may provide substantial information in localizing the disc involved, especially if the findings correlate with dermatome distribution of the sensory disturbances. The most useful diagnostic aid is the disc distention test. If properly done, it will reproduce the patient's pain pattern and definitely establish the level of the lesion.

Many of the patients, if adequately and conscientiously treated by conservative measures, will be relieved of their symptoms or will reach a plateau of improvement which they accept and to which they adjust. If conservative measures fail, operative treatment is indicated. This group, as a whole, also is rewarded by a high incidence of satisfactory results. The operation of our choice is excision of the disc and interbody fusion through the anterior approach.

VENTROLATERAL AND MIDLINE LESIONS

These lesions are associated with cervical myelopathy, and the character and severity of the syndrome they evoke depend upon their size, location and duration. Ventrolateral lesions encroach upon the nerve root and the lateral aspect of the spinal cord adjacent to it, whereas midline lesions intrude upon the central aspect of the anterior portion of the cord (Fig. 6-4).

Ventrolateral lesions produce all the manifestations accompanying nerve root compression; pain is not a significant symptom. The chief radicular motor signs are weakness and loss of tone and volume of the muscles of the upper extremity, particularly the deltoid, triceps and biceps. There may be atrophy of the muscles of the hand; usually there are no sensory disturbances. Larger lesions implicating the cord may produce pyramidal tract signs and spasticity or even an incomplete Brown-Séquard syndrome. The clinical picture mimics intrinsic diseases of the spinal cord, especially amyotrophic lateral sclerosis. The diagnosis can only be made by utilizing all the diagnostic aids available to us; in these cases, myelography provides valuable information. Radiologic examination should be complete, including anteroposterior, lateral and oblique views (Fig. 6-5).

Midline lesions usually produce no signs of nerve root compression, but both lower extremities are primarily affected, although there may be some involvement of both upper extremities.

The extent of involvement of the cervical spine in these lesions varies considerably; radiological examination must include anteroposterior, lateral and oblique views and also lateral flexion and extension views. It may reveal spondylosis of only one, several or all the motor units. The fibrosis and osteophyte formation associated with severe disc degeneration may be sufficient to limit movements in the affected unit markedly (Fig. 6-5 *A* and *B*). On the other hand, if osteophyte formation is minimal, there may be excessive motion amounting to instability of the motor unit. Excessive motion is readily demonstrated in lateral views taken in extreme flexion and extension. Not infrequently, a markedly unstable cervical

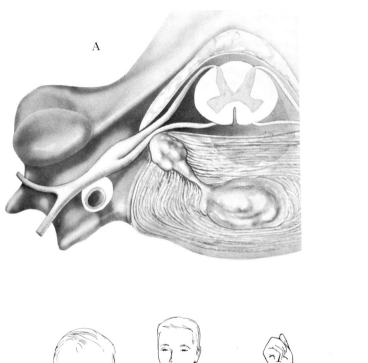

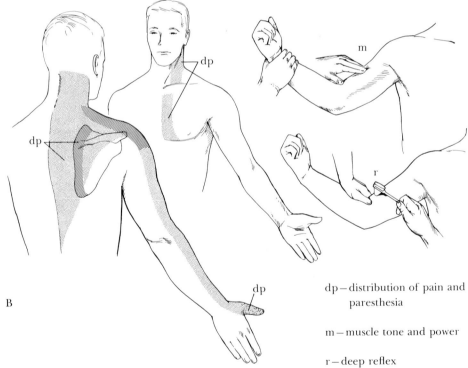

dp — distribution of pain and
        paresthesia

m — muscle tone and power

r — deep reflex

Figure 6-3   *A*, Compression of the nerve root by nuclear tissue at its site of exit from the spinal canal. *B*, Involvement of the C6 nerve root.

C

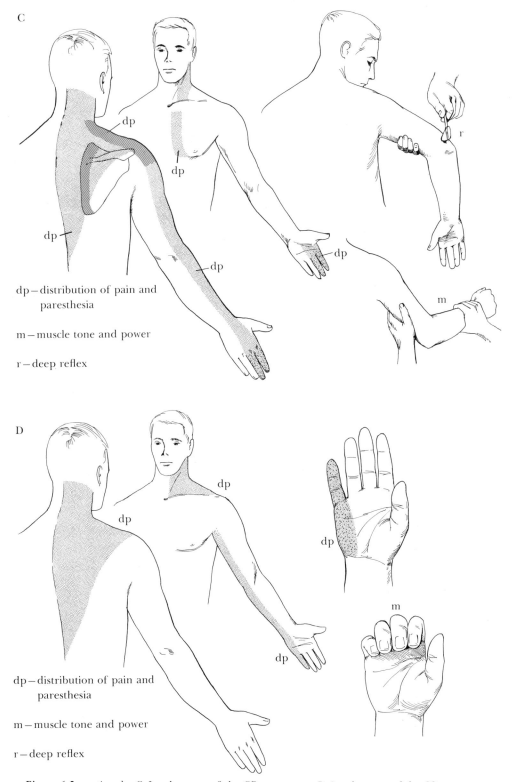

dp – distribution of pain and
     paresthesia

m – muscle tone and power

r – deep reflex

D

dp – distribution of pain and
     paresthesia

m – muscle tone and power

r – deep reflex

Figure 6-3, *continued.* C, Involvement of the C7 nerve root. D, Involvement of the C8 nerve root.

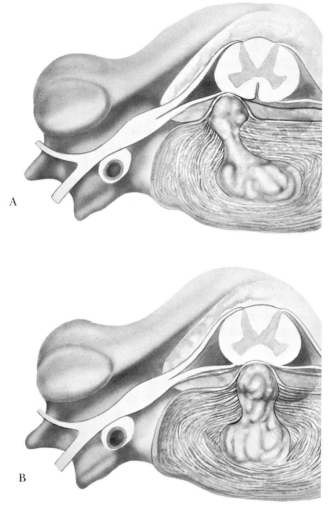

A

B

Figure 6-4   *A*, Ventrolateral lesions encroaching upon the nerve root and lateral aspect of the cord. *B*, Midline lesions encroaching on the central anterior portion of the cord.

vertebra is found just rostral to a fixed segment of the cervical spine or to a block vertebra; the intervertebral disc between the hypermobile vertebra and the fixed segment of the cervical spine may or may not exhibit evidence of collapse (Figs. 6-6 and 6-7). It will be recalled that the spinal canal may be congenitally narrow.[1, 2, 8, 13] When the sagittal diameter is reduced, spondylosis of minimal severity is capable of compressing the cord.

With degeneration and collapse of the intervertebral disc the adjacent vertebrae tend to approximate each other, producing a telescoping effect and accentuation of the cervical lordosis. When the lower lamina slips under the inferior edge of the lamina above, the ligamentum flavum bulges into the spinal canal and may encroach upon the dorsal surface of the spinal cord. Hence it is obvious that the sagittal diameter of the canal may be reduced by ventral and dorsal encroachments which are capable of compressing both the ventral and dorsal aspects of the cord.

As in ventrolateral lesions, myelography in midline lesions is a very important diagnostic tool and should be performed in all cases. It not only provides information regarding the extent and severity of the spondylotic process but it also may uncover other lesions, such as tumors, which may be responsible for the myelopathy. If the myelographic findings indicate that the degree of spondylosis of the cervical spine is minimal and cannot be considered as the etiologic factor responsible for the myelopathy, then it becomes obvious that degenerative diseases of the spinal cord must be given serious consideration. All patients in whom evidence of myelopathy is present and degenerative disease of the spinal cord is suspected should have a study of the dynamics and composition of the spinal fluid. Some patients with cervical spondylosis may show no change in the flow of the cerebrospinal fluid when the head is in the neutral position, but, when the head is hyperextended, a block in the flow of the fluid may occur. In fact, in some patients, Queckenstedt's test may be negative when the head is in the neutral position but positive in either flexion or extension.

The total protein of the cerebrospinal fluid usually is slightly increased in cervical spondylosis but never reaches the levels observed in intraspinal tumors.

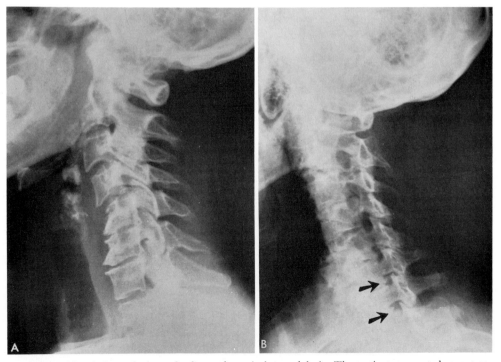

Figure 6-5 *A,* Lateral view of advanced cervical spondylosis. The patient presented symptoms consistent with ventrolateral lesions compressing the nerve roots and the lateral aspect of the cord. *B,* Oblique view reveals marked constriction of the foramina and large posterior osteophytes projecting into the foramina.

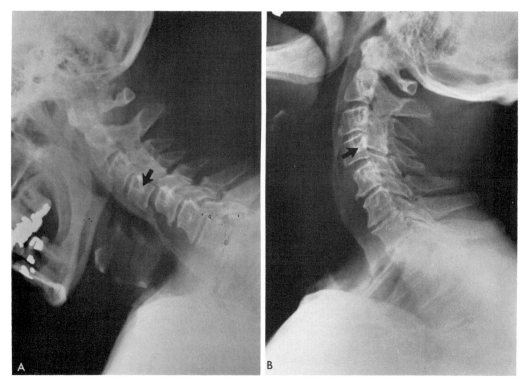

Figure 6-6 Hypermobility of C4 on C5. *A*, The spine is flexed. *B*, The spine is extended. The motor units C5-C6 and C6-C7 are fixed by advanced degenerative changes. The C4-C5 level was responsible for the symptoms, which were relieved by fusing this level.

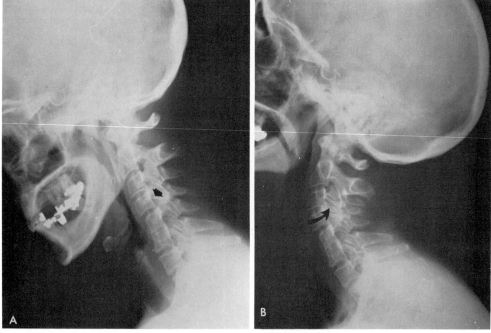

Figure 6-7 Hypermobility of C4 on C5. *A*, The spine is flexed. *B*, The spine is extended. Observe the congenital malformation of the C5-C6 motor unit comprising a block vertebra. Fusion of the C4-C5 level relieved the patient's pain.

Anterior

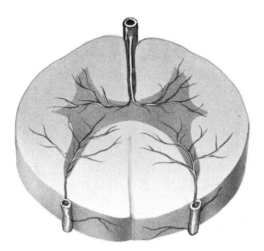

Posterior

Figure 6-8 Circulation of the spinal cord in the cervical region. Note that the anterior spinal artery supplies the anterior portion of the cord.

The surgeon needs all the data that can be accrued in order to plan the surgical approach. Also, this information permits the surgeon to formulate some idea of the result the patient can expect. The best results are attained in patients in whom one or two motor units are involved and in whom cord myelopathy is of short duration. On the other hand, if the lesion has been acting for many years producing irreversible changes in the cord, surgical treatment is debatable. Even in the face of serious neurologic deficits, if the myelopathy still shows evidence of progression, some substantial benefits can be derived from operative intervention. Cervical spondylosis associated with midline lesions or adhesions in and around the root sleeves may cause thrombosis of the anterior spinal artery and its radicular branches, producing local ischemia of the anterior horn cells of the spinal cord (Fig. 6-8). The resulting clinical picture is not unlike that of chronic poliomyelitis or progressive muscular atrophy. Surgery in these cases is questionable.

INVOLVEMENT OF THE VERTEBRAL ARTERY IN CERVICAL SPONDYLOSIS

Not infrequently, patients with cervical spondylosis complain of attacks of giddiness, syncope and weakness in the extremities associated with drop-attacks on certain movements of the head. These symptoms are the results of vertebrobasilar ischemia caused by obliteration of the lumens of the vertebral arteries. It will be recalled that the vertebral arteries enter the bony channels in the transverse processes of the cervical

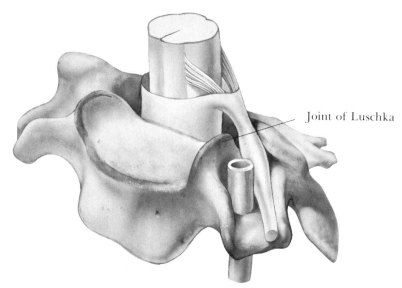

Joint of Luschka

Figure 6-9 At the level of the joint of Luschka the vertebral artery lies just in front of the cervical nerve root.

vertebrae at the level of the sixth cervical vertebra and emerge from the channels in the atlas; then they pursue a medial course and enter the foramen magnum. Also, it should be remembered that the vertebral artery is in close relationship to the joints of Luschka and at this point the artery lies just anterior to the cervical nerve root (Fig. 6-9). The osteo-phytes and fibrocartilaginous tissue associated with spondylosis may en-croach on the vertebral artery and displace it laterally. In advanced spondylosis the vertebral arteries are markedly distorted (Figs. 6-10 and 6-11).

Normally, rotation of the head may produce, on the side to which the head is turned, transient impairment of the blood flow in the artery from the sixth to the second cervical vertebra levels and in the opposite artery at the level of the transverse process of the atlas. It becomes apparent that, in the presence of spondylosis, the blood flow must be reduced or even obliterated if the arteries are encroached upon and that circulation is even further impaired when the vertebral and carotid arteries are atheroma-tous. Arteriograms taken with the head erect and in full rotation to either side will disclose both the degree of distortion in the arteries and the presence of atheromatous changes.[6, 12] According to some reported cases, if the arteries are primarily compressed by spondylotic changes and the atheromatous changes are only minimal, the patient's symptoms can be relieved in a large measure by decompression of the arteries as they pass through the channels in the transverse processes of the cervical vertebrae. We have never performed this operation.[1, 5, 8, 12]

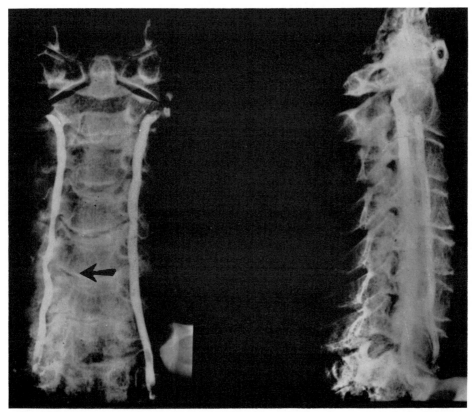

Figure 6-10 Cervical spine affected by severe spondylosis; the vertebral arteries have been injected with an opaque material. Observe the tortuosity of the arteries (particularly the left artery) caused by osteophyte proliferation in the region of the joints of Luschka.

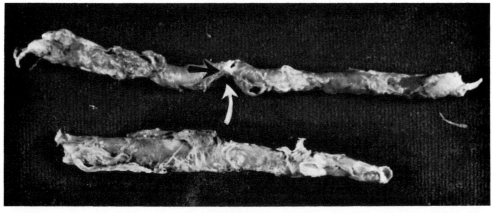

Figure 6-11 Vertebral arteries removed from a cervical spine affected by severe spondylosis. Note the large indentation of the artery at the top caused by osteophytes in the region of the joint of Luschka at the C5-C6 level.

OPERATIVE PROCEDURES

Excision of the Disc and Interbody Fusion (Anterior Approach)

This operation has now been generally accepted and needs no defense provided it is employed in selected cases. In our experience, few of the conditions of the cervical spine that are caused by degeneration of the discs and which need operative treatment cannot be managed by this method. There are many advantages and few disadvantages. The most advantageous features are: (1) The source of the pathological process, the disc, can be readily excised in its entirety; hence, pain is immediately relieved and the patient is insured against future recurrences of disc extrusions. (2) The interbody bone graft restores the height of the disc space, thereby bringing into normal alignment all the components of the motor unit. If subluxation of the apophyseal joints has occurred it is now corrected. (3) The intervertebral foramina are opened providing more room for their contents. (4) The interbody graft wedged between the rostral and caudal vertebrae immediately stabilizes the motor unit. (5) The operation can be performed from C2 to T1; however, at the extremes of the cervical column (C2, C3, C4, C7 and T1) the exposure may be more

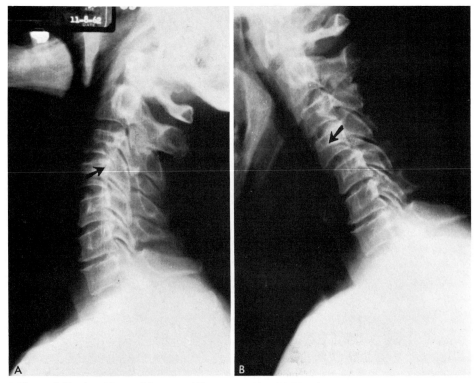

Figure 6-12 A subluxated hypermobile motor unit (C4-C5) above a fixed segment of the spine (C5-C6 and C6-C7). *A*, The spine is flexed. *B*, The spine is extended.

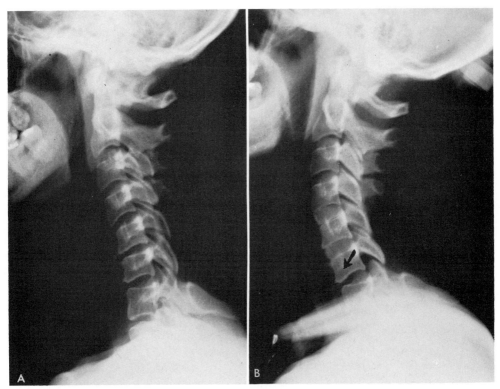

Figure 6-13 *A*, Instability of the cervical spine produced by extensive laminectomies. *B*, This patient (same as in *A*) had the C4-C5 and C5-C6 levels stabilized by anterior body fusions; the C6-C7 unit was not included in the fusion. Note the resulting increased instability at the C6-C7 level.

difficult to attain than in the midportion. (6) Any instability of the motor unit associated with subluxation and hypermobility of a cervical vertebra is immediately corrected. (7) The best results are attained when one or two levels are fused; this length of fusion is applicable to the greater majority of patients with cervical disc disease needing surgery.[3, 4, 11] (8) A solid bony fusion is attained in a relatively short period of time (six to eight weeks) and the postoperative period of convalescence is likewise relatively short.

The few disadvantages are: (1) The possibility of inflicting damage to the anterior surface of the cord and the nerve roots is real; it can occur and has occurred. (2) Insertion of large interbody grafts may exert undue pressure on the discs above and below, predisposing them to degeneration. (3) In patients with porotic bones the grafts may sink into the vertebral bodies. (4) Bone grafts may extrude anteriorly and injure the esophagus; (one patient who was referred to us had spit out a piece of bone three weeks after operation). (5) This operation makes impossible the exploration of the spinal canal and the cord at other levels.

We employ the anterior approach in the following conditions:

1. Acute or chronic cervical disc protrusions or extrusions encroaching on a cervical nerve root.

2. Lesions primarily involving the cervical intervertebral disc which

fail to respond to conservative measures; essentially these produce the so-called "discogenic syndrome."

3. Spondylosis of the cervical spine with associated myelopathy which does not involve more than three discs.

4. Subluxation of motor units associated with marked instability (Fig. 6-12).

5. Instability of the cervical spine following extensive laminectomies with violation of the apophyseal joints and the pedicles (Fig. 6-13).

We employ the anterior operation as described by Robinson and Smith[10] If the excision of the disc is complete, all but a few fibers of the posterior longitudinal ligament are removed. If the uncinate joints are carefully cleaned out with a small angled curette, there is no need to expose further the anterior aspect of the spinal canal or the intervertebral foramina.

Anesthesia

The operation can readily be performed under local anesthesia. Those using local anesthesia claim that by having the patient awake and able to respond to pain stimuli, location of the disc responsible for the syndrome is easily identified. These claims are undoubtedly true. However, we use endotracheal anesthesia. The tube in the trachea is a good reminder of the proximity of the esophagus and trachea. Caution must be exercised when the tube is introduced into the trachea. The neck must not be hyperflexed or hyperextended; in these positions, in the presence of anterior and posterior ridges on the walls of the spinal canal, much harm may be done to the cord, particularly in cases with myelopathy. But damage to the cord may also occur in patients without myelopathy or extensive spondylosis. A case to illustrate this point is that of a woman, 42 years old, with a discogenic syndrome of long standing caused by degeneration of the C5-C6 disc. Considerable difficulty was encountered by the anesthetist in the insertion of the tube. In spite of the advice given not to hyperextend or hyperflex the neck, the patient was put through these extreme movements. Upon exploring the C5-C6 interspace no disc material was found within the annulus; this was one of the first cases approached through the anterior route and the events that had occurred did not become evident until the patient recovered from the anesthesia; she had a typical Brown-Séquard syndrome. The nucleus pulposus had been retropulsed through a rent in the annulus into the spinal canal.

Position of the patient

The patient is placed in the supine position and a small sandbag (or folded towel or sheet) is placed beneath his neck. The neck is extended just a few degrees and never hyperextended. We approach the spine from the left side, therefore, the head is turned slightly to the right. (The spine may just as readily be approached from the right side.) (Fig. 6-14.)

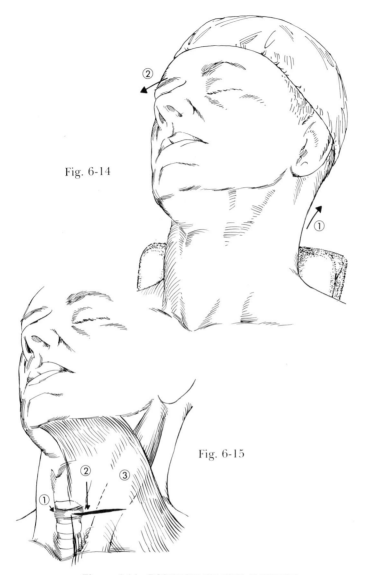

Fig. 6-14

Fig. 6-15

Figure 6-14   POSITION OF THE PATIENT

1. Place a folded towel beneath the interscapular region to hold the head in slight hyperextension.
2. Turn the head slightly to the right (15 to 20 degrees).

Figure 6-15   TRANSVERSE INCISION

1. Locate by palpation the cricoid cartilage opposite C5-C6 for orientation.
2. Make the incision in a skin crease opposite the desired level beginning at the midline and extending laterally for 3 to 3½ inches across the belly of the sternocleidomastoid muscle.
3. Cut the platysma in the same line as the skin incision.

INCISION

Either a vertical or transverse incision can be made depending upon the number of vertebrae to be fused. We employ the transverse incision if one or two levels are to be fused and the longitudinal incision if more than two. The cervical spine from C2 to T1 can be approached through these incisions.

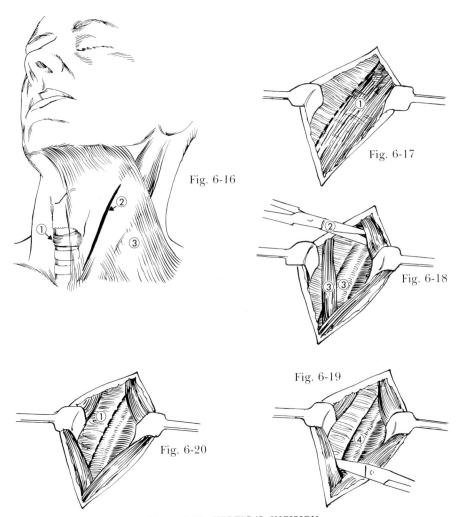

Fig. 6-16

Fig. 6-17

Fig. 6-18

Fig. 6-19

Fig. 6-20

Figure 6-16   *VERTICAL INCISION*

1. Locate by palpation the cricoid cartilage opposite C6 for orientation.

2. Make the incision along the anterior border of the sternocleidomastoid muscle, 2 inches above and 2 inches below the desired level.

3. Cut the platysma in the same line as the skin incision.

NOTE: For both the transverse and the longitudinal incisions the following steps are the same.

Figure 6-17   *EXPOSURE DOWN TO THE PRETRACHEAL FASCIA*

1. Divide longitudinally the anterior layer of the cervical fascia along the anterior border of the sternocleidomastoid muscle.

Figure 6-18

2. By scissor dissection mobilize the anterior margin of the sternocleidomastoid muscle and gently retract the muscle laterally.

3. Now the carotid sheath and the omohyoid muscle are visualized.

Figure 6-19

4. By blunt dissection develop the interval medial to the carotid sheath and retract the omohyoid muscle medially.

Figure 6-20   *EXPOSURE OF THE INTERVERTEBRAL DISC*

1. Make a small longitudinal incision in the pretracheal fascia.

TRANSVERSE INCISION.   For orientation, the cricoid cartilage is felt; it lies directly opposite the C5-C6 disc. The skin incision is made in one of the skin folds at the desired level. It begins at the midline and extends laterally for 3 to 4 inches, crossing the belly of the sternocleidomastoid muscle. The platysma muscle is cut in the same line as the skin incision (Fig. 6-15).

VERTICAL INCISION.   First the cricoid cartilage is palpated, designating the level of the C5-C6 disc. A longitudinal incision is made along the border of the sternocleidomastoid muscle 2 inches above and 2 inches below the desired level; the platysma muscle is cut in the same line as the skin incision (Fig. 6-16).

EXPOSURE DOWN TO THE PRETRACHEAL FASCIA

The following steps of the operation apply to both the transverse and vertical incisions. The anterior layer of the cervical fascia along the anterior border of the sternocleidomastoid muscle is divided longitudinally. By scissors dissection the anterior margin of the muscle is mobilized and gently retracted laterally, bringing into view the carotid sheath and the omohyoid muscle. By blunt dissection the interval medial to the carotid sheath is developed, and the omohyoid muscle is either cut or retracted laterally (Figs. 6-17, 6-18, and 6-19).

EXPOSURE OF THE INTERVERTEBRAL DISC

A small longitudinal incision is made in the pretracheal fascia, and with the index finger the retropharyngeal space is developed for the full length of the incision. The floor of the wound is exposed by retracting the trachea, esophagus and the thyroid gland medially and the carotid sheath laterally. The prevertebral fascia is seen as a glistening sheath covering the vertebral bodies, the anterior longitudinal ligament and the longus colli muscles. The intervertebral disc is clearly seen through the prevertebral fascia (Figs. 6-20, 6-21, and 6-22).

The following precautions should be taken at this stage of the operation: (1) When dividing the pretracheal fascia, the middle thyroid artery should be isolated, divided and ligated. (2) In high incisions, in the region of C2 and C3, the superior artery and vein and the superior laryngeal nerve are encountered. Usually they can be displaced proximally without tension, if not, it may be necessary to divide the vessels. (3) In low incisions, in the region of C6 to T1, it may be necessary to divide the inferior thyroid artery and vein. (4) It should be remembered that the recurrent laryngeal nerve descends along the carotid sheath and ascends between the esophagus and trachea; precaution should be taken not to injure this nerve in low incisions (Fig. 6-23).

IDENTIFICATION OF THE INTERVERTEBRAL DISC

A long, straight needle is inserted into the disc. It penetrates the disc for no more than one-half inch. A radiograph in the lateral view is then

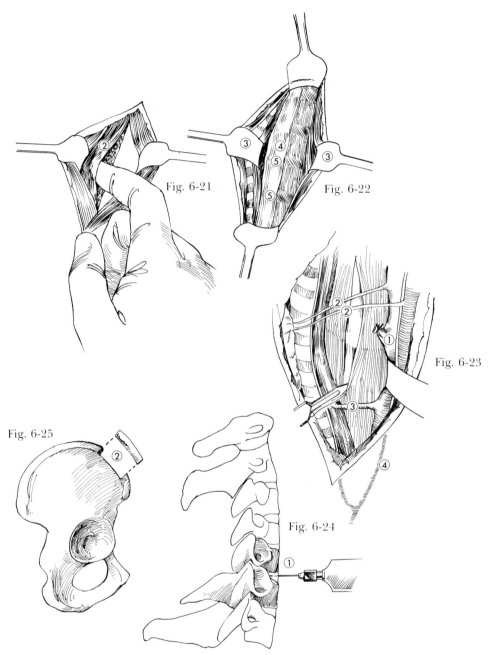

Fig. 6-21

Fig. 6-22

Fig. 6-23

Fig. 6-25

Fig. 6-24

Figure 6-21

2. With the index finger develop the retropharyngeal space for the full length of the incision. This is easily accomplished because the space comprises loose areolar tissue that is readily displaced in any direction.

Figure 6-22

3. Gently retract the thyroid gland, trachea and esophagus medially and the carotid sheath laterally.

4. Now the prevertebral fascia is seen as a glistening sheath covering the vertebral bodies, the anterior longitudinal ligament and longus colli muscles.

5. The intervertebral discs are clearly visualized through the prevertebral fascia.

(*Legend continues on facing page*)

taken. While the film is being developed, the anterior crest of the ilium on the same side is exposed and a block of bone is removed from the iliac crest. It comprises the full thickness of the ilium. Usually the block of bone is approximately 1½ to 2 inches long and 1 inch wide. From it will be cut the bone plugs to be used in the fusion. Generally, by the time the wound over the iliac crest is closed, the radiographs are developed and, from the position of the needle, the level of the exposed disc is determined (Figs. 6-24 and 6-25).

EXCISION OF THE PATHOLOGICAL DISC

By blunt dissection the longus colli muscles are stripped from the anterolateral surfaces of the vertebrae and the discs, and are displaced laterally. At this point, particular care must be taken not to injure the sympathetic chains running through the longus colli muscles. A flat blade retractor ½ to ¾ inches wide) is hooked under the longus colli muscles and the muscles are displaced laterally. With an electrocautery, the anterior longitudinal ligament and the superficial fibers of the annulus fibrosus are divided transversely for the entire width of the disc (Figs. 6-26 and 6-27). At this point, it should be pointed out that by the use of the electrocautery the field is rendered bloodless. There is no need to preserve the edges of the divided prevertebral fascia. If the bone graft is fitted snugly between the vertebrae, the chances of extrusion or displacement of the graft are practically nil.

With a long handled scapel (No. 11 blade) the deep fibers of the annulus are cut across the entire width of the disc. While an assistant makes steady manual traction on the head (one hand is under the chin of the patient and the other under the occiput) with the neck in just a few degrees of extension, a curette is inserted into the disc space and some of the loose fragments are scooped out. Since traction to open up the disc space is not needed at all times we prefer manual traction to continuous traction with a head halter (Figs. 6-28 and 6-29).

After the loose, superficial fragments are scooped out of the disc space, a vertebra spreader is placed deep in one side of the disc space and opened widely. All of the disc tissue is removed with curettes and pituitary forceps, first on one side and then on the opposite side of the disc space. Visualization of the entire disc space is adequate so that every remnant of

---

Figure 6-23   CAUTION

1. When dividing the pretracheal fascia look for the middle thyroid vein, divide and ligate it.
2. In high incisions (C2 and C3) the superior thyroid artery and vein and the superior laryngeal nerve are encountered; displace them proximally. Occasionally it may be necessary to divide the vessels.
3. In low incisions (C6-T1) it may be necessary to divide the inferior thyroid artery and vein.
4. In low incisions don't injure the recurrent laryngeal nerve. Remember, it descends along the carotid sheath and ascends between the esophagus and trachea.

Figure 6-24   LOCALIZATION OF THE INTERVERTEBRAL DISC

1. Insert a fine straight needle in the disc and take a lateral x-ray.

Figure 6-25   REMOVAL OF BONE PLUG

2. While the x-ray film is being developed, remove a block of bone from the anterior iliac crest. The piece of bone should comprise the full thickness of the crest of the ilium.

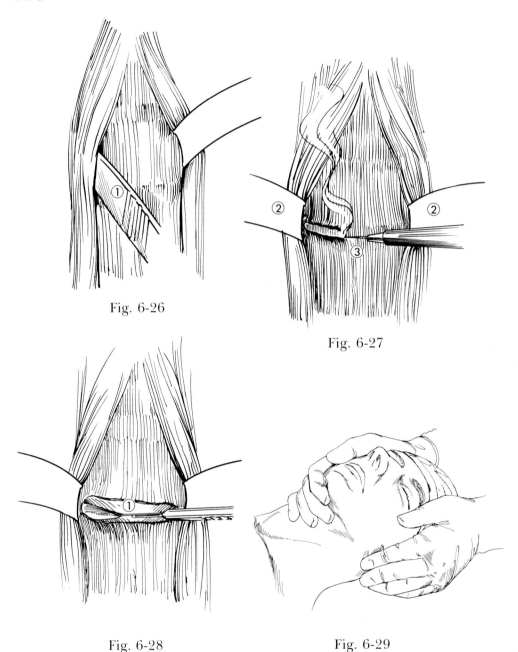

Fig. 6-26

Fig. 6-27

Fig. 6-28   Fig. 6-29

Figure 6-26 *EXCISION OF THE AFFECTED INTERVERTEBRAL DISC*

1. By blunt dissection, without traumatizing the sympathetic chains, mobilize and displace the longus colli muscles laterally, directly opposite the disc to be removed.

Figure 6-27

2. Hook a flat blade retractor ($\frac{1}{2}$ to $\frac{3}{4}$ inches wide) under the muscles.
3. With the electrocautery coagulate and divide transversely the tissues directly over the intervertebral disc.

NOTE: By using the electrocautery the field is rendered bloodless. There is no need to preserve the edges of the divided pretracheal fascia. If the bone block to be inserted fits snugly between the vertebrae, the chances of extrusion or displacement of the graft are practically nil.

(*Legend continues on facing page*)

disc tissue can be removed, including the articular plates, down to the subchondral bone of the contiguous vertebrae. With a small angled curette, the uncinate joints on either side of the disc space are also curetted clean. When this step is finished, the intervertebral space is devoid of any soft tissue, and the anterior fibers of the posterior longitudinal ligament are readily seen. Also the entire circumferential peripheries of both vertebrae are free of any remnants of soft tissue. The interspace is now flushed out with the saline solution and is ready to receive the bone graft (Fig. 6-30).

INSERTION OF THE BONE GRAFT

From the iliac bone previously removed, a block of bone is fashioned and tailored so that the width of the graft equals the interspace between the longus colli muscles, and the height should be such that it fits snugly between the two vertebral bodies. The anterior and lateral aspects of the graft consist of cortical bone.

While an assistant makes steady traction on the head with the neck in the neutral position, the graft is introduced into the disc space and gently tapped into position so that its anterior surface lies just behind the anterior margins of the two vertebrae (Fig. 6-31).

Traction is then released and the head brought into a position of slight flexion.

When the retractors are removed the wound edges fall into place; only the edges of the platysma muscle, the subcutaneous layer and the skin need to be approximated. Fine nylon interrupted sutures make an excellent closure for the skin (Fig. 6-32).

At the end of the operation the patient is fitted with a 2½- to 3-inch felt collar and returned to his room (Fig. 6-33).

POSTOPERATIVE CARE

The patients are fairly comfortable after surgery and are allowed out of bed on the second day. As a rule, they need very little medication except for some sedatives. Most patients experience immediate relief of their pain. They are discharged from the hospital in five to seven days; before leaving the hospital the sutures are removed and they are fitted with a light cervical brace which they wear for six to eight weeks at which time the fusion is usually solid (Fig. 6-34). Now the brace is removed and

---

Figure 6-28   REMOVAL OF THE DISC

1. With a scapel cut the annulus fibrosus across the entire width of the disc.

Figure 6-29

2. Have an assistant make strong manual traction on the head to open up the disc space.

NOTE: Traction is made with the neck only slightly hyperextended. I prefer manual traction to continuous traction with a head halter because it can be applied and released as desired. If the fusion is performed to stabilize dislocations and fracture-dislocations, skeletal traction (15 pounds) is maintained at all times during the operation. The weights can be increased if widening of the disc space is desired.

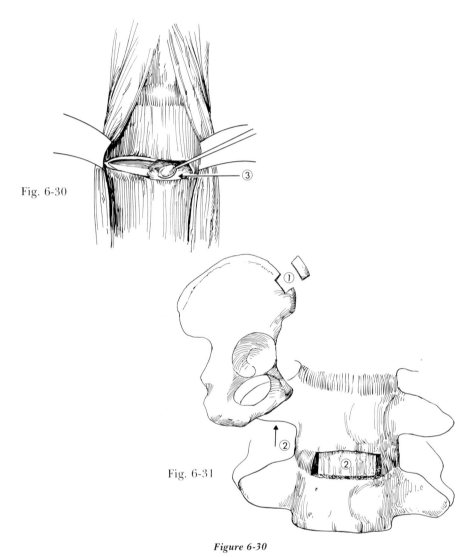

Fig. 6-30

Fig. 6-31

Figure 6-30

3. With a curette remove the entire disc piece by piece. Also remove the articular plate above and below down to subchondral bone.

NOTE: Curved curettes of varying sizes facilitate removal of disc material from the uncovertebral joints.

Figure 6-31   INSERTION OF BONE GRAFT

1. Cut out a bone block from the iliac bone previously removed.

NOTE: The width of the graft should be same as the width of the intervertebral space exposed between the longus colli muscles; the height of the graft should be such that it fits snugly between the two vertebral bodies. The graft should have cortical bone on both sides.

2. While manual traction is applied, to open the disc space, gently tap the graft into position.

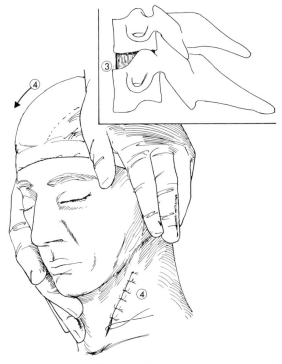

Figure 6-32

3. The anterior surface of the graft should be behind the anterior margins of the vertebrae.

4. Bring the head to a slightly flexed position and close the wound in layers. There should be no need to place a drain in the wound.

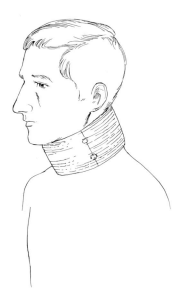

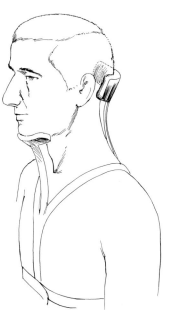

Figure 6-33 Felt collar fitted to patient at the end of the operation.

Figure 6-34 Cervical brace worn for six to eight weeks at which time the fusion is, as a rule, solid.

replaced with a felt collar holding the head in the neutral position. Also, at this point isometric exercises for the neck muscles are started and increased daily as the patient's tolerance increases. After a period of ten to 14 days the soft collar is removed; at first for several hours each day, and then for increasing periods, so that within ten to 14 days the collar is discarded.

These patients can return to light work within two to three weeks and to heavy work in six to eight weeks. Radiographs are taken before they leave the hospital and at intervals of every three weeks thereafter, until solid bony arthrodesis is attained. These patients are not discharged at this time but requested to return for re-evaluation every three to four months for the next year.

Laminectomy and Posterior Spine Fusion

In cases with widespread spondylosis with myelopathy, simple laminectomy is a valuable procedure to decompress the spinal cord. This is particularly true if there is radiological evidence of a congenitally narrow spinal canal and evidence of posterior indentations of the cord. On the other hand, attempts to mobilize the spinal cord by dividing the dentate ligaments, or even several nerve roots, in order to gain access to anterior excrescences for the purpose of removing them, have been uniformly disastrous; the neurologic deficit invariably becomes worse. In these cases, the spinal cord is stretched tightly over the anterior, hard, bony transverse ridges at the levels of the intervertebral discs. The cord is further strapped in a fixed position by the dentate ligaments and the nerve roots whose sheaths may be enmeshed in a mass of adhesions. Such a cord is extremely vulnerable to even the slightest manipulation, particularly so if its blood supply is already severely compromised by the pathological process.

If a laminectomy is decided upon in these cases it should be adequate so that the cord is completely decompressed; this may mean the removal of the laminae of three, four, five or even more vertebrae. In performing the operation the laminae must be removed in such a fashion that not the slightest pressure is made on the spinal cord.

There is considerable controversy as to whether the dentate ligaments should be cut and the dura opened. We do not believe that these procedures are necessary for a satisfactory result. Moreover, it is doubtful if facetectomy or removing the pedicles is essential. To us it seems more logical to remove the laminae of as many vertebrae as necessary to insure adequate decompression of the spinal cord, to extend the laminectomy as far lateral as possible but not beyond the articular facets and to fuse the affected segments of the spine. This approach to the problem achieves the three steps necessary for recovery: (1) the cord is decompressed, (2) the stability of the spine is insured and (3) a successful arthrodesis terminates the spondylotic process and favors resorption of the anterior and posterior osteophytes. If the magnitude of the operation precludes doing a posterior spine fusion, then an anterior spine fusion can be performed as a subsequent operation.

Fig. 6-35

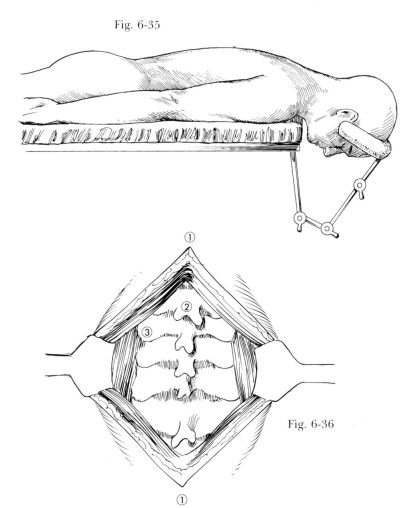

Fig. 6-36

Figure 6-35   Patient is in the prone position with the head supported by a headrest; the head is fixed to the rest so that the neck is slightly flexed.

Figure 6-36   EXPOSURE OF POSTERIOR ELEMENTS

1. Make a longitudinal midline skin incision over the spinous processes of the vertebrae beginning one vertebra above and one below the proposed fusion area.

2. Deepen the incision to the tips of the spinous processes in the same line as the skin incision.

3. By sharp subperiosteal dissection expose the laminae and carry the dissection laterally to the margins of the apophyseal joints.

Technique of Laminectomy and Posterior Spine Fusion

This procedure should be the team effort of a neurosurgeon and an orthopedic surgeon. We prefer endotracheal anesthesia.

POSITION OF THE PATIENT

The patient is placed on the operating table in the prone position, with the head supported by a headrest which gives ample room for the anesthetist to administer to the patient. The head is fixed to the headrest so that the neck is slightly flexed (Fig. 6-35).

INCISION AND EXPOSURE

A longitudinal midline skin incision is made over the spinous processes of the cervical vertebrae beginning one vertebra above and one below the proposed fusion area (Fig. 6-36). Deepen the incision to the tips of the processes and with a sharp periosteal elevator expose the laminae subperiosteally. Carry the dissection laterally to the lateral margins of the apophyseal joints. If the dissection is entirely subperiosteal, very little bleeding occurs. At this point, by packing and the use of the electrocautery, complete hemostasis should be attained. It is important at this stage of the operation to identify the vertebrae. Usually this can be done readily since the fifth cervical vertebra has the last bifid spinous process and the seventh the longest. But the anatomy in this region is not always constant. The most accurate method is to insert a pin into the tip of one of the spinous processes and take a lateral radiograph. Next, with a flat, sharp bone cutter remove the spinous processes at the bases of the vertebrae which are to be included in the fusion area (Fig. 6-37).

LAMINECTOMY

This part of the operation is executed with great caution; the lower jaw of the rongeurs used to bite off the laminae must not at any time make any pressure on the underlying cord. The laminae are removed as far laterally as the apophyseal joints (Fig. 6-38).

POSTERIOR SPINE FUSION

This is the method of Robinson and Southwick[10] used in flexion and extension injuries of the cervical spine.

Starting with the most rostral vertebra to be included in the fusion area, a thin osteotome is inserted into the joint space and turned slightly on its side to open the space. The tip of a sucker is inserted into the joint space to hold the facets apart. A hole is drilled through the inferior facet into the joint space and a No. 20 stainless steel wire is passed through the drill hole and drawn out through the distal part of the apophyseal joint. This procedure is performed first on the apophyseal joints of one side and then on those of the opposite side (Fig. 6-39).

The posterior iliac crest of one of the ilii is exposed subperiosteally and two long stout bone struts are removed. The length of the grafts are equal to the distance from the superior margin of the most proximal vertebra to the inferior margin of the lamina of the most distal vertebra. The bone struts are placed over the posterior and lateral aspects of the apophyseal joints and anchored tightly in place by the wires (Fig. 6-40).

The patient's condition may not permit doing a posterior spine fusion after the laminectomy is completed. In this event, the spine should be stabilized later through the anterior approach. A fusion from C3 to C7 can be achieved through the anterior route.

Immediately following the operation the patient is fitted with a cervical brace. The patient is allowed out of bed in five to seven days; the brace is worn at all times until the fusion is complete, which may be four to six months after the operation.

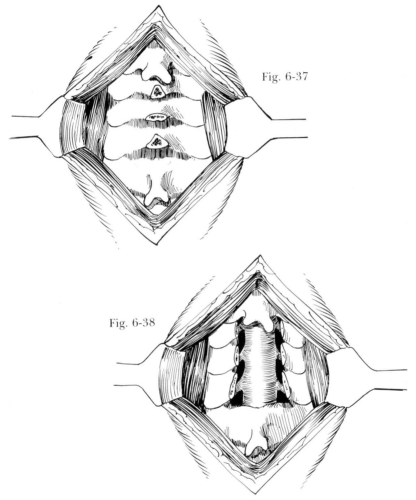

Figure 6-37   With a flat bone cutter remove at their bases the spinous processes of the vertebrae to be included in the fusion area.

Figure 6-38   Remove the laminae of the vertebrae to be included in the fusion area as far laterally as the apophyseal joints.

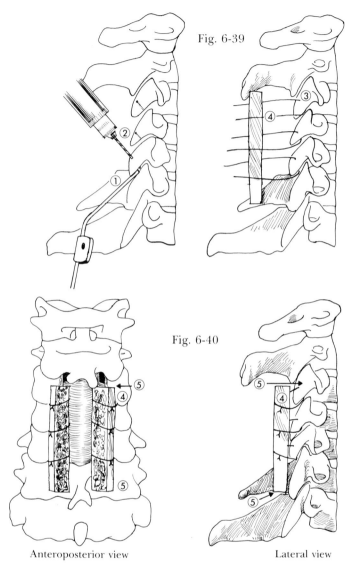

Fig. 6-39

Fig. 6-40

Anteroposterior view   Lateral view

Figure 6-39 WIRING OF VERTEBRAE

1. Spread the articular processes with a narrow, thin osteotome and then insert the tip of a small, surgical sucker into the interval.

2. With a 7/64 inch drill make a hole through the inferior facet of the vertebra above; the drill points obliquely downward.

3. Pass a No. 20 stainless steel wire through the drill hole.

NOTE: This procedure is performed on the inferior processes of all the vertebrae to be included in the fusion area.

Figure 6-40 SEATING OF BONE GRAFTS

4. Pass the wires around the cortical-cancellous grafts (obtained from the posterior iliac crest) and secure them snugly against the facet joints.

5. The grafts extend from the top of the laminae of the most proximal vertebra to the bottom of the laminae of the most distal vertebra.

PSEUDARTHROSIS

Pseudarthrosis may occur following anterior or posterior fusions. In our experience, the incidence of pseudarthrosis was higher in the spines with anterior interbody fusions. In fact, we have never had a pseudarthrosis in our posterior spine fusions. As will be shown in the section following, 12 per cent of all patients with anterior fusions developed pseudarthrosis. Fortunately, very few were symptomatic. When pseudarthrosis occurs and is symptomatic, regardless of whether it is in an anterior or posterior fusion, we are of the opinion that repair should be done through the anterior approach. The procedure is relatively simple, it is less traumatic to the patient, and the convalescent period is smoother.

REPAIR OF PSEUDARTHROSIS (ANTERIOR APPROACH)

If the pseudarthrosis lies in a posterior fusion, the repair is effected by performing a fusion between the two vertebrae involved. An anterior spine fusion is performed in the same manner as that described following excision of the vertebral disc (see p. 112). If the pseudarthrosis lies in an interbody fusion, one of two repairs may be performed through an anterior approach depending on the local findings.

The repair should be done through an anterior incision on the side opposite that of the first operation. By so doing, less scar tissue is encountered in exposing the cervical spine. The affected level is exposed in the same manner as previously described for uncomplicated anterior fusions. If the intervertebral space is adequate and will accept a graft after all debris within it is removed, the subchondral bone of both vertebrae is curetted clean of all cartilage and fibrous tissue and a new bone plug is inserted as previously described.

If the interspace is very narrow and will not accept an adequate graft, the interspace can be spanned with a longitudinally placed graft which sits in a groove in the vertebral bodies and bone chips are packed in the interspace.

Technique of Anterior Fusion (Bailey and Badgley)

The anterior aspect of the cervical spine is approached through a vertical incision made on the nonoperated side as previously described. (See p. 114).

After the disc space is identified, the prevertebral fascia is divided longitudinally in the midline and with a sharp periosteal elevator it is stripped from the anterior surfaces of the vertebral bodies above and below the pseudarthrosis. With a sharp, fine osteotome a trough is cut in the bodies $1/2$ in. wide and $3/16$ in. in depth, extending from the near top of the upper vertebra to the bottom of the lower vertebra. All fibrous tissue is removed from the interspace and packed with cancellous bone. A graft obtained from one of the anterior iliac crests is tailored to fit the

Text continues on page 133.

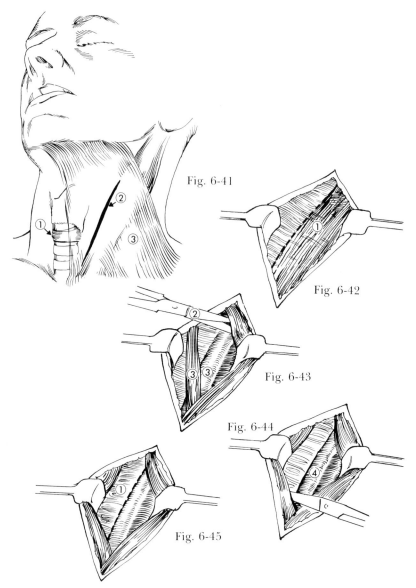

Fig. 6-41

Fig. 6-42

Fig. 6-43

Fig. 6-44

Fig. 6-45

Figure 6-41   INCISION

1. Locate the cricoid cartilage; this is opposite the sixth cervical vertebra.
2. Make an incision along the anterior border of the sternocleidomastoid muscle, 2 inches above and 2 inches below the affected level.
3. Cut the platysma in the same line as the skin incision.

Figure 6-42   EXPOSURE DOWN TO THE PRETRACHEAL FASCIA

1. Divide longitudinally the anterior layer of the cervical fascia along the anterior border of the sternocleidomastoid muscle.

Figure 6-43

2. By scissor dissection mobilize the anterior margin of the sternocleidomastoid muscle and gently retract it laterally.
3. Now the pulsating carotid sheath and the omohyoid muscle are visualized.

Figure 6-44

4. By blunt dissection develop the interval medial to the carotid sheath.

Figure 6-45   EXPOSURE OF THE ANTERIOR ASPECT OF THE VERTEBRAL BODIES

1. Make a small incision in the pretracheal fascia.

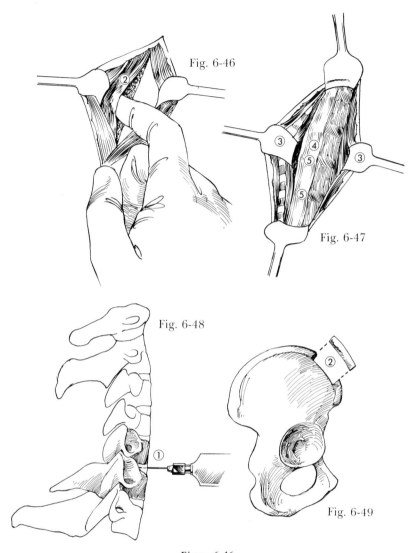

Fig. 6-46

Fig. 6-47

Fig. 6-48

Fig. 6-49

Figure 6-46

2. With the index finger develop the retropharyngeal space for the full length of the incision.

Figure 6-47

3. Retract the thyroid gland, trachea and esophagus medially and the carotid sheath laterally.

4. The prevertebral fascia is seen as a glistening sheath covering the vertebral bodies, longitudinal ligament, discs and longus colli muscles.

5. The intervertebral discs are clearly visualized through the prevertebral fascia.

Figure 6-48   *LOCALIZATION OF VERTEBRA*

1. Insert a fine straight needle in a disc space and take a lateral x-ray.

NOTE: The site of the lesion, such as in a dislocation, may be recognized at this stage of the procedure by characteristics of the disc, which may be mushy and bulging.

Figure 6-49

2. While x-ray film is being developed, take a block of bone from the anterior crest of the ilium; it should comprise the full thickness of the crest.

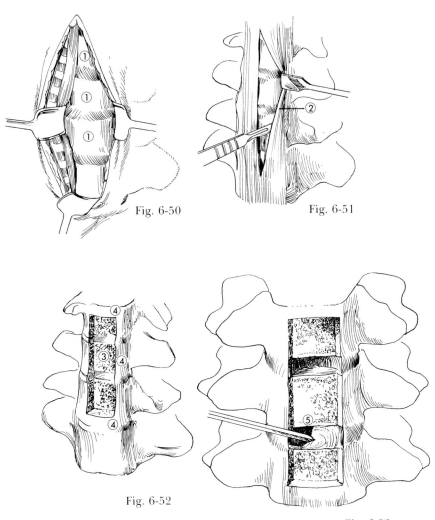

Fig. 6-50

Fig. 6-51

Fig. 6-52

Fig. 6-53

Figure 6-50 PREPARATION OF THE GRAFT BED

1. Identify the vertebrae to be included in the fusion.

Figure 6-51

2. Incise longitudinally and in the midline the prevertebral fascia and with a sharp elevator reflect the fascia off the vertebral bodies.

Figure 6-52

3. Cut a trough in the anterior aspects of the vertebral bodies, ½ inch in width and ³/₁₆ inch in depth.

NOTE: Use a fine sharp osteotome or an electric dental drill or saw to cut the trough.

4. The trough in the end vertebrae spans three-quarters of the vertical height of each vertebra and spans the entire vertical height of the middle vertebra.

Figure 6-53

5. Clean out the disc spaces with a pointed rongeur to a depth of approximately ½ inch.

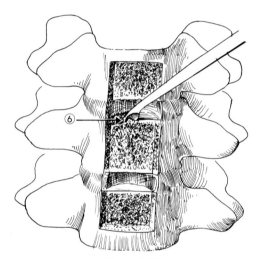

Figure 6-54

6. With a sharp curette remove the articular cartilage off the articular plates down to subchondral bone.

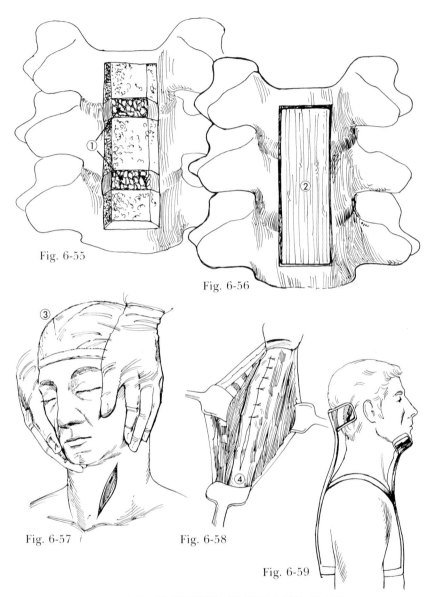

Fig. 6-55

Fig. 6-56

Fig. 6-57

Fig. 6-58

Fig. 6-59

Figure 6-55   PLACEMENT OF THE BONE GRAFT

1. Pack fine cancellous bone chips in the open disc spaces.

Figure 6-56

2. Cut the graft so that it fits snugly in the trough.

Figure 6-57

3. Now bring the neck to the neutral or slightly flexed position. This position firmly seats the graft in its bed.

Figure 6-58

4. Approximate the edges of the prevertebral fascia over the graft.

Figure 6-59   Apply a cervical brace which must be worn four to six months.

NOTE: Take x-rays every four to six weeks to determine stage of fusion.

trough and then mortised into it. With interrupted sutures, the prevertebral fascia is closed over the bone graft (Figs. 6-41 to 6-58).

Immediately after the operation is completed, a light cervical brace is applied (Fig. 6-59). The patient is ambulated in five to seven days. Fusion should be solid in four to six months, at which time the brace is discarded and isometric exercises for the cervical muscles are instituted.

REFERENCES

1. Brain, L.: Some unsolved problems of cervical spondylosis. Brit. Med. J. 5333:771-777, 1963.
2. Burrows, E. H.: The sagittal diameter of the spinal canal in cervical spondylosis. Clin. Radiol. 14:77-86, 1963.
3. Cloward, R. B.: New method of diagnosis and treatment of cervical disc disease. Clin. Neurosurg. 8:93-132, 1962.
4. DePalma, A. F.: Study of the cervical syndrome. Clin. Orthop. 38:135-141, 1965.
5. Gortuai, P.: Insufficiency of vertebral artery treated by decompression of its cervical part. Brit. Med. J. 5403:233-234, 1964.
6. Hutchinson, E. C. and Yates, P. O.: Cervical portion of vertebral artery: Clinico-pathological study. Brain 79:319-331, 1956.
7. Keggi, K. J., et al.: Vertebral artery insufficiency secondary to trauma and osteoarthritis of the cervical spine. Yale J. Biol. Med. 38:471-478, 1966.
8. Payne, E. E. et al.: The cervical spine. An anatomicopathological study of 70 specimens (using a special technic) with particular reference to the problem of cervical spondylosis. Brain 80:571, 1957.
9. Robinson, R. A. and Smith, G. W.: Anterolateral cervical disc removal and interbody fusion for cervical disc syndrome. Johns Hopkins Hosp. Bull. 96:223, 1955.
10. Robinson, R. A. et al.: Surgical approaches to the cervical spine. Instruc. Lect. Amer. Acad. Orthop. Surg. 17:299-330, 1960.
11. Robinson, R. A., et al.: The results of anterior interbody fusion of the cervical spine. J. Bone Joint Surg. 44-A:1569-1586, 1962.
12. Sheehan, S. et al.: Vertebral artery compression in cervical spondylosis. Arteriographic demonstration during life of vertebral artery insufficiency due to rotation and extension of the neck. Neurology 10:968, 1960.
13. Smith, G. W. and Robinson, R. A.: The treatment of certain cervical spine disorders by anterior removal of the intervertebral disc and interbody fusion. J. Bone Joint Surg. 40-A:607-662, 1958.
14. Stookey, B.: Compression of spinal cord and nerve roots by herniation of nucleus pulposus in cervical region. Arch. Surg. 40:417-432, 1940.
15. Wolf, B. S. et al.: Sagittal diameter of bony cervical spinal canal and its significance in cervical spondylosis. J. Mt. Sinai Hosp. New York 23:283-292, 1956.

Chapter 7

HYPEREXTENSION INJURIES OF THE SOFT TISSUES OF THE CERVICAL SPINE

The ever-increasing number of acceleration and deceleration injuries of the cervical spine, sustained in automobile accidents, makes it almost mandatory that these injuries be considered separately, as a special group. First, the acute pathologic process encountered in hyperextension injuries is discussed, and next, the clinical picture the patients present.

MECHANISM OF INJURY

The mechanism producing the injuries is essentially one of prolongation and hyperextension of the neck (Fig. 7-1). In the typical, uncomplicated, rear-end mechanism the head pursues a backward and downward course producing extreme hyperextension of the neck; it is then projected forward to a position of extreme flexion and, finally, it returns to the neutral position. It is during the period of severe hyperextension that damage is inflicted upon the structures of the neck. In its backward course the head encounters no barrier to confine or restrict the forces of prolongation and hyperextension acting on the neck. This is not true of flexion mechanisms in which the forces are restrained when the chin strikes the anterior chest wall or in lateral mechanisms when the head strikes the shoulder. In these two latter mechanisms the arcs of motion are well within the normal range of motion of the cervical spine, hence, the injuries sustained are minimal in intensity. In the simple form of rear-

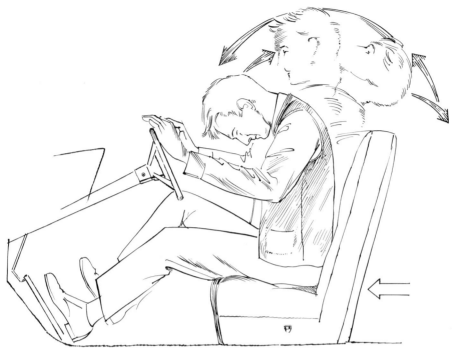

Figure 7-1 The mechanism causing injuries to the soft tissues of the cervical spine is essentially one of prolongation and hyperextension of the neck. The neck is then severely flexed, and finally the neutral position is assumed.

end collisions no passive force is applied to the head, so that there is rarely any disruption of the osseous elements, but rather only involvement of the soft tissue structures. However, other existing factors may complicate the rear-end collision mechanism. These may be congenital or acquired in nature. The acquired factors are essentially those produced by degenerative changes in the cervical spine; they may be responsible for irreversible changes and prolonged disability.

There is very little in the literature dealing with the basic pathologic lesions sustained by the soft tissues of the neck at the time of a rear-end collision. Nevertheless, one can infer what has occurred by the clinical manifestations that a victim presents. Also, McNab has clearly shown in animals subjected to hyperextension mechanisms that certain specific lesions result depending upon the intensity of the forces applied to the neck.[8]

INJURIES SUSTAINED BY THE SOFT TISSUES ANTERIOR TO THE CERVICAL SPINE

MUSCLES

In addition to providing its motor control, the muscles of the neck are the chief stabilizers of the cervical spine and, as a group, provide

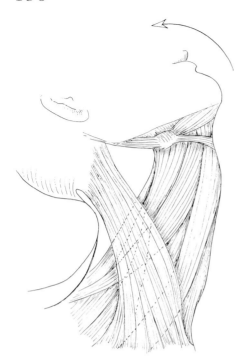

***Figure* 7-2**   When the cervical spine is subjected to severe hyperextension forces, the anterior muscles of the neck may be severely stretched and some muscle fibers may be torn.

protection of the underlying vital structures. When caught off guard and subjected to severe hyperextension forces, the anterior muscles, particularly the sternocleidomastoid, the scaleni and longus colli muscles, may be severely stretched and some of their fibers even torn (Fig. 7-2). This accounts for the severe muscle spasm and limitation of motion that the victims frequently present 12 to 48 hours after the accident. Also, it accounts in a large measure for the pain and tenderness at the root of the neck. If one side of the neck is involved more than the other, the patient may exhibit the typical features of torticollis.

ESOPHAGUS AND TRACHEA

The muscle strata of the esophagus may be stretched or torn, producing hemorrhage and edema in the retropharyngeal space (Fig. 7-3). The trachea may be likewise injured. This acute pathology readily explains the symptoms of dysphagia and hoarseness that the victims frequently present.

LONGUS COLLI MUSCLES AND THE SYMPATHETIC CHAIN

It should be remembered that on either side of the anterior surface of the cervical column are the sympathetic chains running over the longus colli muscles (Fig. 7-4). As previously noted, severe hyperextension injuries may stretch and tear the muscle fibers; this must also be true of the

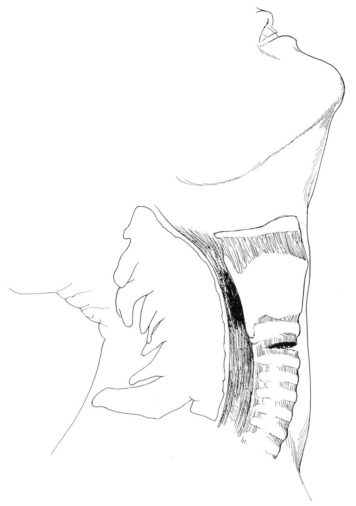

Figure 7-3   Hyperextension and prolongation of the cervical spine may stretch and even tear the muscular stratum of the esophagus; the trachea may be injured.

sympathetic chains. The resulting hemorrhage and edema further implicate the sympathetic nerve fibers. This accounts for the bizarre manifestations which the victims frequently exhibit such as nausea, blurring of vision, dizziness, nystagmus, deafness, tinnitis and occasionally dilation of one pupil. These are symptoms resulting from involvement of the cervical sympathetic nerve fibers.

INJURY TO THE INTERVERTEBRAL DISCS

The stability of the cervical spine is largely dependent upon the intervertebral discs which constitute strong bonds between the vertebral bodies (Fig. 7-5). There is sufficient clinical and radiological evidence indicating that the intervertebral discs may be severely injured by hyper-

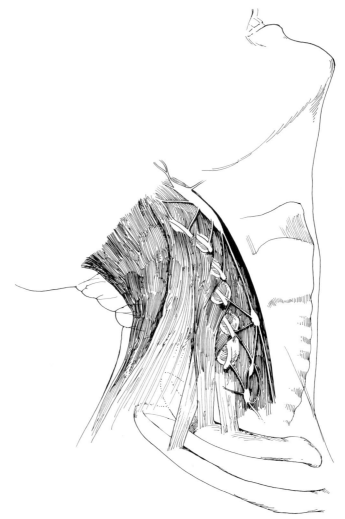

Figure 7-4 Hyperextension and prolongation of the cervical spine may severely stretch or even tear the longus colli muscles and the sympathetic chains which are immediately related to the muscles.

extension mechanisms of the neck. The observations made by Bailey[1] and Forsyth[5] clearly depict the types of lesions of the discs that may be encountered. Also, McNab's animal experiments fortify these observations.[8] We have demonstrated the specific lesions many times at the operating table.

During a severe hyperextension injury, the disc may be severely crushed and the anterior longitudinal ligament attenuated or ruptured. In some instances, within a few days, the disc bulges anteriorly (Fig 7-6). This new configuration may be discernible in roentgenograms taken to show soft tissue contrast (Fig 7-7). In a recent review of 146 cases which came to surgery, 23 patients exhibited discs with this early abnormality.

Following a crushing injury, the disc gradually undergoes degeneration and, within several months, an increasing diminution in height of

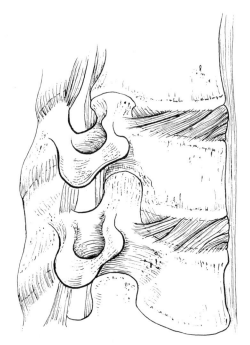

Figure 7-5   Under normal conditions the cervical disc is the most important single stabilizing structure between any two vertebrae.

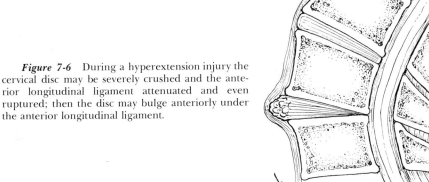

Figure 7-6   During a hyperextension injury the cervical disc may be severely crushed and the anterior longitudinal ligament attenuated and even ruptured; then the disc may bulge anteriorly under the anterior longitudinal ligament.

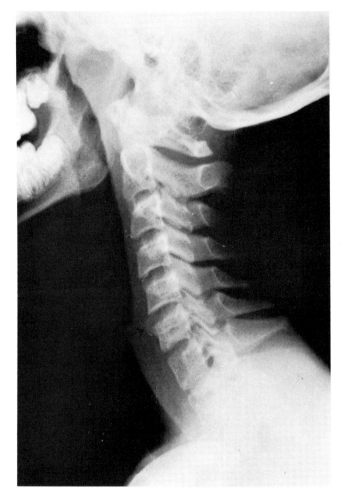

Figure 7-7 Bulging of the C5-C6 disc. This finding was discernible in a 17-year-old female three weeks after a hyperextension injury.

the disc occurs. Serial radiographs taken every four to six weeks may reveal this phenomenon. We have had occasion to follow these progressive phases of disc implication in 11 patients (Fig. 7-8).

More profound lesions may occur to the intervertebral disc than the one just described. If severe forces are applied to the neck in hyperextension-acceleration injuries the anterior longitudinal ligament may rupture; this may be followed by an avulsion of the disc from either the cephalic or caudal vertebra. As noted by Bailey,[1] the line of cleavage may occur between the disc and the articular plate of the vertebra or between the articular plate and the cancellous bone adjacent to the plate (Fig. 7-9). In addition to being associated with disruption of the prevertebral fascia, anterior longitudinal ligament, longus colli muscles and their overlying sympathetic chains, such lesions must also be accompanied by large retropharyngeal hematomas. Radiographs, as a rule, give no clue to the

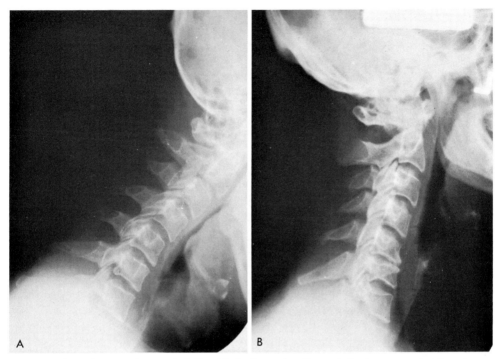

Figure 7-8 Degenerating cervical disc. (*A*), Radiographs of a cervical spine two weeks after a hyperextension injury; the C5-C6 disc appears normal. (*B*), The same cervical spine as it appeared ten months later. Observe the progressive degeneration of the intervertebral disc.

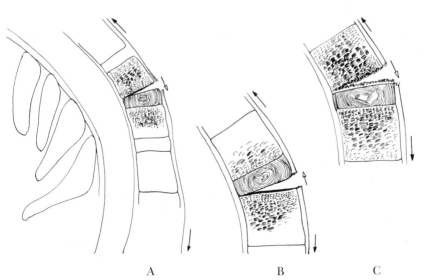

A   B   C

Figure 7-9 Types of injuries of the intervertebral disc following severe hyperextension injuries. In addition to rupture of the anterior longitudinal ligament: (*A*) the intervertebral disc may be avulsed from the proximal articular plate; (*B*) it may be avulsed from the distal plate; (*C*) it may be detached together with the articular plate from the cancellous bone immediately adjacent to the plate.

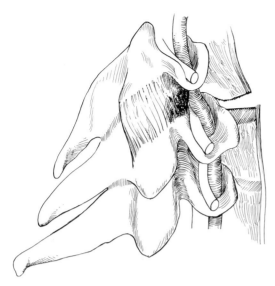

Figure 7-10 Following disruption of the anterior attachments of the disc, in hyperextension injuries, the contents of the intervertebral foramina of the affected motor unit may be severely compressed.

severity of these pathologic lesions, except that as time passes the disc spaces show some diminution in height. Occasionally, the separation can be visualized in radiographs, particularly in flexion and extension views. This radiological diagnosis was made in four of our patients. In the past four years, we have demonstrated this lesion in 17 patients who were subjected to anterior cervical fusions many months after the injury. It was interesting to note the ease with which the discs could be separated from the vertebrae by simply using a blunt dissector, indicating that following separation of the discs healing between the discs and the adjacent vertebral plates was inadequate. The nucleus pulposus was readily removed as large, fragmented, fibrotic segments.

With wide disruption of the attachments of the intervertebral discs, hemorrhage and edema must also implicate the soft tissue elements surrounding the intervertebral foramina, resulting in compression of the nerve roots in the foramina and of the vertebral artery which lies in close proximity to the foramina (Fig. 7-10). This readily explains the symptoms of radiculitis and sympathetic manifestations which frequently accompany these injuries.

SUBLUXATIONS OF THE CERVICAL VERTEBRAE

If the mechanism just described is carried one step further, a vertebral body having lost its moorings to an intervertebral disc could easily be displaced backward for varying distances and then resume its normal anatomical alignment with the body below. However, in its backward migration, subluxation of the apophyseal joints must also occur, resulting in tearing of their capsular ligaments. At this point, it is essential to point out that the spinal cord is firmly fixed in the canal by the dentate ligaments and that the nerve roots and the vertebral arteries with their investing chains of sympathetic fibers are held in rigid bony canals (Fig. 7-11). Any deformation of the cervical column, even if momentary, may

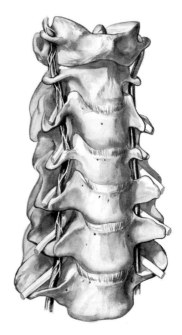

Figure 7-11 Observe that the vertebral arteries and their chains of sympathetic nerve fibers and the nerve roots are contained in rigid bony canals.

result in actual compression or stretching of these important structures (Fig. 7-12). The inflammatory process resulting from such deformations may be an added factor, producing constriction of the nerve roots, the vertebral artery and the sympathetic fibers.

CHRONIC PATHOLOGIC LESIONS

Up to this point, only the acute basic pathologic lesions have been discussed. However, clinical experience reveals that the initial injury may

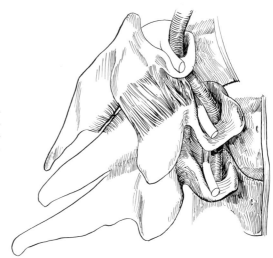

Figure 7-12 Deformation of the cervical column causes compression and stretching of its vital contents (cord, vertebral arteries, sympathetic fibers and nerve roots).

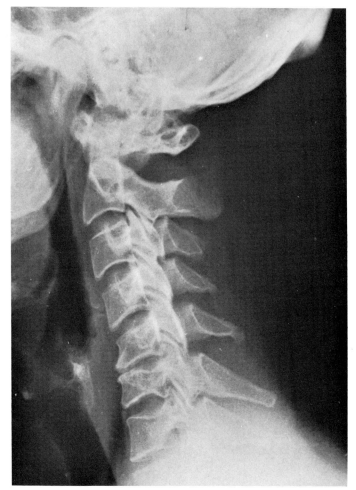

Figure 7-13 Degeneration of a single disc (C5-C6) following a hyperextension injury. Observe the narrowing of the disc space and the formation of peripheral osteophytes on the adjacent surfaces of the fifth and sixth cervical vertebrae.

be followed by months or even years of disability. Therefore, one must assume that in these cases, following the acute pathology, a reparative process sets in that is characterized by the formation of scar tissue and adhesions enmeshing the nerve roots, the vertebral artery and sympathetic chains; this process produces constriction and irritation of these structures. Also, the detached disc may not attain firm anchorage to the vertebral body and undergoes degeneration and it may even be extruded. This sets the stage for the formation of osteophytes at the peripheries of the involved vertebral bodies. These osteophytes may assume a circumferential configuration and involve the joints of Luschka which form the anteromedial boundaries of the intervertebral foramina. At this site, they may cause narrowing of the lumen of the foramina. Similar changes may occur around the margins of the apophyseal joints which form the posterolateral boundaries of the foramina. These osteophytes narrow the foramina or may even impale the contents of the foramina and the nearby vertebral artery. Inadequate healing of a disc to a vertebral body may result in excessive hypermobility of the involved vertebra; this in itself is sufficient for protracted disability. Occasionally this instability may be detected in radiographs when taken with the neck in positions of extreme flexion or extension. If the injury occurs in a normal spine, the changes described are usually limited to one, and occasionally two, segments. Radiologically, the remaining cervical column appears normal (Fig. 7-13).

PATHOLOGY FOLLOWING REAR-END COLLISION IN THE PRESENCE OF DEGENERATIVE CHANGES OF THE CERVICAL SPINE

After the fourth decade, degenerative alterations in the cervical spine are frequently encountered and, with each successive decade, there is a progressive increase in the severity of the changes and the number of segments involved.[6, 9] In the presence of these abnormalities, even minimal violence is capable of producing severe symptoms and, as a rule, the patients manifest protracted and often recalcitrant syndromes. The clinical picture varies with the nature of the pre-existing lesions and the nature of the injury.

Also; something should be said of the bizarre personalities that many victims of rear-end collisions present. In an attempt to explain these changes, the patients have been labeled hysterical or suffering from traumatic or litigation neurosis. It is our opinion that many of us have put too much emphasis on the role that litigation plays on the effectiveness of treatment.[3] Also, it is our belief that many of us are guilty of underestimating the severity of the pathology resulting from rear-end collisions; hence, the varied and bizarre complaints of many patients are taken too lightly. This attitude is passed on to the suffering patients who then become anxious, mentally disturbed and emotionally unbalanced. Many of these unfortunate patients are passed on to psychiatrists for psychiatric evaluation. On more than one occasion, we have seen anxiety and apprehension replaced by mental calm when time was taken to explain to the patient that there were definite organic reasons for the presenting symptoms and that relief was not out of reach.

Besides failure of an adequate evaluation of the pathologic condition, another factor may be responsible for bizarre behavior problems in patients involved in rear-end collisions. The personality structure of the patient may be altered by cerebral concussion sustained at the time of the accident. Many patients give a history of momentary loss of consciousness or an explosive sensation in the head at the time of the accident. After the accident, they complain of vertigo, a sensation of confusion, frontal headaches, insomnia and irritability. Concussion can result from sudden mechanical deformation and pressure on the frontal and temporal lobes when, during backward acceleration of the head, the forward movement of the brain is restrained by the anterior vault of the skull. With forward acceleration of the head, the occipital portion of the brain may suffer

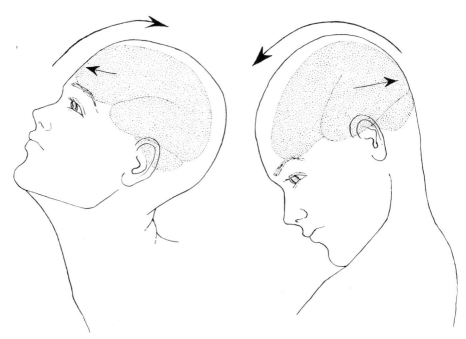

Figure 7-14 Concussion may occur from sudden deformation and pressure on the frontal and temporal lobes during hyperextension injuries.

concussion (Fig. 7-14). Concussion can also be produced by the action of acceleration and deceleration forces acting on the brain. The experimental work of Denny-Brown and Russell supports this belief.[2] Therefore a plea is in order that we take a new look at this disorder, that we try to understand and adequately evaluate the basic pathologic process present and that we be more sympathetic with these unfortunate patients.

CERVICAL SYNDROME OF HYPEREXTENSION

Cervical Spine Injuries

Following uncomplicated hyperextension injuries, the cervical syndrome which evolves depends on many factors, such as the intensity of the forces acting on the cervical spine during the accident, the age of the patient and the presence or absence of other contributory factors, such as degenerative or congenital abnormalities. It was previously stressed that in the presence of such existing alterations of the cervical spine, minimal traumata are capable of initiating severe and recalcitrant syndromes.

The pattern of the syndrome is governed by the level of the cervical spine involved and the degree to which the soft tissue elements are implicated at this level. For example, a syndrome resulting from trauma to the C3-C4 level would differ from one arising from damage to the C6-C7 level. Nevertheless, there are certain features which are common to most syndromes. In the section dealing with the pathology associated with hyperextension injuries, it was pointed out that there is close correlation between the soft tissue injuries and the symptom complex presented. Comprehension of this relationship should provide a logical approach to the management of these injuries.

Acute Clinical Syndrome (Whiplash Injury)

Immediately following a hyperextension injury of the cervical spine, the patient is usually unaware of the magnitude of the injury. At this time he may experience nothing more than some slight discomfort and stiffness in the cervical region. Only rarely is severe pain in the neck with radiation in one or both upper extremities experienced. However, after a period of 12 to 24 hours he begins to realize that something is radically wrong. Pain in the base of the neck is severe and aggravated by motion; motion is restricted and painful; and radiation of pain into the base of the neck, top of the shoulders and in the right or left arm as far as the elbow appears. If there has been stretching and tearing of the tissues of the trachea and the esophagus, hoarseness and dysphagia may be present, and if the sympathetic chain is involved, bizarre symptoms, such as nausea, dizziness, disturbance of vision, earache and even precordial pain may be present. If the vertebral arteries are implicated, either from pressure or spasm, the patient may complain of faintness, giddiness, drop attacks or even periods of unconsciousness. We have seen one elderly patient with complete paralysis of both upper and lower extremities due to pinching of the spinal cord between large posterior osteophytes and a bulging ligamentum flavum following a hyperextension mechanism.

In the early phase of the usual cervical syndrome, the objective findings are fairly constant. The patient holds his head in a slightly flexed position guarding against any motion in any arc. Occasionally, he presents the clinical picture of torticollis. There is evidence of spasm of the anterior and posterior muscles of the neck and of one or both of the trapezius muscles. Active and passive motion is restricted and painful, and pressure over the base of the neck elicits tenderness. Generally, the neurologic examination is negative; however, we have observed in several patients dilation of one pupil due to sympathetic stimulation. Radiological examination, at this time, is usually negative except that, in some instances in which a disc has been severely traumatized, anterior bulging of the disc may be demonstrable.

After a seven- to ten-day period, the acute symptoms begin to subside and a more crystallized clinical pattern appears depending upon the level of the cervical spine implicated. Spasm of the cervical muscles decreases and motion increases. However, in many instances, hyperextension and rotation to one or the other side may be restricted and painful for many months. The patient now can discern specific areas of pain and tenderness and, as a rule, these depend upon the cervical nerve root involved. It was previously pointed out that considerable overlap of segmental distribution of cervical nerves exists, so that specific pain and sensory patterns can not always be depended on to single out the nerve root or roots responsible for the syndrome. Nevertheless, in spite of this possible overlap, in most instances, the pattern of radicular pain and sensory manifestations is fairly consistent with the nerve root or roots involved. Therefore, knowledge of the anatomic distribution of the cervical nerve roots is helpful in determining the level of the cervical spine affected.

Pain is most frequently referred to the root of the neck, the occipital and mastoid regions, the top of one or both shoulders, to the superomedial angle and vertebral borders of the scapula and to the anterior aspect of the chest wall. Occasionally, pain is referred to the triceps area and to the extensor or flexor surfaces of the forearm. As previously recorded, if the sixth nerve root is involved, pain may radiate along the outer aspect of the shoulder and arm to the thumb; the biceps reflex may be diminished or absent. If the seventh root is implicated, the pain also radiates to the top of the shoulder and the outer aspect of the arm, but in this pattern, pain and numbness involve the index finger and, to a lesser extent, the middle finger. The triceps may be weak and its reflex diminished or abolished (Fig. 6-3).

Involvement of the eighth nerve root is the least common and causes pain along the inner aspect of the upper arm along the ulnar border of the hand into the little finger. Further help in identifying the root involved is the knowledge that each major muscle or group of muscles is supplied by a dominant nerve root. For example, the deltoid muscle by C5, the biceps by C6 and the triceps by C7. Any change in power, tone or reflex responses in these muscles points to the nerve root involved (Fig. 6-3).

So far we have discussed the pattern of the symptom complex that appears following hyperextension injuries, but these same patterns of varying intensities may appear spontaneously or as the result of occupational stresses in cervical spines exhibiting degenerative changes. The syndrome following a hyperextension injury is the result of a sudden disruption of tissues, especially the discs, causing hemorrhage and edema which compress the contents of the intervertebral foramina; whereas the syndrome associated with degenerative changes is the result of disintegration of the discs, with or without extrusion of nuclear material, accompanied by a hyperplastic process characterized by the formation of scar tissue, osteochondral spurs and adhesions which enmesh the nerve roots, vertebral arteries and the sympathetic chains. In a hyperextension injury, if healing of the acutely disrupted tissues is not complete, the patient will present, in time, the same symptom complex as that associated with degenerative changes in the cervical spine but not initiated by acute trauma. Also, eventually the affected segment of the cervical spine will show narrowing of the traumatized disc and hypertrophic changes of the adjacent vertebrae (Fig. 7-13).

MANAGEMENT OF FRESH HYPEREXTENSION INJURIES

It is our belief that the most important facet of conservative treatment is rest of the cervical spine. Rest should be prolonged and continuous in order to permit adequate healing of torn tissues and complete recession of the reparative process. This is best achieved by the wearing of a cervical collar which holds the head in a position of slight flexion. The collar should be worn day and night and should be removed only for toilet purposes. It should be worn for four to six weeks. In the event that there is severe muscle spasm and pain, the patient should be put to bed for seven to ten days in order to relieve the neck of the weight of the head. Traction during this phase of the treatment is contraindicated, particularly if a disc has been severely traumatized or detached from one of the adjacent vertebral bodies. The patient should be instructed to use, when in the recumbent position, a pillow of sufficient thickness to support the head in a position of slight flexion. During this period of treatment, radiant heat and analgesics will add to the patient's comfort.

After the third week, the acute symptoms will have subsided sufficiently to institute isometric exercises (see page 95). This is an essential part of the program because within a period of three weeks the cervical musculature will lose considerable tone and power. After the fourth week, the collar should be removed several hours each day and the program of exercises intensified. The collar should be discarded at the end of seven or eight weeks but worn at night for several months. Another important facet of this program is the teaching of the patient in the use of his neck. The head, at all times, should be held in the slightly flexed position and all painful arcs of motion should be avoided, particularly that of hyperextension. This attitude of the head and neck should be maintained throughout all daily activities. If the patient should experience an aggravation of his symptoms, the collar should be reapplied for several days.

Some of the trigger points of pain and tenderness, especially those in the regions of the superomedial aspect of the scapula and along the vertebral border of the scapula, can often be relieved by injection of a local anesthetic agent. Also, the local injection of hydrocortisone into the tissues overlying the laminae of the cervical segment involved is often effective in relieving pain and muscle spasm.

Finally, the patient should be made aware of the fact that his symptoms, regardless of how bizarre they seem, have an organic background and that conscientious and prolonged therapy is necessary. If this is done, the patient's apprehension will lessen and he will be more cooperative. Failure to do this increases the patient's apprehension and he begins making the circuit of physicians and allied medical therapists, including the psychiatrist, in order to obtain relief.

RESULTS OF CONSERVATIVE MANAGEMENT

In spite of a rigid and conscientious conservative program for the treatment of cervical syndromes, regardless of the etiological factors involved, our results are far from satisfactory. This is best illustrated in a study performed by us several years ago in which all patients with a cervical syndrome seen over a period of five years were included; all patients were followed for at least one year.[3] The initial treatment in most of these patients was not instituted by us, but after they came under our care the average period of treatment for the group was 13 weeks. In this group there were 386 patients; 311 of these were treated conservatively. Of the 311 patients we were able to obtain a follow-up study on 255. Of these, 74 patients, or 29 per cent, of the group obtained complete relief; 126, or 49 per cent, were improved and 55, or 22 per cent, were not improved.

OPERATIVE MANAGEMENT OF THE CERVICAL SYNDROME CAUSED BY HYPEREXTENSION INJURIES

From the study noted above it becomes obvious that methods other than those available to us in a conservative regimen must be employed in order to relieve many patients of pain and disability. This brings us face-to-face with the surgical approach to this problem. Having failed to obtain an acceptable result with conservative measures, the question arises, When is surgical intervention indicated? Surgical intervention is indicated only when the status quo reached by the patient is unacceptable and intolerable. We must remember that many patients are capable of making and are willing to make those necessary adjustments which will render the situation tolerable; or, in other words, they can live with their disability.

SELECTION OF THE LEVEL INVOLVED

Having made the decision to approach the problem surgically, the next problem of major importance is the selection of the level or levels affected. A careful study of the clinical pattern of the syndrome together with the x-ray findings are sufficient in many instances to establish the site or sites of trouble. However, these two diagnostic aids leave a considerable margin of error; this can be lessened by the disc distention test (see page 90). This test gives, by far, more information than discography, myelography and electromyographic studies, diagnostic aids which we no longer employ routinely.

RADIOGRAPHIC FEATURES

There are certain radiographic features which are useful in determining the disc involved.

1. Bulging of the disc—This is noted in some patients after hyperextension injury and indicates severe crushing of a disc and rupture or attenuation of the anterior longitudinal ligament and the annulus fibrosus (Fig. 7-15).

2. Separation of the disc from the vertebral bodies—This lesion is not often or readily discernible by x-ray but in a few instances it is demonstrable. We have observed this lesion preoperatively in four patients. It occurs after severe hyperextension injuries.

3. Rapidly collapsing disc—After hyperextension injuries, the x-rays may fail to show any evidence of pathology; however, serial x-rays taken

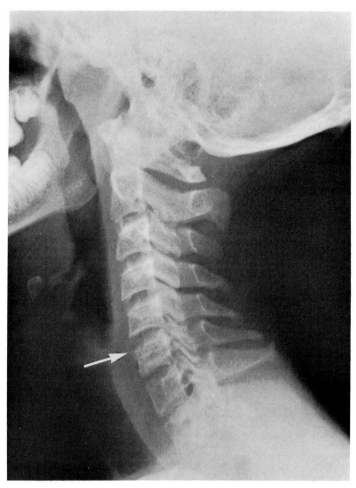

Figure 7-15 Anterior bulging of disc at the C5-C6 level. This lesion was demonstrable three weeks after injury; the patient is 17 years old.

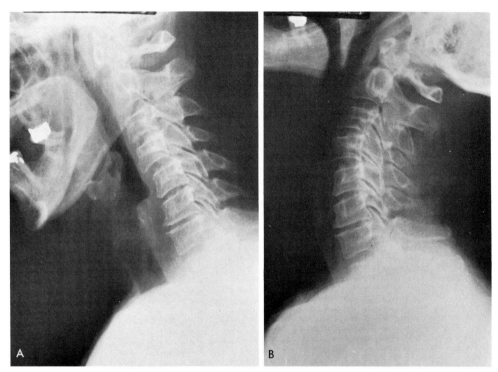

Figure 7-16   Hypermobility of the cervical spine at the C4-C5 level; the segments C5-C6 and C6-C7 are fixed by degenerative changes. (*A*). The cervical spine is flexed. (*B*), It is extended.

every four to six weeks may reveal a progressive diminution in the height of an involved disc. We have observed this phenomenon in 11 patients (Fig. 7-8).

4. Hypermobility of a vertebra above or below a fixed cervical segment—In the presence of a fixed segment of the cervical spine, whether of degenerative or congenital origin, the vertebra above or the one below may become hypermobile. Symptoms may arise from this level with or without injury (Fig. 7-16).

5. Deformation of a vertebral body—Rounding of the anterior margin of a cervical body may be the clue pointing to the disc immediately above as the pathologic level. This deformation is undoubtedly due to the hypermobility of the vertebra above (Fig. 7-17).

OPERATIVE TECHNIQUE—ANTERIOR CERVICAL SPINE FUSION

Excision of the affected disc or discs and fusion of the adjacent vertebrae through the anterior approach has proven to be a valuable procedure for the relief of this type of cervical syndrome. The technique employed is the same as that performed for cervical spondylosis requiring operative intervention and is described in the section, Operative Treatment of Cervical Disc Disease.

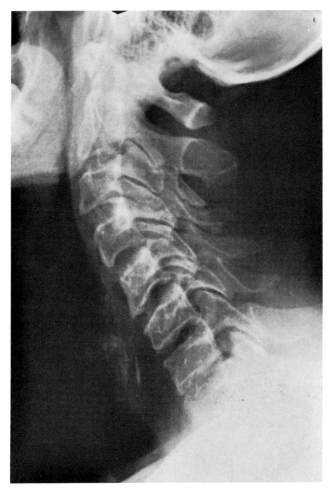

Figure 7-17 Rounding of the anterosuperior margin of C6 probably caused by hypermobility of C5 on C6. Fusion of the C5-C6 level relieved the patient's symptoms.

REFERENCES

1. Bailey, R. W.: Observations of cervical intervertebral-disc lesions in fractures and dislocations. J. Bone Joint Surg. 45-A:461-470, 1963.
2. Denny-Brown, D. and Russell, W. R.: Experimental cerebral concussion. Brain 64:93-164, 1941.
3. DePalma, A. F.: Study of the cervical syndrome. Clin. Orthop. 38:135-141, 1965.
4. Forsyth, H. F. et al.: The advantages of early spine fusion in the treatment of fracture-dislocation of the cervical spine. J. Bone Joint Surg. 41-A:17-36, 1959.
5. Forsyth, H. F.: Extension injuries of the cervical spine. J. Bone Joint Surg. 46-A:1792-1797, 1964.
6. Friedenberg, Z. B. et al.: Degenerative changes in the cervical spine. Anatomy study. J. Bone Joint Surg. 41-A:61-70, 1959.
7. Frykholm, R.: Lower cervical vertebrae and intervertebral discs. Surgical anatomy and pathology. Acta Chir. Scand. 101:345-59, 1951.
8. Macnab, I.: Acceleration injuries of the cervical spine. J. Bone Joint Surg. 46-A:1797-1799, 1964.
9. Silberstein, C. E.: The evolution of degenerative changes in the cervical spine and an investigation into the "joints of Luschka." Clin. Orthop. 40:184-204, 1965.

Chapter 8

COMPLICATIONS AND RESULTS OF OPERATIVE TREATMENT FOR CERVICAL SPINE DISEASE

COMPLICATIONS

Many complications may occur while performing disc excision and anterior interbody fusion. Some are minor, such as transient hoarseness and dysphagia due to local postoperative edema, and some are more serious complications, such as lacerations of the esophagus, tears of the large vessels, puncture of the pleura and laceration of the spinal cord. All of these complications, and particularly the more serious ones, are avoidable, and their occurrence is directly related to the surgeon's competence. We do not mean to imply that serious complications never occur in the hands of skillful and dexterous surgeons, because we are very cognizant that they do. But it is important to appreciate that the anterior approach to the cervical spine is fraught with many dangers and should not be taken lightly.

The posterior approach to the spine is safer for the patient as long as the operative procedure is limited to the exterior of the posterior neural elements. Exposure of the spinal cord is another matter, particularly if the procedure is being performed to decompress a spinal cord with myelopathy associated with cervical spondylosis. It has been pointed out previously that in these circumstances the cord is very vulnerable and even the slightest manipulation may be followed by catastrophic results. This area is not to be invaded by the uninitiated, for it is a delicate situation for even the most experienced surgeon.

In our series of cases, we were fortunate enough to have no serious complications in the patients subjected to operation on the posterior aspect of the spine. However, it should be noted that these patients, as a group, had a more stormy postoperative period than patients with anterior operations. They experienced more pain, their convalescence was more protracted, and in many the posterior incision healed in such a fashion that it was far from being cosmetically acceptable.[3, 4]

In the group of patients subjected to disc excision and anterior spine fusion there were some minor complications. Many patients experienced varying degrees of hoarseness and dysphagia which were transient in nature and disappeared within a few days. These sequelae were undoubtedly the result of local postoperative edema. There was no instance of permanent injury to the recurrent laryngeal nerve.

Several patients awoke from the anesthesia with a Horner's syndrome; this complication too was transitory except in two patients in whom the condition can now be acknowledged permanent. There were no postoperative infections or hemorrhages. There was one injury to the spinal cord; this was not the result of surgical instrumentation. Retropulsion of nuclear material occurred while the patient was being intubated for an endotracheal anesthesia. The patient developed a Brown-Séquard syndrome which was still evident two years after the surgery.

There were other complications of disc excision and interbody fusion through the anterior approach; these will be considered in the section dealing with the results of this procedure.

RESULTS

What was previously recorded about end results in disc surgery of the lumbar spine is applicable to end results of surgery on the cervical spine. There is one exception: fusion of the lower lumbar spine over the past six or seven decades has proven to be an excellent operative procedure for instability and other diseases affecting this region. This is not true of anterior body fusion in the cervical spine. The immediate postoperative results of anterior fusion of the cervical spine are indeed satisfactory; what the results will be 20 years after fusion is another matter. The so-called "long-term end result studies" now appearing in the literature reveal considerable variation in the published results.[1, 4, 6, 7, 8] In the critical analysis of any report, many factors bear on the end results, and each in its own right may contribute to a good or a poor result. The judgment of no two surgeons is the same in the selection of patients. In meeting the challenge of a specific situation, each surgeon is best able to sense his own level of performance, which may be entirely different from that of another surgeon facing the same conditions. The patient poses a wide spectrum of variables, such as age, social and economic status, motivation and duration of the disease, which affect the end results. With regard to the term "end result" as it applies to studies on disc surgery and interbody fusion on the cervical spine, acknowledgment must be made that the end point is still far out in the future and any judgment on the ultimate worth of the operative procedure is, at this time, only speculative.

On the other hand, so-called end result studies are most important in all disciplines. They provide the meeting ground for comparisons of ideas, attitudes and even essential basic knowledge of the subject of the study. It must be acknowledged that the one who derives the most from such a study is the surgeon from whom the report stems. It's a fair estimate of his capabilities to meet a certain challenge.

Results of Conservative Treatment

With the aforementioned qualifications relative to the worth of end result studies, the results and observations noted in two separate studies conducted by us are included here. When these are compared with similar investigations, they parallel the observations of some and differ from others. The first study relates the results obtained in a group of patients treated conservatively.[3]

CLASSIFICATION OF PATIENTS

This group comprised 311 patients ranging in age from 19 to 61 years. Strangely enough, the number of females exceeded the males; there were 166 (53 per cent) females and 145 (47 per cent) males. These patients were seen over a period of five years and all patients were followed for at least one year. All these patients had cervical disc disease of varying degrees, ranging from implication of one disc to all discs. The average period of treatment was 13 weeks. Of the 311 patients, we were able to re-evaluate 255. The essential features of the conservative treatment were rest of the cervical spine, as produced by the wearing of a cervical collar, and the institution of isometric exercises as soon as they were tolerated.

The levels most commonly involved, in the order of frequency, were the C5-C6 level (56 per cent), the C4-C5 level and the C6-C7 level.

RESPONSE TO CONSERVATIVE TREATMENT

The response to treatment was placed in one of three categories: (1) complete relief, (2) improved and (3) no improvement. Only 74 patients (29 per cent) were completely relieved; 126 (49 per cent) were improved

Table 8-1 *Response to Conservative Treatment*

	No.	%
Complete Relief	74	29
Improved	126	49
Not Improved	55	22

Table 8-2 *Litigation and Effectiveness of Treatment*

	174 Patients Uninvolved in Litigation (%)	81 Patients Involved in Litigation (%)
Complete Relief	25	37
Improved	52	35
Not Improved	23	28

and 55 (22 per cent) were not improved (Table 8-1). From these data it is obvious that the overall results from conservative treatment are far from being acceptable.

THE ROLE OF LITIGATION

The patients were divided into two groups: (1) those not involved in litigation and (2) those involved in litigation. In the first group there were 174 patients and in the second 81. Of those not involved in litigation, 25 per cent were completely relieved; 52 per cent were improved and 23 per cent were not improved. Of those involved in litigation, 37 per cent were completely relieved; 35 per cent were improved and 28 per cent were not improved (Table 8-2). The data of both groups do not differ significantly. It becomes apparent then that many of us have put too much emphasis on the role that litigation plays in the effectiveness of treatment.

Evaluation of Anterior and Posterior Cervical Fusion

During the same five-year period, 75 patients with anterior or posterior cervical spine fusions were available for evaluation. Seventeen had posterior fusions and 58 had anterior fusions; 53 patients had multiple levels fused and 22 had one level fused. In the group with anterior fusions, 73.9 per cent were rated excellent, 15.2 per cent as improved and 10.7 per cent as poor. On the other hand, in the group with posterior fusions, 34.7 per cent were rated excellent, 34.7 per cent as improved and 27.6 per cent as poor (Table 8-3). Although this surgical series is small, it does suggest the superiority of the anterior over the posterior fusion. This observation is confirmed in a much larger series of anterior spine fusions which will be discussed later.

Table 8-3 *Results of Anterior and Posterior Fusions (75 Patients)*

	Anterior Fusions (58)	Posterior Fusions (17)
Excellent	73.9 %	34.7 %
Improved	15.2 %	34.7 %
Not Improved	10.7 %	27.6 %

Disc Excision and Anterior Interbody Fusion

The operative treatment of degeneration of the cervical intervertebral disc has become a focus of interest for both the orthopedic surgeon and neurosurgeon during the past decade. Despite the frequency with which this operation is being performed, there is a dearth of information available on the long-range results of this form of therapy. In the hope of improving the surgeon's perspective in this area, the authors have carefully reviewed their cases involving surgery in the cervical spine so that the surgeon can better anticipate the quality of result he can expect and the factors which affect the result.

CLASSIFICATION OF PATIENTS

Of 246 cases of anterior interbody fusion performed up to the time of publication, 156 were chosen for study because their postoperative period was one year or more. Follow-up periods of less than one year were felt to be invalid because of the frequently noted changes in symptomatology during the first postoperative year. Of the 156 patients suitable for study, 146 were able to return for complete followup evaluation including interview, physical examination and roentgenographic examination of the cervical spine. Each patient was examined by an orthopedic surgeon other than the operating surgeon. In this series, the ratio of males to females was approximately 1:2. The age ranged from 17 to 62 years. The number of months postoperative was from 12 to 53 months, the average being 27 months. The duration of symptoms before operation ranged from two months to 20 years with an average of 2.8 years.

INDICATIONS FOR SURGERY

Essentially there was only one indication for surgery, namely, failure to relieve the patient of neck and arm pain by the orthodox methods of conservative treatment.

GRADING SYSTEM FOR THE RESULTS

It is difficult if not impossible to arrive at a system of grading based on objective findings in cervical spine surgery. Neither the indications nor the goals of cervical disc surgery are related to abnormal physical findings but rather to the relief of pain. It is toward the relief of pain that the reviewer must turn his attention, and unfortunately the relief of pain is highly subjective. Changes in arcs of motion or in minor neurologic abnormalities were of little consequence to the patient and indeed he was rarely aware of them. For this reason, the system which evolved in this study was based entirely on subjective findings. The results were graded excellent, good, fair and poor. "Excellent" included those patients with no complaints referable to the cervical spine and who had resumed all their normal activities. "Good" comprised patients who had occasional discomfort in the cervical spine but whose symptoms did not interfere with their

Table 8-4   *Level of Fusions (309 levels fused)*

Level	No.	%
C2-C3	2	0.7
C3-C4	17	5.5
C4-C5	113	36.5 ⎫
C5-C6	125	40.4 ⎬ 76.9
C6-C7	51	16.5
C7-T1	1	0.4

daily activities. "Fair" encompassed those patients who still experienced neck and arm pain but the intensity of this pain was markedly less than before operation. In these individuals, the overall activity was impaired to some degree. "Poor" included those patients who noted no improvement or who were worse as compared to their condition prior to surgery. This rating system is not unlike that used to report most of the other large series of cervical disc operations in the literature.

LEVELS FUSED

In 146 patients, 309 levels were fused from the C2-C3 level to the C7-T1 level (Table 8-4). The C4-C5 level was fused 113 times (36.5 per cent) and the C5-C6 level was fused 126 times (40.4 per cent). Thus, 76.9 per cent of the number of levels fused were at the C4-C5 and C5-C6 levels. It is interesting to speculate that the high incidence of disc degeneration at these levels may be related to the higher mobility at these levels as compared to those above and below.

RESULTS AS RELATED TO NUMBER OF LEVELS FUSED

The striking observation made was that as the number of levels fused increased, the number of satisfactory results decreased. The highest incidence of satisfactory results was obtained when one level was fused, whereas the lowest incidence was noted when three levels were fused (Table 8-5). All rules have exceptions and in this series two patients who had four disc spaces fused were rated as having good results. This trend was also noted by Robinson.[7]

Table 8-5   *Relationship of Number of Levels Fused and Results*

No. of Levels Fused	1	2	3	4
% of Total Group	*19.3*	*56.9*	*22.5*	*1.3*
Excellent	21.4	18.1	6.1	
Good	50	45.8	36.4	
Fair	25	25.3	45.4	
Poor	3.6	10.8	12.1	

Table 8-6   *Patient Evaluation*

	No.	%	
Excellent	23	15.6 ⎱ 60.5	⎱
Good	66	44.9 ⎰	89.6 Satisfactory
Fair	43	29.1	⎰
Poor	14	10.4	

PATIENT EVALUATION

A rating of excellent or good was achieved by 60.5 per cent of the total group. If excellent, good and fair results are considered satisfactory, then 89.6 per cent fall into this category. There were 10.4 per cent poor results (Table 8-6). Reviewing the various series of disc operations reported in the literature, one finds great variation in the quality of results, from 100 per cent and 97.5 per cent improved at one extreme to 65 per cent improved at the other extreme. In general, as one carefully examines these reports it is apparent that the most glowing reports are based on poor quality of follow-up evaluation; that is to say, they are based solely on results of a written questionnaire rather than a personal interview and physical examination.[1, 2, 5, 6, 7, 8]

COMPARISON OF PATIENTS WITH AND WITHOUT TRAUMA

The patients in this series were divided into two groups: (1) those with a spontaneous onset of symptoms and (2) those with a history of trauma initiating their symptoms (Table 8-7). The only significant difference between two groups is that the average age in the group associated with trauma is slightly lower than that associated with a spontaneous onset of symptoms. The incidence of satisfactory results was essentially the same for both groups: 91.3 per cent in the former and 87.3 per cent in the latter.

In those cases with a traumatic onset of symptomatology, an automobile accident was the initiating factor in 55.4 per cent. The ratio of rear-end collisions to front-end collisions was 2.4:1.

Table 8-7   *Results as Related to Trauma*

	Spontaneous Onset		Traumatic Onset	
% of Total Series		37.4		62.6
Average Age		44 years		41.8 years
Results (%):				
E	63.7 ⎰	20.1 ⎱	58.7 ⎰	13.0 ⎱
G		43.6 ⎰ 87.3		45.7 ⎰ 91.3
F		23.6 ⎰		32.6 ⎰
P		12.7		8.7

Table 8-8   *Fusion Results in Extensive Degenerative Disease*

	(20 Patients — 13.6% of Series)
Results	%
Excellent	5 ⟩ 30 ⟩ 80 Satisfactory
Good	25
Fair	50
Poor	20

PATIENTS WITH EXTENSIVE DEGENERATIVE CHANGES

Patients with extensive degenerative changes in the cervical spine were studied as a group. It was interesting to note that patients in this category had three or more levels fused and, as previously noted, the incidence of satisfactory results is far below that observed in patients who had only one or two levels fused. This group comprised 20 patients or 13.6 per cent of our total series (Table 8-8). In the fair and good categories were 75 per cent of the patients and only five per cent were rated excellent.

Pseudarthrosis

A detailed discussion of the failures will be discussed later, but in this group, 16 cases disclosed one or more pseudarthroses. It became apparent that in the cervical spine, as in the lumbar spine, a higher incidence of pseudarthrosis occurs in long fusion areas.

A diagnosis of pseudarthrosis was made when there was demonstrable motion between the spinous processes above and below an operated disc level in the lateral flexion-extension roentgenogram of the cervical spine. Generally this finding was associated with absorption of the bone graft. In only two instances the grafts remained intact but failed to produce a solid fusion (Fig. 8-1).

A pseudarthrosis may occur after a solid fusion has been achieved. However, in the majority of the cases with pseudarthrosis, fragmentation and absorption of the graft followed by development of the pseudarthrosis occurred early in the postoperative period.

Pseudarthrosis does not preclude a satisfactory result (Table 8-9). Of

Table 8-9   *Fusion Results in Pseudarthrosis*
(16 patients — 10.9% of series)

	No.	**%**
Results		
Excellent	1	6.2 ⟩ 93.5 Satisfactory
Good	5	31.2
Fair	9	56.1
Poor	1	6.2

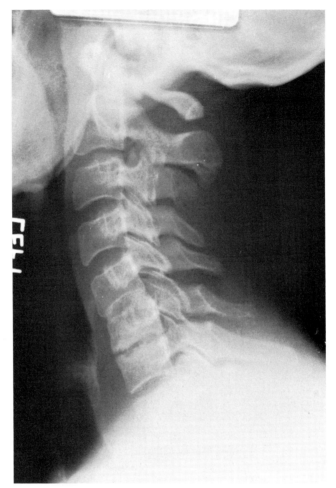

Figure 8-1 Pseudarthrosis in a two-level fusion. Observe the complete absorption of the bone graft at the C6-C7 level.

the 16 cases of pseudarthrosis, one was graded excellent, five were graded good, nine were graded fair and one was graded poor. Thus 15 of the group were graded as satisfactory. This lack of correlation between a solid bony fusion and good results was also noted by Robinson.[7]

In relating the incidence of pseudarthrosis to the number of levels fused, it was found that the highest incidence of pseudarthrosis was found in the group with three levels fused (Table 8-10).

Table 8-10   *Levels of Fusion*
in Pseudarthrosis (16 patients)

2-Level Fusion 7
3-Level Fusion 8
4-Level Fusion 1

Another interesting observation was the location of the pseudarthrosis in multiple-level fusions. Seven patients with a two-level fusion developed a pseudarthrosis. In four of these patients the pseudarthrosis was present at the lower level and in three it was present at both levels. Eight patients with three-level fusions exhibited pseudarthrosis. In these, pseudarthrosis was present at the distal level in six and the middle level in two. The highest incidence of pseudarthrosis was at the C5-C6 level, comprising 74 per cent of the pseudarthroses at all levels.

ABSORPTION OF THE BONE GRAFTS

Fragmentation and partial absorption of the bone grafts was observed in 26 patients; 14 of the 26 developed a pseudarthrosis (Fig. 8-2). The remaining 12 achieved a solid fusion. Taking these as a group, regardless of whether a fusion was attained or not, four were rated excellent, nine good, twelve fair and one poor (Table 8-11). A satisfactory

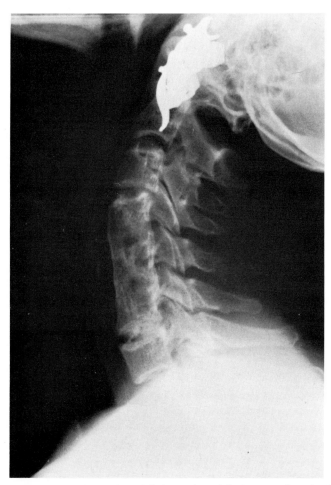

Figure 8-2 Fragmentation and partial absorption of the bone graft at the C6-C7 level. This is a three-level fusion.

Table 8-11 *Absorption of Grafts (26 patients)*

Result	%		
Excellent	15.3	49.9	96 Satisfactory
Good	34.6		
Fair	46.1		
Poor	3.8		

result was achieved in 96 per cent and an excellent or good result in 49.9 per cent.

EXTRUSION OF THE GRAFT

Extrusion of the graft occurred in four instances. In all cases a solid fusion was eventually achieved (Fig. 8-3). However, the interval of time to obtain this fusion result was greatly prolonged. After the fusion became solid, the symptoms gradually disappeared. In one patient, symptoms persisted for six months before improvement. This observation indicated that a fusion will occur between two vertebral bodies after removal of the disc and curettage of the articular surfaces of the vertebra, but the time

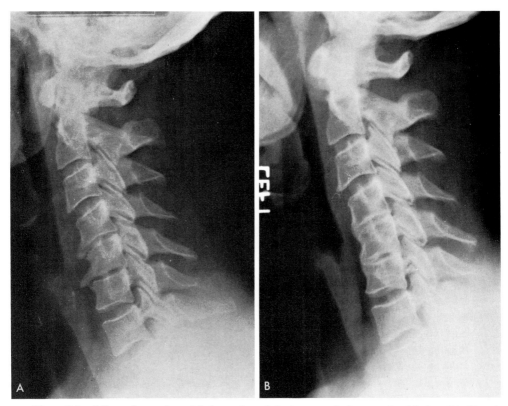

Figure 8-3 *A*, Extrusion and partial absorption of the bone grafts in a two-level fusion (C4-C5 and C5-C6). Note the collapse of the disc space. *B*, Solid fusion was obtained in spite of extrusion and partial absorption of the bone grafts. Fusion was achieved in eight months.

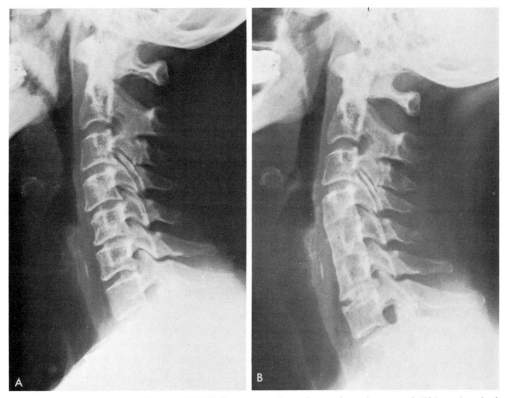

Figure 8-4   *A*, Observe that the C6-C7 disc appears by radiographs to be normal. This patient had a two-level fusion (C4-C5 and C5-C6). *B*, Degeneration of the disc below the fusion area (C6-C7) occurred within 18 months after fusion of the two levels above.

period to achieve this result is much greater than when a bone graft is inserted between the vertebrae. In general, if the graft is not extruded or absorbed, a solid fusion occurs in six to 12 weeks.

DEGENERATION OF THE DISC ABOVE OR BELOW THE FUSION

Roentgenographic evidence of degeneration of the disc above or below the fused segment of the cervical spine is not a rare finding. These alterations may occur in discs which appear roentgenographically normal or degenerated. In this series, 14 patients exhibited this phenomenon. This sequela may or may not be associated with a recurrence of symptoms. Three of the 14 patients noted a recurrence of neck or arm pain. All were relieved by fusion of the newly affected level. Further passage of time will be necessary before the true incidence of this phenomenon can be observed (Figs. 8-4 and 8-5).

ABSORPTION OF POSTERIOR AND ANTERIOR OSTEOPHYTES

Following a solid fusion, the fate of pre-existing posterior and anterior osteophytes is unpredictable. In our series, 58 per cent of the cases

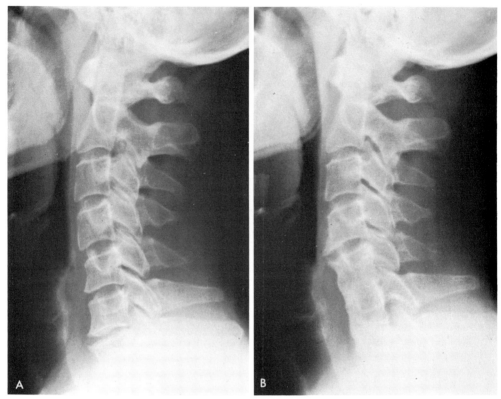

Figure 8-5   *A*, Observe that the C4-C5 disc appears normal. *B*, Degeneration of the disc above the fusion area (C4-C5) occurred within two years after fusion of the C5-C6 and C6-C7 levels.

with posterior osteophytes revealed roentgenographic evidence of complete or partial resorption. Forty-two per cent of the total series showed no demonstrable change. It was interesting to note that following successful fusion the presence or absence of posterior osteophytes is not related to the final result. In those patients who developed a pseudarthrosis, the osteophytes persisted or increased in size (Figs. 8-6, 8-7, and 8-8). Following successful fusion, anterior osteophytes always disappeared.

CAUSES OF FAILURE

Having reviewed the late complications of disc excision and anterior interbody fusion, it is appropriate to list the causes of failure. These are: (1) extrusion of the graft, (2) degeneration of a disc above or below the fusion area, (3) fusion at the wrong level, (4) failure to fuse all the levels producing symptoms, (5) absorption of the bone graft, (6) pseudarthrosis, (7) arachnoiditis and chronic scarring of the nerve roots. This latter complication of cervical spondylosis must be considered because, if the function of the nerve fibers in the root is disrupted completely, the neurologic deficit is permanent. The fibrosis, which may involve a nerve root and its sheath, may be extensive; also, if the radiculopathy is associated with

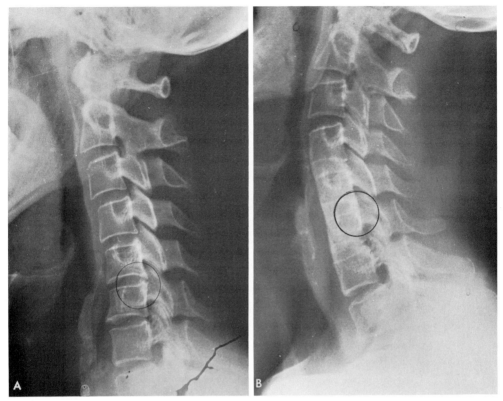

Figure 8-6   Absorption of posterior osteophytes following fusion. *A*, Note the posterior osteophytes on the surfaces of the C5 and C6 vertebrae before fusion of the C5-C6 level. *B*, Complete absorption of the posterior osteophytes at the C5-C6 level after fusion. This radiograph was taken 15 months after the fusion was performed.

myelopathy, the prognosis is poor and these factors contribute to the failure of any form of treatment. A final cause for failure is (8) selection for surgery of a highly emotional patient with a pronounced functional overlay. Careful evaluation of the patient's objective findings and weighing them against the degree of functional overlay are most essential. Many of these patients have definite organic reasons for their symptoms and should be actively treated, for if they get relief their functional element may decrease or even disappear. This is not true in patients in which the functional overlay completely dominates the clinical picture. These patients are made worse by any type of surgery.

If one surveys the entire spectrum of diseases of the intervertebral discs, from the cervical to the lumbosacral region, it soon becomes obvious that much information has accumulated in the past three decades. The clinical, physical and mechanical properties of the disc are better understood; and the role that these factors play in the basic pathologic processes affecting the disc is explicable. Clear models of the different syndromes associated with cervical and lumbar disc diseases have been evolved and accepted.

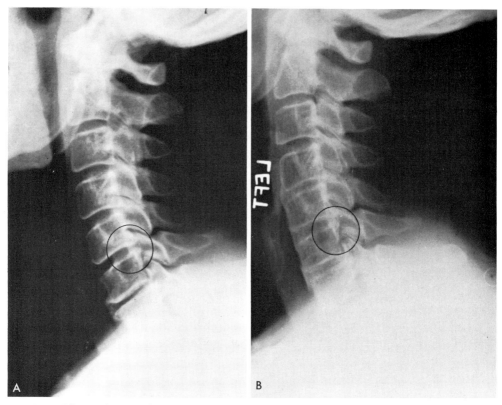

Figure 8-7 Persistence of posterior osteophytes following fusion. *A*, Observe the posterior osteophytes at the C5-C6 level and the anterior osteophytes at the C6-C7 level. *B*, Eighteen months after fusion the posterior osteophytes at the C5-C6 level still persisted; the anterior osteophytes at the C6-C7 level have disappeared. This patient was symptom free.

Certain concepts of treatment have been developed which, although still controversial, are not empirical but are based on a knowledge of the basic pathologic process acting on the disc. Ingenious surgical methods and techniques of treatment have been designed and refined; and although their proper indications are still in a state of turmoil, the turbulence is subsiding gradually and in the near future the waters should be calm.

Much has been achieved in and contributed by the field of radiology; and from all current evidence even greater new developments and refinements of old methods are about to explode on us in the near future. We have better comprehension of the cervical syndromes associated with radiculopathy as to cause, course, response to treatment and prognosis.

Yet, in this spectrum there are gray, and even some black, areas. We are still ignorant of the pathogenesis of disc disease. Whether the pathologic process is related to the process of aging, heredity or developmental error is not known. What is the catalyst for the process and how is it evoked?

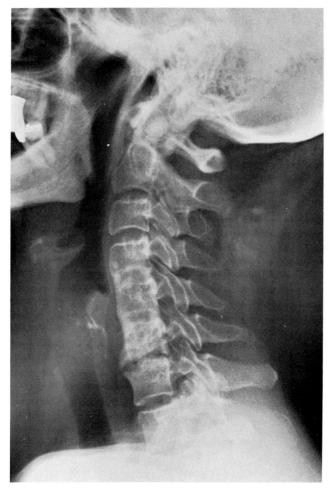

Figure 8-8 Formation of posterior and anterior osteophytes at the level of a pseudarthrosis (C6-C7). This patient had a three-level fusion (C4 to C7).

Do we really understand myelopathy, its true pathogenesis, its course, its prognosis, its end point? Do we really know all the ways that myelopathy may manifest itself?

These and many other queries are as yet unanswered. However, there is reason to believe that many of these questions will be answered in the near future. Never in the history of medicine has a more intensified effort been made to solve the basic fundamental problems which relate to disease states. The answer may be forthcoming from one or a combination of many scientific areas—biochemistry, biophysics, genetics and many others. Our young men in these fields are indeed fortunate to be part of and to participate in a movement which within a few decades may change our entire concept of disease states and which may put the emphasis on prevention rather than on treatment, evolving an entirely new and different approach to the problems of the intervertebral disc.

REFERENCES

1. Cloward, R. B.: Surgical treatment of traumatic cervical spine syndromes. Wiederherstellungschir. u. Traum. 7:148-185, 1963.
2. Connolly, E. S. et al.: Clinical evaluation of anterior cervical fusion for degenerative cervical disc disease. J. Neurosurg. 23:431-437, 1965.
3. DePalma, A. F.: Study of the cervical syndrome. Clin. Orthop. 38:135-141, 1965.
4. DePalma, A. F. and Cooke, A. J.: Results of anterior interbody fusion of the cervical spine. Clin. Orthop. 60:169-185, 1968.
5. Dereymaeker, A. and Mulier, J.: La fusion vertébrale par voie ventrale dans la discopathie cervicale. Rev. neurol. 99:597-616, 1958.
6. Herzberger, E. E. et al.: Treatment of cervical disc disease and cervical spine injury by anterior interbody fusion. A report on early results in 72 cases. Zbl. Neurochir. 23:215-227, 1963.
7. Robinson, R. A.: The results of anterior interbody fusion of the cervical spine. J. Bone Joint Surg. 44-A:1569-1586, 1962.
8. Stuck, R. M.: Anterior cervical disc excision and fusion: Report of 200 consecutive cases. Rocky Mountain Med. J. 60:25-30, 1963.

Chapter 9

CLINICAL SYNDROME OF THE THORACIC INTERVERTEBRAL DISC

Protrusions of the intervertebral disc in the area of the thoracic spine assume greater significance than would be expected from their relatively rare incidence. The reason for this is that their confusing clinical picture frequently leads to delays in diagnosis, which markedly hamper the efficacy of surgical intervention and allow for irreversible damage to the thoracic cord. With today's modern techniques, early surgical intervention is frequently followed by a favorable postoperative course, much unlike the dreaded situation of past decades. Far too often, however, patients are diagnosed as late as one to two years after the onset of their symptomatology, having been treated for a variety of visceral disorders, when signs of advanced cord compression are present. Results at this stage are frequently of limited value to the patient.

It is difficult to assess the frequency of thoracic disc degeneration in the population as a whole but certain inferences can be drawn from ratios of thoracic disc operations to total disc operations. Love and Keefer report an incidence of two to three per 1000.[2] Other authors have reported an incidence varying from one to ten per 1000 for thoracic disc herniations. Thoracic disc degeneration appears predominantly in males, those in their fifth decade being most often affected. Tovi and Strang report that approximately one-quarter of their cases of thoracic disc degeneration occurred at the eleventh space and more than one-half of all protrusions have involved the ninth, tenth and eleventh spaces.[3]

171

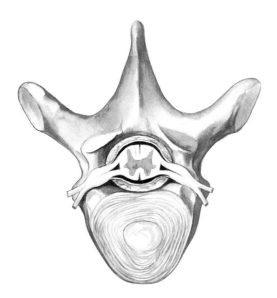

Figure 9-1 Illustration demonstrating relationship of thoracic cord to neural canal. Note the lack of leeway between neural and osseous structures.

HISTORY

An understanding of the symptoms and physical findings of thoracic disc degenerations requires comprehension of the anatomic relationship in this area between the thoracic disc and the spinal cord. The relatively small dimensions of the neural canal in this area and the relatively small amount of leeway between the thoracic disc and the cord should be recalled (Fig. 9-1). One can divide posterior disc herniation into certain anatomic groups depending upon their location, that is, central, central-lateral and lateral (Fig. 9-2). Approximately one-half of disc protrusions fall into the central group, the remainder being divided into either the central-lateral or lateral categories.

Lateral herniation of the nucleus will produce a root compression syndrome, with unilateral pain limited to one or two dermatomes. Central and central-lateral discs involve the long tracts to varying degrees depending on their location. Symptoms involve both the back and lower extremities. Sphincter control may be lost with central protrusion.

Pain is the most common presenting symptom. Most commonly the pain is dorsal or dorsolumbar in location. The back pain is frequently associated with a segmental, radicular type of pain that may be either unilateral or, less frequently, bilateral in nature. When the symptomatology evolves as a unilateral situation the clinical picture tends to be one of slow progression, whereas a bilateral onset of symptomatology is more likely to progress rapidly and irreversibly. Trauma appears to be a precipitating factor in approximately one-third of the cases.

Sensory symptoms, particularly numbness, are frequent components of the thoracic disc syndrome. The numbness will usually begin peripherally in the lower extremities and spread centrifugally. The sensory changes may be unilateral at onset and later may become bilateral. A sense of unsteadiness and an ataxic gait may also be present. Hyperesthesia or paresthesia are less frequently noted by these patients.

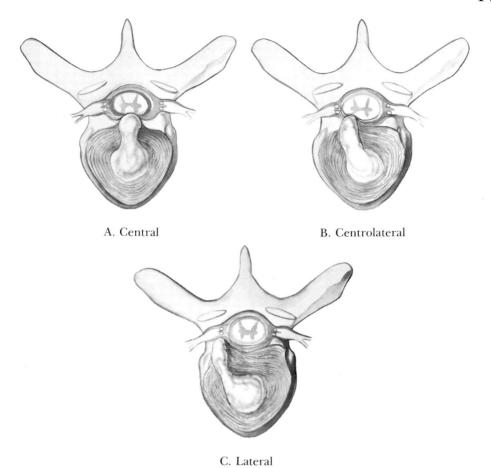

A. Central   B. Centrolateral

C. Lateral

Figure 9-2 *A*, Central thoracic disc herniation with implication of cord. *B*, Centrolateral thoracic disc herniation with implication of cord and root. *C*, Lateral thoracic disc herniation with implication of root.

Visceral symptoms referable to the bowel or bladder are frequently noted in thoracic disc syndromes when cord pressure is present. The complaints may vary from urinary retention or incontinence to bowel constipation or incontinence.

As the long tracts become involved, weakness of one or both legs may become noticeable. Motor weakness progresses at a variable speed, usually affecting the peripheral part of an extremity first. More often a spastic rather than a flaccid type of paresis is present.

PHYSICAL FINDINGS

Certain nonspecific findings are present with thoracic disc herniation which are of little help in localization of the area of pathology. Limitation of motion, paravertebral muscle spasm and scoliosis are all seen in this disorder. As compression of neural structures becomes more marked, neurologic deficits, which help to accurately localize the level of the lesion, may become apparent.

In regard to sensory findings a unilateral or, less frequently, bilateral sensory level may be apparent. An ataxic gait and a positive Romberg test are less frequently noted. Sensory disturbances have been absent in only ten per cent of some series.[3]

Motor and reflex changes are noted at a later stage in the progression of this clinical syndrome than sensory changes. As motor weakness develops the quadriceps and Achilles reflexes usually become increased on the side of the weakness; less often the flaccid type of paraparesis or paraplegia is present. It is frequently noted that there is an absence or diminution of the lower abdominal reflexes. The plantar response may be extensor or flexor.

As previously noted the chronological development of symptomatology is usually pain, then sensory disturbance, weakness and, last, visceral abnormalities.

RADIOGRAPHIC EVALUATION

Routine roentgenograms of the thoracic spine frequently demonstrate narrowing of the affected disc space, irregularity of the disc space, osteophyte formation and calcification. Tomograms may be necessary in order to demonstrate calcification when this is not marked. Myelography should be performed to accurately localize preoperatively the level of pathology and help to demonstrate a lesion which may be mimicking a disc, such as a tumor. A complete or partial block is frequently noted at the level of the affected disc. If lumbar myelography demonstrates a complete block it may be necessary to investigate the area above this block through cisternal myelography. An excellent review of the problems of roentgenography with thoracic disc degeneration has been presented by Baker, Love and Uihlein.[1]

DIFFERENTIAL DIAGNOSIS

Pain in the thoracic spine with or without radiation into the chest and abdomen can be caused by thoracic discs as well as a plethora of other pathologic entities. As in most other areas, it is most often an error of omission in our thinking process which leads to a missed diagnosis of a thoracic disc. If one carefully considers the diagnosis of a thoracic disc, performs a complete neurologic examination, and, if indicated, a myelogram, he will most assuredly make the correct diagnosis. If this entity is not entertained however, one may be easily led astray.

Rheumatoid or ankylosing spondylitis affecting the thoracic spine frequently gives rise to sensations of pain and stiffness in this area. The history of arthritis is usually of help in differentiation between these entities. Often, but not always, the serologic tests for rheumatoid arthritis are positive. In many instances routine roentgenograms demonstrate the characteristic calcification of the longitudinal ligaments in ankylosing spondylitis and help to elucidate the picture. Early in the course of the disease, however, x-rays may be negative.

Malignant tumors, either intraspinal or extraspinal, may give rise to dorsal spine pain mimicking a thoracic disc. Myelography will usually differentiate nondiscogenic space-taking lesions even in the presence of a complete block through the use of a cisternal myelogram. The search for extraspinal tumors must include good quality x-rays of the thoracic spine, chest, rib cage and mediastinum. Frequently planograms of suspicious areas in the mediastinum are required.

Relatively recently an entity known as the costovertebral joint syndrome has been delineated; this condition can produce pain in the thoracic spine radiating unilaterally in a radicular fashion. This is secondary to inflammation in a costovertebral joint. Tenderness is noted directly over the affected costovertebral joint and can be relieved by injection of an anesthetic agent directly into this joint.

Visceral abnormalities are known to produce dorsal spine pain with or without radiation. In the gastrointestinal tract, posterior perforating ulcers and pancreatitis as well as malignancies affecting the posterior abdominal wall can produce extremely confusing symptomatology. Lesions affecting the genitourinary system can also produce radicular pain closely mimicking lower thoracic disc syndromes. In the cardiovascular realm ischemic conditions of the myocardium as well as aortic aneurysms can be productive of symptoms suggestive of thoracic disc disease.

Disc space infections are usually found in a younger age group than are disc herniations. Disc space infections present a unique roentgenographic appearance outlined in the chapter on pathology of the intervertebral disc. It should be recalled that this infection may be present without significant alteration in temperature or white cell count.

Fractures and dislocations in the thoracic spine do not usually present a difficult diagnostic challenge as their appearance is readily evident on routine x-ray examination of the thoracic spine if they are carefully looked for.

Herpes zoster may present as radicular pain with or without a midline component but within a relatively short period of time will make itself evident with the appearance of a typical vesicular rash along a radicular distribution.

REFERENCES

1. Baker, H. L., Jr., et al.: Roentgenologic features of protruded thoracic intervertebral discs. Radiology 84:1059-65, 1965.
2. Love, J. G. and Kiefer, E. J.: Root pain and paraplegia due to protrusions of thoracic intervertebral disks. J. Neurosurg. 7:62-69, 1950.
3. Tovi, J. D. et al.: Thoracic intervertebral disc protrusions. Acta Chir. Scand. Suppl. 267:1-41, 1960.

Chapter 10

OPERATIVE TREATMENT OF THORACIC DISC DISEASE

The management of thoracic disc lesions is entirely different than that of cervical and lumbar disc lesions. In general, unless there is a cauda equina syndrome or progressive motor deficits, the treatment of cervical and lumbar discs is conservative. On the other hand, there is no place for conservative treatment in thoracic disc lesions. If anything can be done for these patients, it is always in the realm of surgery. Unfortunately, the irony of the situation is that many patients with lumbar disc lesions are subjected to surgery far too often and far too soon; whereas, many patients with lesions of the thoracic spine, who should be operated on as soon as possible, come to surgery far too late. There are reasons for this paradoxical situation. The clinical picture of thoracic lesions is protean in nature and may mimic many other lesions, particularly intrinsic diseases of the spinal cord. Up to this time, a syndrome characteristic of thoracic disc lesions has not been evolved. This is in contrast to the cervical and lumbar disc lesions which can be readily recognized because of their clear, sharply delineated syndromes. Even more important is the fact that treating physicians and surgeons lack, in their thinking process, awareness of thoracic disc lesions. Until this entity, thoracic disc lesion, is consistently included in the differential diagnosis there is little hope that the current situation as it relates to diagnosis and treatment of these lesions will change.

The great variability of thoracic disc lesions is due to the nature of the pathology which in turn is governed by the size, location and duration of the disc protrusion. It was previously pointed out that truly lateral lesions produce radicular pain, whereas central lesions implicate the long tracts, and central-lateral lesions may involve the long tracts and also compress the nerve roots. Although pain is associated with over 65 per cent of the cases, in the remaining cases there may be no pain. When pain is absent, there is little to differentiate disc lesions from spinal cord tumors or intrinsic cord disease. The size of the lesion also plays a major role in the character of the presenting clinical picture. Large lesions not only compress the cord but also may obliterate the blood supply to a segment of the cord producing a vascular myelopathy. When this occurs, portions of the cord above and below the disc lesion may be affected, so that clinical manifestations, such as sensory levels, do not correspond to the level of the pathologic disc. Also, the thoracic portion of the cord is very vulnerable to any space-occupying lesion. It was previously recorded that the thoracic cord lies in the smallest part of the spinal canal and is fixed by the nerve roots and dentate ligaments. In the presence of a large disc protrusion there is no room for displacement of the cord, and the dentate ligaments hold it tightly against the protrusion. The resulting tension is another factor capable of impairing the already compromised blood supply to the cord. Some very interesting and unusual findings have been encountered upon exploring the cord: the disc may erode the anterior dura; a spicule of the disc may actually penetrate the anterior aspect of the cord; hematomyelia of the cord may occur as well as posterior infarction of the cord at the level of the protrusion; the cord may be stretched and deformed over the protrusion with areas of necrosis and edema.[1, 4, 5]

That these lesions are missed more often than they are diagnosed is evident from statistical reviews. The average time period from the onset of symptoms to the time of surgery is approximately two years.[4, 5] In one series of cases, the diagnosis was made preoperatively in only 11 cases (27 per cent) out of 41.[4, 5] To complicate the situation further, plain radiographs give very little significant information, except for occasional calcification in the disc affected, but this is not pathognomonic of disc protrusion. Although it is difficult to make any early clinical diagnosis, myelography, properly done, will reveal a space-occupying lesion requiring surgical intervention in almost 100 per cent of the cases. Unfortunately, again because of the lack of awareness in most instances, myelography is not done until late in the course of the disease.

The indication for operative intervention in thoracic disc lesions is clear; once the diagnosis is established the only treatment that may benefit the patient is removal of the protrusion and decompression of the cord. There are no contraindications except poor general health in a patient already debilitated by the disease. It should be remembered that thoracic disc lesions are progressive; a patient not operated on can only get worse. The episodic nature of the disease punctuated by appearances of remissions is very misleading and should not influence the decision to operate.

SURGICAL CONSIDERATIONS

Operative treatment for thoracic disc lesions is fraught with many hazards for the patient and with much disappointment for both the surgeon and the patient.[4, 6, 7] The operation should be performed by a neurosurgeon knowledgable in the anatomy of the region and in the variable pathologic processes he may encounter. There is no doubt that in many instances the outcome of the operation depends entirely on the knowledge, judgment and skill of the surgeon.

The objectives of operative intervention are clear. They are: (1) to remove the protrusion, (2) to halt further progression of cord dysfunction, (3) not to traumatize the cord or compromise further its blood supply at the site of injury and (4) to restore any motor or sensory deficits. As yet, there is no general agreement as to how these goals can best be achieved. Some surgeons favor a hemilaminectomy, others a complete laminectomy, and still others the lateral approach. It would seem that any of these procedures can be used provided they are applicable to the nature of the pathologic lesion.

The lateral approach is essentially an extension of costotransversectomy. It provides only limited exposure of the dura and is totally inadequate for an extensive exploratory operation. It becomes apparent that it is appropriate only when the preoperative diagnosis is definitely established.[2]

Most surgeons prefer extensive laminectomy of three or four laminae if necessary. This provides adequate exposure of the cord; but the laminae must be removed with the utmost caution in order to avoid crushing the cord against an unyielding protrusion. It is well recognized that the changes which take place in a cord compressed by a disc protrusion render it extremely vulnerable to even the slightest surgical trauma. It may be necessary to remove even the pedicle on the side of the lesion if more lateral exposure is desirable. If an extensive exploration must be done the lateral approach makes it impossible.

Most surgeons favor opening the dura in order to evaluate adequately the state of the cord. Visible areas of necrosis are ominous and any manipulation of the already damaged cord is very likely to induce further changes. For this reason, some only advocate simple decompression of the cord without making an attempt to remove the protrusion.[3] In order to mobilize the cord and permit access to the protrusion, the dentate ligaments may be sectioned bilaterally; some surgeons do not hesitate to section two or three spinal roots in order to facilitate exposure of the lesion.[8] Removal of the protrusion by the intradural route is far less traumatic to the cord than removing it extradurally; furthermore, any manipulation of the cord is under direct visual control.

Having exposed the nuclear mass, a decision must be made as to its disposition. Logue[3] favors leaving the mass in situ if the cord shows areas of focal necrosis; any attempt to tamper with the cord, no matter how gently it is done, may induce rapid progression of the neurological deficits. The same is true if the lesion consists of a hard bony transverse ridge under the cord. On the other hand, if the protrusion is rounded and soft and the cord shows no gross abnormal changes it should be removed.

The extradural approach is certainly indicated if the disc is readily accessible in the lateral position.[2]

Regardless of the operative techniques employed, thoracic disc lesions as they currently come to the surgeon's attention carry a grave prognosis and a high morbidity. The best results are attained in cases recognized very early with a small lesion and no degenerative changes in the cord. There is a close correlation between the severity of the preoperative neurological deficit and the postoperative results. Usually the operative results are very discouraging in patients with severe neurological deficits. Good results can be expected in patients with root pain alone or in combination with only minimal cord compression.[3, 8]

ARTHRODESIS

Spine fusion following removal of the disc protrusion is indicated only if the posterior articular joints or the pedicles have been violated. This can be determined at the time of operation on the disc. Because it is desirable, in most instances, to leave the laminectomy site uncovered, the fusion should be done by laying cancellous bone across the transverse processes of the vertebrae involved. The bone is readily obtained from one of the posterior iliac crests.

Technique of Arthrodesis

With a sharp periosteal elevator, strip all soft tissues from the apophyseal joints and continue the dissection laterally until the transverse processes are exposed. First, carry out the dissection on one side, then on the other. Using a sharp periosteal elevator or osteotome, denude the transverse processes of all soft tissues.

By subperiosteal dissection, expose one of the posterior iliac crests and remove long slabs of cancellous bone. Place the strips of cancellous bone across the posterior surface of the exposed transverse processes. Also pack iliac bone along the lateral aspects of the vertebrae and across the apophyseal joints. Upon closing the wound, care should be taken to avoid displacing the bone slabs and also to prevent bone chips from dropping on the cord.

When the patient becomes ambulatory he should wear some form of back support; a Taylor brace is adequate. The brace is worn until there is radiological evidence of a solid bony fusion.

REFERENCES

1. Fisher, R. G.: Protrusions of thoracic disc. The factor of herniation through the dura mater. J. Neurosurg. 22:591-593, 1965.
2. Hulme, A.: The surgical approach to thoracic intervertebral disc protrusions. J. Neurol. Neurosurg. Psychiat. 23:133-137, 1960.
3. Logue, V.: Thoracic intervertebral disc prolapse with spinal cord compression. J. Neurol. Neurosurg. Psychiat. 15:227-241, 1952.
4. Love, J. G. and Kiefer, E. J.: Root pain and paraplegia due to protrusions of thoracic intervertebral disks. J. Neurosurg. 7:62-69, 1950.

5. Love, J. G.: Thoracic disc protrusions, J.A.M.A. 191:627-631, 1965.
6. Mixter, W. J. and Barr, J. S.: Rupture of intervertebral disc with involvement of spinal canal. N. Eng. J. Med. 211:210-215, 1934.
7. Müller, R.: Protrusion of thoracic intervertebral disks with compression of spinal cord. Acta Med. Scand. 139:99-104, 1951.
8. Tovi, J. D. et al.: Thoracic intervertebral disc protrusions. Acta Chir. Scand. Suppl. 267:1-41, 1960.

Chapter 11

SALIENT CLINICAL FEATURES OF LUMBAR DISC LESIONS

The only truly constant feature of the clinical syndrome of lumbar disc lesions is the great variability of the signs and symptoms, not only from patient to patient but in the same patient. This confusion can be clarified only if one appreciates the progressive nature of the disease and correlates the clinical manifestations with both the different phases of the pathologic process in the disc and the changes which occur in the surrounding tissues. In addition, it is most important to remember that the response of patients to the same stimuli is quite variable. Other factors that vary the clinical picture are the site of the lesion and the nerve roots involved, the size of the extrusion and the anatomical peculiarities of the spinal canal as to size and shape. It will be shown that in the early phases of the disease the clinical features are related directly to derangement of the intervertebral disc and its effect on the adjacent nerve roots; but, toward the end of the pathologic process, the clinical picture is clouded by the secondary changes that occur in the motor unit as a whole. These changes may even dominate the clinical syndrome and, in themselves, show considerable variability. In spite of all the factors that can obscure the true nature of the lesion, in the majority of patients the correct diagnosis and the localization of the lesion can be arrived at. This entails a careful analysis of the patient's history and of the subjective and objective characteristics that the patient presents. In our judgment, a diagnosis of a lumbar disc lesion can be made in most instances by a careful study of the clinical syndrome. However, a true appreciation of the presenting clinical features necessitates comprehension of their methods of production. In addition, there are some diagnostic tools and tests which are most helpful in confirming the diagnosis or in eliminating the probability of other lesions; when indicated, these should be utilized.

HISTORY

Injury

Injury is a very variable feature in the history of lumbar disc lesions. The majority of patients associate the disease with a specific injury. Not infrequently, the patient may portray a vivid account of the mechanism of the injury and the sudden appearance of symptoms. Some individuals deny any previous injury to the low back region; others recall an incident that occurred days or weeks before the onset of the severe symptoms, without correlating the injury with the presenting clinical manifestations; still others closely recognize the association of the presenting syndrome to a previous trauma because what had been considered a minor low back strain gradually and progressively developed into a serious, incapacitating back disorder. It may require some subtle probing on the part of the physician to elicit a history of trauma prior to the onset of symptoms. It is safe to state, however, that in some instances an acute, severe attack of low back pain instituted by some form of trauma is usually preceded by some prior discomfort or dull ache in the lumbar region. This is particularly true and characteristic of the early phases of degeneration of the nucleus pulposus when the annulus fibrosus is still intact; however, with degeneration of the annulus, trivial trauma may precipitate an attack. Nevertheless, a large group of patients deny, and the physician is unable to elicit, a history of trauma.

The mechanisms and severity of injuries capable of initiating an acute lumbar disc syndrome also show wide variations. In young adults, before biochemical abnormalities begin in the nucleus or in the very early phase of this process, a violent flexion injury is required to cause retropulsion of the nucleus. Although these cases are indeed rare, they do occur. Generally, the discs above the L4-L5 level are involved and the result is usually catastrophic. In the lumbar spine a massive nuclear extrusion compressing the cauda equina suddenly and severely results in partial or complete paralysis and loss of sphincter function. These lesions are true emergencies. With an abnormally small spinal canal, compression may be caused by a large, bulging, dorsal protrusion under the posterior longitudinal ligament, pressing the cauda equina against the laminae. As pointed out, during the intermediate stage of nuclear disintegration trivial traumata, such as stooping to pick up a small object, stepping off a curb, sneezing or coughing, may precipitate a severe attack. Not infrequently the patient volunteers the information of feeling a "sudden snap" in the lower back or of experiencing the sensation of "something tearing" in the back. These phenomena are undoubtedly caused by sudden rupture of the defective annulus due to a sudden rise in the tension in the nucleus and backward displacement of nuclear material.

Pain Patterns

As in the cervical syndrome, the pain patterns observed in the lumbar disc lesions are varied and may be very confusing. However, mechanisms for the production of the different types of pain have been postulated and confirmed by experimental and clinical observation that, if understood, are helpful not only in determining the cause and site of origin of a specific mode of pain but also in instituting the appropriate therapeutic measures. In general, pain in the lumbar region alone or associated with pain in the lower extremities is the result of stimuli applied to the mesodermal structures of the spine or to the nerve roots either within the dural sac or after they emerge from the dura. Based on the site of origin, pain can be classified as scleratogenous or dermatogenous pain.

SCLERATOGENOUS PAIN

As previously pointed out, this type of pain results when mesodermal tissues are stimulated by noxious agents. The mesodermal structures involved, such as ligaments, tendons, periosteum and periarticular tissues, are closely related to the skeleton. These tissues are very sensitive to pain; the pain evoked is described as being deep, dull, aching pain and poorly localized. Although it is constant, its intensity varies markedly depending on the character of the stimulation and the structure affected. It is associated with widespread radiation and exhibits no lines of delineation which would limit it to a well-defined region. This type of pain has no cutaneous distribution but is confined to the deep structures. Radiation is to the mesodermal elements connected to the skeleton; these elements are of the same embryonic origin as the mesodermal tissues initially stimulated. The area of radiation is designated the sclerotome, in contrast to the cutaneous area of pain distribution, called a dermatome, which follows irritation of a nerve root (Figs. 11-1 and 11-2). Not infrequently, when the mesodermal tissues are severely stimulated the pain may be accompanied by a vasovagal response such as sweating, nausea, decrease in the blood pressure and even collapse.

After the initial stimulation, radiation of pain does not occur immediately but may be delayed, sometimes for several hours. From the point of origin it radiates distally without a break in continuity; the extent and spread of the pain is in direct proportion to the intensity of the initial stimulation at the site of origin.

In the lower back, during the early phase of disc degeneration and before nerve root implication, this mechanism may be responsible for the deep-seated pain in the lumbar region which later may radiate into one or both extremities. The pain in the lower extremities is vague, ill defined and without cutaneous component. With rest the intensity of the pain lessens, but with excessive activity it becomes more pronounced. No motor, sensory or reflex alterations occur. The same mechanism explains the low back syndrome after disorganization of the disc and the normal dynamics of the motor unit are seriously impaired.

During the intermediate phase of disintegration of the disc, a large

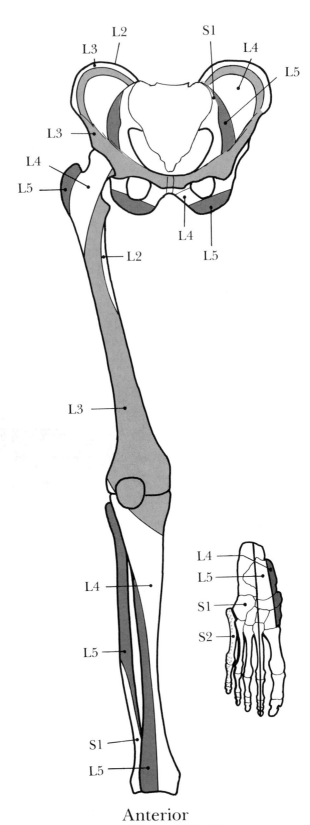

Anterior

Figure 11-1 Patterns of the sclerotomes.

184

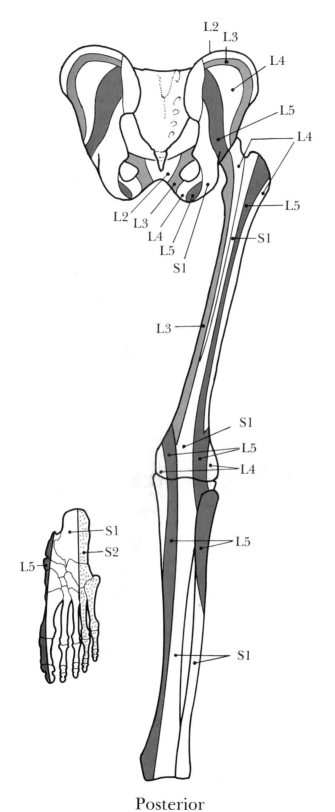

Posterior

Figure 11-1 Continued.

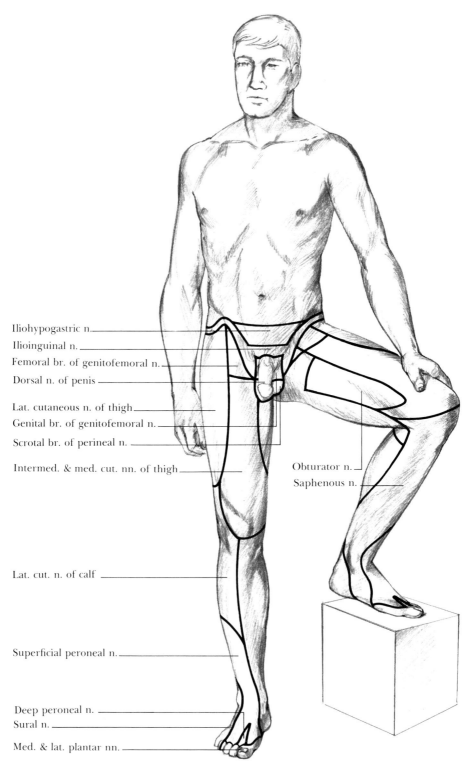

Iliohypogastric n.

Ilioinguinal n.

Femoral br. of genitofemoral n.

Dorsal n. of penis

Lat. cutaneous n. of thigh

Genital br. of genitofemoral n.

Scrotal br. of perineal n.

Intermed. & med. cut. nn. of thigh

Obturator n.

Saphenous n.

Lat. cut. n. of calf

Superficial peroneal n.

Deep peroneal n.

Sural n.

Med. & lat. plantar nn.

Figure 11-2 Patterns of the dermatomes.

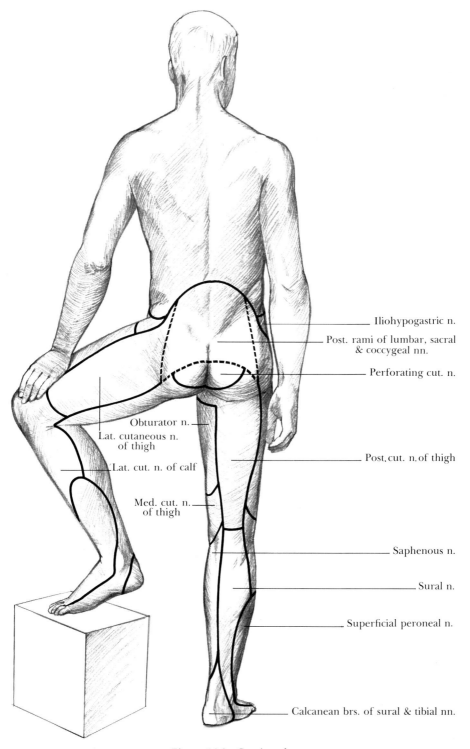

Figure 11-2 Continued.

bulging dorsal protrusion without contact with the nerve roots may produce severe low back pain by this mechanism. In these cases, the annulus fibrosus and the posterior longitudinal ligament are severely stretched by the nucleus pulposus. Also, when an extruded fragment of nuclear material becomes suddenly impacted between the vertebral rims, the sudden, ensuing back pain may be explained by this same mechanism.[1] It should be understood that in lumbar disc lesions, scleratogenous pain and pain due to direct irritation of the nerve roots may co-exist.

DERMATOGENOUS PAIN

This pain is more readily understood. There are two types of dermatogenous pain, "fast" and "slow." Fast pain, characteristically, is sharp, lancinating and clearly localized to a specific cutaneous area. Stimulation evokes an immediate response and appreciation of pain disappears as soon as the stimulation ceases. Slow pain is very much different; it is vague, dull aching with no clear localization. The response to stimulation is delayed and not immediate, and adaptation is poor. It spreads to a wide skin area but the area is poorly defined. Stimulation of a nerve root by contact, traction or pressure may produce both fast and slow pain; however, the predominant type depends on the nature and duration of the stimulus.

The composition of a nerve root comprises nerve fibers of varying diameters (from 0.5 to 10.0 μ); also the conduction speed of the fibers shows greater variability (0.6 to 90.0 m. per second).[4] Experimental and clinical evidence indicates that, in general, the larger fibers are concerned with the motor and proprioceptive systems and the smaller fibers with skin sensation. To the larger fibers of the latter group belong touch, pressure and fast pain; while to the smaller fibers belong temperature and "slow" pain. These groups of nerve fibers respond to various stimuli quite differently. In general, a mechanical stimulus produced by rapidly applied pressure will stimulate the proprioceptive and touch fibers, causing paresthesias, and the fast pain fibers. On the other hand, when pressure is slowly applied, causing a physiological blocking of the fibers, the motor, proprioceptive and touch fibers are affected first and next the temperature and slow pain fibers.[5]

Until recently the onset of radicular pain associated with acute lumbar disc lesions was not clear, and many controversial opinions have been set forth to explain this phenomenon. However, the work of Smyth and Wright[9] has shed some light on this problem. Their experiments conclusively reveal that pressure on a lumbar nerve root will produce radicular pain identical to that experienced by the patient before the removal of the extruded nuclear material which was in contact with a nerve root. Also, that an affected nerve root is far more sensitive than a normal root. The longitudinal extension of the pain was in direct proportion to the amount of pressure on the root. This last observation may explain the great variation in the longitudinal extent to which a dermatome may be involved. Extrusions making only minimal contact with a nerve root produce pain which radiates only a short distance along the dermatome, whereas those exerting great pressure produce a full-blown pressure to an affected nerve root. This observation is of great clinical importance because it provides an explanation for the presence of sciatica without gross extrusion of nuclear material. Simple minimal bulging of a disc may be the only stimulus needed to evoke a sciatic syndrome. It is not uncommon to explore the lumbar spine of a patient presenting a classical picture of sciatica and find no protrusion, yet the nerve root appears injected, slightly swollen and irritable. This last observation also clarifies the bizarre phenomenon of recurrence of sciatica shortly after removal of extruded disc material in a patient who had been completely relieved of symptoms by the operation. At this point it should be remembered that the inelastic nerve roots under normal conditions are free and are capable of adapting themselves to the movements of the limbs and spine. It was previously pointed out that the range of movement of the nerve roots is from 2 to 8 mm.[3, 7, 8, 10] Following removal of extruded material, the hypersensitive nerve root may be tethered by reactionary fibrosis. This together with the traction made on the sensitive nerve root by movements of the spine and limbs may be the stimulus to initiate the reappearance of sciatica.

The exacerbation of pain by raising the extended leg (straight leg raising) is further evidence of the effects of traction on a sensitized nerve root firmly bound down to a nuclear extrusion. Normally, the extended leg can be raised 30 to 40 degrees before the nerve roots begin to move along the intervertebral foramina, and the leg can be raised to 90 degrees without discomfort to the patient, except some tension in the posterior structures of the back and leg as the leg approaches the end of the arc.[2] When a disc lesion is present, the arc of movement in the affected leg is markedly diminished or may be nil. If the leg is forced beyond the extremes of this limited arc, the patient experiences severe pain in the back and leg. This is particularly true of lesions of the L4-L5 and L5-S1 discs. The explanation for the limitation of movement is simple enough; the maneuver makes traction on the sensitive root (usually the L5 or S1 nerve root), which, at this time, is compressed or displaced by a nuclear protrusion and bound down by a local reactionary process. Stretching of the irritable root is the stimulus which causes an exacerbation of the radicular pain. Exacerbation of pain may also be produced by raising the extended leg on the unaffected side. Normally, raising the leg on one side causes the lumbar roots on the opposite side to move out of the foramina for a short distance and to slide towards the midline. In the presence of a disc lesion, straight leg raising on the unaffected side makes traction on the affected root of the opposite side and thereby stimulates the involved nerve root (Fig. 12-16).[3, 7, 8, 10]

In summary, it may be briefly stated that the disruption of a disc and the subsequent deranged mechanics of the motor unit are accompanied by deep, dull aching pain with wide radiation and poor localization. The pain radiates to structures of mesodermal origin (muscles, tendons, ligaments and periosteum) which are innervated by nerve fibers from nerve roots of the same embryonic level as the affected disc. This is scleratogenous pain which radiates to a scleratome. True radicular, or dermatogenous, pain is superficial and localized to a specific cutaneous region; there

are two types of pain, fast and slow. Dermatogenous pain is sharp, lancinating and well-delineated on a cutaneous area called a dermatome; each
nerve root has its specific dermatome, although there is some overlap.
The work of Smyth and Wright clearly shows that dermatogenous pain
can be evoked by minimal pressure, or even touch, on a nerve root and
that sensitized nerve roots are more responsive than normal nerve roots.[9]
Any form of pressure, tension or traction within certain limits on a nerve
root, regardless of its source, can produce radicular pain, and the extension of pain along a dermatome will depend upon the intensity of the
stimulus. If the limits are exceeded, the root no longer functions. Severe
compression of a nerve root also causes loss of root function; pain disappears and there is evidence of motor and sensory deficits.

It should be recalled that the end point of the pathologic process in
the disc is complete disruption of the motor unit. The secondary changes
that occur in the intervertebral joint per se and the posterior articular
joints mimic degenerative arthritis or osteoarthritis of other joints. Also the
pain produced by the disorganized motor unit is in all respects similar to
that observed in degenerative arthritis. The pain is more or less localized
to the affected region of the spine. Its intensity varies considerably and is
affected by such factors as rest, activity and weather changes. Characteristically, inactivity produces stiffness and soreness, whereas activity tends to
alleviate these symptoms. However, overactivity invariably increases the
intensity of the pain.

Finally, something must be said about the character of the pain
associated with spinal cord lesions. The pain in the back may be insignificant or even lacking, and, although radiation to one or both extremities
may be present, its intensity is never severe. On the other hand, the evidence of implication of neural elements is clearly evident. There are
marked motor deficits such as muscle weakness, atrophy or even paralysis;
sensory alterations are clear and unequivocal, such as impairment or loss of
sensation over the dermatome or dermatomes of the neural segments
involved; and lastly, there are reflex changes. It was pointed out that
cervical myelopathy may cause pain to the anterior aspect of the thighs,
subcostal areas and the buttocks; the pain is poorly localized. There also
may be present motor impairment of the lower extremities such as muscle
atrophy, weakness and loss of stability of the lower limbs. Impaired
sphincter function may also exist.

Level of Disc Lesion

It is general information that the discs most commonly involved in
the lumbar spine are the L5-S1 and the L4-L5 discs. Implication of the
L3-L4 level is not common; however, there is evidence that lesions at this
level are more frequent than generally appreciated. Lesions at the L1-L2
and L2-L3 levels are indeed rare and are more prone to occur in young
adults subjected to violent flexion of the spine.

Double Lesion

Disc lesions occurring at two levels are not a rare finding (eight to ten per cent). However, only one may be responsible for the presenting syndrome. Usually they occur at successive levels, most frequently at the L4-L5 and the L5-S1 levels.

ONSET OF THE LUMBAR DISC SYNDROME

Careful analysis of the history of many patients reveals that the manner in which the syndrome is first initiated varies widely. Nevertheless, several crystal-clear patterns evolve which are so characteristic that a diagnosis of a lumbar disc lesion can often be made from its mode of onset. The following patterns are recorded in their order of frequency.

1. Diffuse constant pain in the back

The most common onset is characterized by a diffuse continuous pain in the lower lumbar region which comes on gradually and is punctuated by periods in which the pain increases in intensity. These periods of exacerbation of pain may or may not be initiated by some excessive flexion strain of the lumbar spine. Generally, the pain is mechanical in nature; it is relieved by rest and aggravated by activity. As a rule, in spite of the severity of the pain, most patients are capable of carrying on with their usual activities; rarely is the pain of such intensity that the patient is totally incapacitated. However, from time to time, we encounter a patient whose emotional instability and intolerance to pain is such that, particularly during the periods of exacerbation, the pain renders him completely incapacitated.

This mode of onset is typical of the period of early degeneration of the nucleus before sequestration of the nuclear material occurs and before the degenerative process in the annulus is so advanced that it can no longer prevent herniation of nuclear particles. It also is encountered in the terminal phases of the disease when there is complete disorganization of the motor unit and the reparative process is not yet sufficiently advanced to stabilize the affected segment. As the pathologic process in the nucleus and annulus progresses, permitting nuclear extrusion, the symptom complex just described is often complicated by bouts of sciatica which may be gradual or sudden in onset. This, of course, may occur in the early or late stages of nuclear degeneration.

2. Sudden severe pain

This manner of onset is initiated by sudden displacement of nuclear material. The patient is seized by severe agonizing pain in the low back region which, in many instances, is completely incapacitating. Generally, the patient exhibits an abnormal posture due to severe muscle spasm; the lumbar spine is flexed; the lumbar curve is flattened or reversed; the trunk may be listed to one side. The patient, if capable, moves about slowly and cautiously. Any movement of the trunk exacerbates the pain, whereas rest relieves it. Fortunately, the acute symptoms tend to abate within a few days, but in some cases not for several weeks. Although this may be the first manifestation of disc disease, if careful inquiry is made, a history of some previous back discomfort can usually be elicited.

3. SCIATIC PAIN WITHOUT BACK PAIN

This symptom complex varies widely. Generally it occurs when a nuclear sequestrum comes in contact with one of the nerve roots. In a small percentage of patients, the attack comes on suddenly and the pain radiates the full length of the limb along the dermatome of the involved nerve root. In a large percentage of these patients the pain comes on slowly, often felt as an ache in one of the buttocks, and gradually spreads distally. In some patients, it is localized to the posterior or posterolateral aspect of the thigh, depending on whether the S1 or L5 root is implicated; in some, it may extend as far as the calf or lateral aspect of the lower leg, or to the sole of the foot, or to the dorsum of the outer three toes—again, depending on the nerve root affected. From time to time, the presenting complaint is pain limited to a small but specific area such as the buttocks, the back of the thigh, the calf or the sole of the foot. In rare instances, the pattern of spread of the pain may be reversed; it may begin in the calf or sole of the foot and gradually spread cephalward (Fig. 11-3).

Characteristic of this type of pain is the fact that change of posture of the trunk or of position of the limb brings no relief, and that rest, as a rule, does not diminish its intensity. Increased intra-abdominal pressure produced by coughing and sneezing markedly increases the severity of the pain. Patients with a severe attack walk with the hip and knee slightly flexed and place the foot slowly on the floor. This is done in order to prevent any undue traction of the nerve root which normally occurs when the extended leg is flexed at the hip. On the other hand, some of the patients exhibit no external malfunction; there is no back pain, no muscle spasm. Back motion is free and unrestricted, and the patients are able, in most instances, to carry on their daily activities. As pointed out, this type of onset usually occurs when a nuclear extrusion makes contact with a nerve root. This phenomenon may occur either during the stage of nuclear sequestration (the intermediate stage) or toward the end of the pathologic process in the nucleus, at which time fibrosis of the disc is the predominant feature, but fragments of nuclear material which may be extruded may still be present. The distance that the pain spreads along a dermatome is directly proportional to the amount of tension and compression to which the root is subjected.

An interesting phenomenon is, from time to time, observed in patients with severe sciatica: the pain may suddenly disappear but the motor and sensory deficits remain. This indicates that the physiologic function of the root is completely interrupted, and must not be misconstrued as evidence that the patient is getting better.

It should also be remembered that any of the patterns of sciatica may

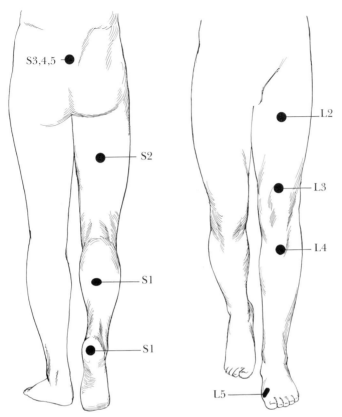

Figure 11-3 Pain may radiate to small, isolated, specific areas along the course of a dermatome.

be initiated by simple contact of a sensitive nerve root without actual herniation of nuclear material. In other words, slight bulging of the annulus without rupture may be sufficient to precipitate a sciatic syndrome by merely touching a hypersensitive root.

4. Back pain with sciatica

In a small percentage of the patients, back pain and sciatica appeared simultaneously. Two clinical types of this syndrome are discernible: in one, the symptoms of back pain and sciatica appear suddenly and simultaneously; in the other, the onset is gradual. The former is generally associated with some sudden flexion stress applied to the lumbar spine causing rupture of the annulus and retropulsion of nuclear material; the latter is consistent with gradual extrusion of the nuclear fragments through the annulus fibrosus. The pain in the back and the sciatica may be of almost equal severity, but in most instances the intensity of one overshadows the other. When pain in both the back and the leg is severe and of sudden onset, the patient may be totally incapacitated and may present a dramatic clinical picture. The pain may be so severe that the affected leg is held in the flexed position and the patient avoids any maneuver that might tend to extend the limb. There is severe spasm of the lumbar paravertebral muscles and frequently a severe list of the trunk (Fig. 12-2).

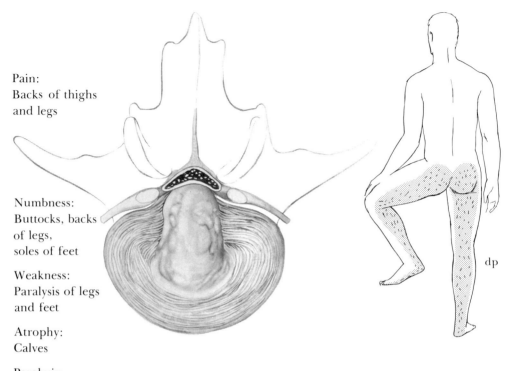

Pain:
Backs of thighs
and legs

Numbness:
Buttocks, backs
of legs,
soles of feet

Weakness:
Paralysis of legs
and feet

Atrophy:
Calves

Paralysis:
Bladder and bowel

Figure 11-4   Massive herniation at the level of the third, fourth or fifth disc may cause severe compression of the cauda equina. Pain is confined chiefly to the buttocks, the back of the thighs and legs. Numbness is widespread from the buttocks to the soles of the feet. Motor weakness or loss is present in the legs and feet with loss of muscle mass in the calves. The bladder and bowels are paralyzed.

5. CAUDA EQUINA SYNDROME DUE TO MASSIVE NUCLEAR EXTRUSION

It was pointed out that severe flexion strains imposed on the lumbar spine may suddenly produce a massive extrusion of nuclear tissue which may severely compromise the cauda equina. This tragic condition may occur in young adults before nuclear changes begin. It may also occur when the pathologic changes in the nucleus and the annulus are far advanced. In this latter situation, the extrusion may be produced by minor trauma. Sudden compression of the cauda equina results in partial or complete paralysis and loss of sphincter function. Early recognition of the lesion and early decompression of the cauda equina is most essential because an interval of a few hours is sufficient to cause irreversible changes in the compressed nerve roots. In the young adult, the lesion is usually found above the level of the L4-L5 disc; but in the older age group, it may occur at any level. The authors have encountered four such cases. In no instance was recovery of the cauda equina complete in spite of adequate decompression. The fact that none of these patients came to surgery under 12 hours after the injury is undoubtedly the factor responsible for the serious ensuing consequences (Fig. 11-4).

VARIABILITY OF THE CLINICAL COURSE

It was pointed out that wide variations are found in the clinical course of lumbar disc lesions. These events not only vary from patient to patient, but they vary in the same patient from one time to another, depending upon the manner of progression of the pathologic process in the disc. This variability is characteristic of lumbar disc lesions, and unless understood, the presenting clinical picture may indeed become very confusing. The most important fact to remember is that the presenting manifestations, at any one moment, represent the patient's response to the precise nature and pathologic condition of the disc. On the other hand, let us not forget that, depending upon the patient's motivation and emotional stability, the response to the same stimuli will also differ from patient to patient.

Character of Recurrent Attacks

In general, following an initial episode of low back pain with or without sciatica, the patient will experience repeated attacks which increase in frequency and severity proportional to the activity of the pathologic process involving the affected intervertebral disc. As the process in the disc advances and reaches the terminal phase of complete fibrosis, the attacks become less frequent and the symptoms less severe.

There may be wide variation in the nature of the attacks; but, broadly speaking, they simulate the various modes of onset previously described with variations in the duration and the severity of the symptoms.

Between attacks, the patient may experience little or no discomfort. The length of the period between attacks is unpredictable; in some patients it may be a matter of weeks, in others months and in others years. Many factors influence the frequency and duration of the attacks and the severity of the symptoms: the phase of the pathologic process in the disc, the role of activity of this process, vulnerability to or protection from unusual flexion forces applied to the spine, the degree of activity of the patient between and during attacks, and the lack of institution of adequate therapeutic measures during and between episodes. On the other hand, it must be remembered that an acute, severe attack may suddenly appear without any provocation and may be initiated by only a trivial incident.

During the early phase of the disc pathology, the patient may experience nothing more than repeated bouts of a dull ache, poorly localized in the lumbar region. He soon realizes that the frequency, severity and duration of the attacks are related to his activity. Also, he learns to respect mild prodromal symptoms by limiting his activity and, by so doing, may even ward off an attack. Not infrequently, the disc lesion in this stage may give rise to no symptoms whatsoever until some traumatic incident occurs initiating the symptom complex.

It is possible for a patient to go through the early phase, bypass the intermediate phase or phase of nuclear extrusions, and go directly into the terminal phase of the pathologic process (Fig. 11-5). These patients may never experience the sharp, lancinating pain associated with sudden rupture of the annulus and the sciatica caused by irritation of a nerve root. This does not imply that patients reaching the final phase of disc

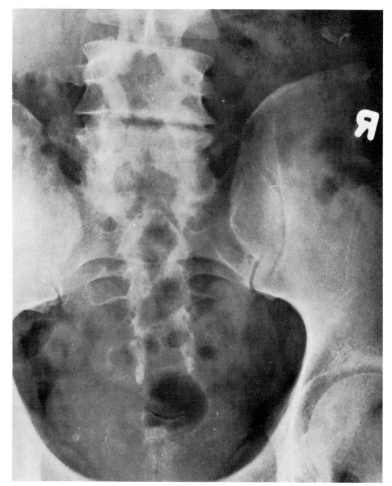

Figure 11-5   Final phase of disc degeneration. The L4-L5 disc is severely collapsed and advanced secondary changes are noted at the vertebral rims. This patient had repeated episodes of backache but never had sciatica.

disintegration never suffer from sciatica. Even during this period, loose fragments of nuclear material which may be extruded through the annulus by a flexion strain of the lumbar spine may still be present. Although rare, this is not an infrequent occurrence in middle aged and elderly individuals. Characteristic of all acute, severe attacks, whether they are ushered in gradually or suddenly or whether they occur in the early, intermediate or final stage of the disease, is the spontaneous diminution or disappearance of the severity of the symptoms. However, the degree of activity of the patient has some bearing on the course of the acute episode. Markedly restricted activity or, better, total rest, tends to hasten the diminution of the severity of the symptoms.

Character of Sciatic Syndrome

Usually patients with low back pain associated with early disc changes will eventually experience repeated attacks of sciatica characteristic of the phase of nuclear extrusions. In the beginning, the episodes of acute back pain associated with rupture of the annulus and the severe, lancinating pain caused by root irritation are relatively frequent and a period is often reached when an episode may be initiated by no obvious cause. The variations in the patterns of sciatica observed in these patients have already been described. At this point, it should be emphasized that the distalward spread of radicular pain along the dermatome of the root involved is in direct proportion to the degree of pressure on and displacement of the root by the nuclear extrusion. In addition to the sharp cutaneous pain, there is also a deep-seated pain in the entire leg. Back and leg pain may coexist but not infrequently one or the other may be present in one attack and the reverse may be true in still another episode; or the clinical picture may be dominated by the severity of either the back or leg pain.

In most patients with sciatica only one leg is involved and in subsequent attacks the sciatica is confined to the same leg. However, this is not true in all patients; in some, both legs are affected simultaneously or at different times during the same attack, or the pain may shift from one leg to the other. A large dorsal nuclear extrusion is capable of compressing simultaneously the roots on either side of the midline. Two nuclear extrusions may be present each involving separate roots. This is indeed rare but from time to time it does occur (Fig. 3-19).

The course of the clinical syndrome associated with the phase of nuclear extrusions may be greatly modified by adequate therapy, chiefly, rest. The frequency and intensity of subsequent episodes can be decreased by conscientious adherence to certain measures designed to protect the back from activities and stresses which tend to precipitate recurrences.

During the terminal phase of disc disintegration, the clinical findings are essentially those of any degenerated and functionally impaired articulation. The pain in the low back, as a rule, is dull and aching in nature; it is relieved by rest and aggravated by excessive activity. From time to time, this period may be punctuated by an episode of sciatica, indicating that some nuclear tissue is still present in the disc space. Finally, when fibrosis of the disc is complete and matured, the symptoms abate or even disappear. It should be remembered that in many instances the terminal stage of fibrosis may not be capable of stabilizing the motor unit; the capsular and ligamentous components of such a unit are lax and provide little or no fixation. Such an unstable motor unit frequently gives rise to back pain.

Character of Motor, Sensory and Reflex Changes

Once a nerve root is involved, its functional deficits tend to be more enduring than the low back symptoms. On the other hand, the patient may not be cognizant of neural changes in the motor fibers until the alterations are far advanced (Figs. 11-6, 11-7, and 11-8).

Motor changes

These comprise weakness or paralysis, loss of tone and loss of mass of the affected muscle group. Rarely is only a single muscle involved; rather,

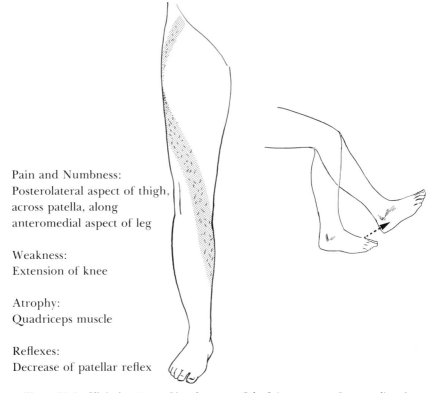

Pain and Numbness:
Posterolateral aspect of thigh,
across patella, along
anteromedial aspect of leg

Weakness:
Extension of knee

Atrophy:
Quadriceps muscle

Reflexes:
Decrease of patellar reflex

Figure 11-6 Clinical pattern of involvement of the L4 nerve root: Sensory disturbances are pain and numbness along the posterolateral aspect of the thigh, across the patella and along the anteromedial aspect of the leg. Motor involvement consists of weakness in extension of the knee and loss of mass of the quadriceps muscle. Reflex changes concern the knee only; the patellar reflex is decreased.

Pain and Numbness:
Anteromedial aspect of
leg and foot

Weakness:
Dorsiflexion of foot
and great toe

Atrophy:
Anterior tibial

Reflexes:
No change

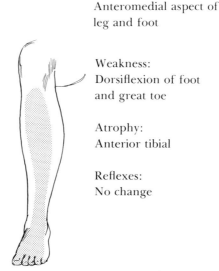

Figure 11-7 Clinical pattern of involvement of the L5 nerve root: Sensory alterations comprise pain and numbness along the anteromedial aspect of the leg and foot. Motor changes are weakness of dorsiflexion of the foot and great toe, and some atrophy of the anterior tibial may be demonstrable. There are no reflex changes.

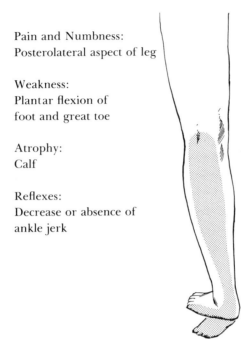

Pain and Numbness:
Posterolateral aspect of leg

Weakness:
Plantar flexion of
foot and great toe

Atrophy:
Calf

Reflexes:
Decrease or absence of
ankle jerk

Figure 11-8 Clinical pattern of involvement of the S1 nerve root: Pain and numbness is present along the posterolateral aspect of the leg. Motor involvement includes weakness of plantar flexion of the foot and the great toe, and atrophy of the calf. Reflex changes concern the tendo-Achilles; the ankle jerk may be decreased or absent.

the entire muscle group supplied by the motor fibers of the affected root is affected. In most patients, the mild motor manifestations are associated with a lumbar disc syndrome of long standing; however, from time to time, the features are so pronounced that they may comprise the chief complaints of the patients. This latter situation is the result of severe compression of the nerve root in the canal or the intervertebral foramen. This interrupts the sensory fibers and deletes pain but leaves in its wake varying gradations or motor deficit ranging from weakness and wasting to complete paralysis of a muscle group. This phenomenon is dramatically emphasized when a massive nuclear extrusion occurs which is capable of compressing the entire cauda equina. As a result of the sudden and severe compression, the patient exhibits paralysis of the lower limbs, widespread sensory deficits and interruption of sphincter function. Varying degrees of motor dysfunction also may occur in the final phase of the process affecting the disc; the nerve root may be firmly bound in situ by dense adhesions or the process may involve the root itself. The resulting motor alterations generally are permanent.

The muscles implicated are usually those of the buttocks, the thigh and the calf. Early in the syndrome, loss of muscle mass and tone are very subtle changes and their detection may be very difficult, requiring unusual acuity and a fine sense of touch on the part of the examiner. At this time, pain is the dominant feature of the sciatica, in contrast to the findings in the later stages of the syndrome, at which point muscle weakness and loss of muscle mass may be the prominent features and the intensity of pain insignificant. Muscle power is best tested by having the affected group act against resistance; the specific manner by which the muscles are tested will be discussed subsequently.

SENSORY CHANGES

Involvement of nerve roots in lumbar disc lesions is, as a rule, associated with varying degrees of sensory changes confined to the cutaneous distribution of the root, the dermatome (Fig. 11-2). Many workers have investigated the patterns of distribution of the specific nerve roots; however, their results show much variation. This is, in part, explainable by the anatomical fact that the exact cutaneous distribution of the lumbar nerve roots varies from individual to individual and that some overlap exists in adjacent dermatomes. In the nerve roots which are most frequently involved in lumbar disc lesions, namely, L4, L5 and S1, this overlap is particularly prevalent.

It becomes apparent that localization of a disc lesion may be difficult and even impossible if the cutaneous distribution of a nerve root was used as the sole means to identify the root affected. Identification of the responsible nerve root can accurately be achieved by establishing correlation between the presenting sensory pattern, the motor elements involved and the localization of the radicular pain. The tests we employ to establish these findings will be discussed later. Besides impairment of sensation due to dysfunction or no function of the sensory fibers of a nerve root, patients frequently complain that they are not aware of the affected leg or that they do not appreciate the exact position of the limb. This is indicative of implication of proprioceptive nerve fibers which may be involved along with the other fibers of sensation.

REFLEX CHANGES

Alterations in a nerve root caused by contact with a nuclear extrusion or irritation by some other noxious agent may produce impairment of the normal tendon reflex phenomenon at the knee and ankle joint. Diminution or absence of the ankle jerk is almost pathognomonic of implication of the S1 or S2 nerve roots. In lumbar disc lesions, the S1 root is most frequently affected, whereas the S2 root is rarely implicated. When the ankle jerk is lost, the level involved in most instances is the L5-S1 disc. However, it should be remembered that occasionally the S1 nerve root may be affected by nuclear extrusion originating above the L5-S1 disc and migrating caudally.

Impairment of the L5 nerve root is not associated with any alterations in the reflex at the knee or ankle. The reflex at the knee is altered but rarely deleted by changes in the L3 and L4 nerve roots. Therefore, the knee jerk is not affected by disc lesions at the L4-L5 and L5-S1 levels.

The behavior of an impaired or lost reflex is fairly characteristic. Even after the nerve root is freed from contact with any abnormal tissue, recovery is very slow and, in some instances, the reflex is permanently impaired or lost. It is not unusual to find only partial recovery two or three years after surgery and to observe no recovery in a large percentage of patients four or five years later.

Exacerbations and Remissions

It was pointed out that the lumbar disc syndrome is periodically punctuated by exacerbations and remissions. In the preceding pages, we attempted to explain the factors responsible for the presenting symptoms and modes of onset by correlating them with various phases and changes that occur in the pathologic process involving the affected disc. However, the causes of exacerbations and remissions cannot always be explained because, in many patients, we are not able to correlate these manifestations with the prevailing pathologic process in the disc. Since many of the phenomena occur during a period of exacerbation and when remission of symptoms are not clear, we can only speculate on the causative factors. Nevertheless, the assumptions made in many areas are reasonably logical.

During the early phase of the changes occurring in the disc and before the annulus ruptures, a sudden increase in nuclear pressure, resulting from excessive activity or flexion strains, may suddenly increase the tension of the fibers of the annulus, producing localized deep pain. With elimination of the abnormal forces and by imposed rest, tension in the disc decreases and the pain diminishes in intensity or disappears.

If the same forces are applied to the lumbar spine when the pathologic process has progressed to the point that the annulus shows advanced degeneration, the annular fibers may tear further, giving rise to a sudden exacerbation of local pain. The fibers of the annulus may rupture, permitting extrusion of nuclear material which, in turn, may contact with a nerve root; not only is the low back pain aggravated but leg pain is added to the clinical picture. In the wake of this disruptive process local edema must follow, implicating not only the local tissues but also the nerve roots. This is another factor which may cause exacerbation of symptoms.

The dramatic, sudden onset of severe low back pain associated with profound disability and the just as dramatic, sudden disappearance of the pain is ingeniously explained by Armstrong.[1] A sudden entrapment of sequestrated nuclear material between the rims of the vertebral bodies is responsible for the severe pain and disability. The impacted disc material "locks" the intervertebral joint. "Unlocking" the joint is effected by one of two methods: by shrinkage of the nuclear sequestrum, or by movement of the vertebrae. The nuclear tissue is then extruded completely beyond the vertebral rims or slips back between the bodies. In either case, the pain suddenly and dramatically disappears. Posterior displacement of the sequestrum may result in radicular pain if it comes in contact with a nerve root. A completely extruded disc can not re-enter or slip in the intervertebral space; the pressure within the space prevents this. On the other hand, an impacted or trapped sequestrum between the vertebral rims may slip back into the intervertebral space.[1]

Diminution or disappearance of radicular leg pain due to pressure and displacement of a nerve root by a sequestrum of nuclear tissue may follow shrinkage of the nuclear mass or a shift in position of the mass in relation to the nerve root. Extrusion of degenerated nuclear tissue occurs repeatedly at irregular intervals; therefore, it is reasonable to assume that the amount of extruded material may increase steadily; this increase in mass may adversely affect the patient's symptoms by making greater pressure on a nerve root.

Other phenomena which have been proposed to explain remissions and alterations of symptoms of radicular pain are: the nerve root may adapt itself to the degrees of pressure and tension exerted on it; the root may change its position in relation to the nuclear sequestrum by slipping to one or the other side and thereby reducing the tension and pressure exerted by the nuclear extrusion; the root may actually lengthen sufficiently to reduce the tension imposed on it.[3]

It was pointed out that the nerve root may become involved in a local inflammatory process which firmly binds the root to the surrounding tissues. The inelastic root is now no longer able to adjust itself to movements of the trunk and limbs. Under these conditions, movements of the trunk and limbs exert undue traction on the affected nerve root. The resulting tension accentuates the intensity of the symptoms.

REFERENCES

1. Armstrong, J. R.: Lumbar Disc Lesions; Pathogenesis and Treatment of Low-Back Pain and Sciatica. 3rd. ed., Baltimore, Williams & Wilkins, 1965.
2. Charnley, J.: Orthopaedic signs in diagnosis of disc protrusion, with special reference to straight-leg-raising test. Lancet 1:186-192, 1951.
3. Falconer, M. A. et al.: Observations on the cause and mechanism of symptom-production in sciatica and low-back pain. J. Neurol. Neurosurg. Psychiat. 11:13-26, 1948.
4. Gasser, H. S.: Pain-producing impulses in peripheral nerves. A. Research Nerv. and Ment. Dis., Proc. (1942) 23:44-62, 1943.
5. Inman, V. T. and Saunders, J. B. de C. M.: Anatomico-physiological aspects of injuries to intervertebral disc. J. Bone Joint Surg. 29:461-475, 1947.
6. Lewis, T., Sir: Pain, New York, Macmillan, 1942.
7. O'Connell, J. E. A.: Sciatica and mechanism of production of clinical syndrome in protrusions of lumbar intervertebral discs. Brit. J. Surg. 30:315-327, 1943.
8. Sjöqvest, O.: The mechanism and origin of Lasèque's sign. Acta Psych. and Neurol. Supp. 46:290-297, 1947.
9. Smyth, M. J. et al.: Sciatica and the intervertebral disc. An experimental study. J. Bone Joint Surg. 40-A:1401-1418, 1958.
10. Woodhall, B., et al.: The Well-leg-raising test of Fajersztajn in the diagnosis of ruptured lumbar intervertebral disc. J. Bone Joint Surg. 32-A:786-792, 1950.

Chapter 12

CLINICAL MANIFESTATIONS
OF LUMBAR DISC SYNDROME

A meticulous and methodical analysis of the presenting signs and symptoms associated with lumbar disc lesions is most essential in order to establish the nature of the pathologic process of the affected disc and to determine the precise disc and nerve root involved. Such an examination should be performed in all patients with pain localized to the lower back with or without radicular pain and in all patients with nerve root irritation, regardless of the cutaneous pattern they present.

In order to cover all the significant points necessary to establish a correct diagnosis, an orderly plan of examination should be conducted. This includes a thorough analysis of the presenting subjective and objective clinical features, with an attempt to correlate these manifestations with the pathologic process in the disc. If the examiner takes time to hear the patient's story and pays particular attention to the behavior of the syndrome, and if he carefully analyzes the patient's complaints, the subjective evidence alone may be more than sufficient to make the correct diagnosis and to pinpoint the localization of the disc lesion and the specific nerve root affected. There are many methods of examination which, if conscientiously performed, will give the necessary information to establish the diagnosis. The plan that we prefer is to critically analyze first the subjective features and, second, the objective manifestations of the presenting clinical picture. If, as the result of our examination, we feel that other diagnostic aids, such as special x-ray views, cineradiography, electromyography or myelography, are necessary to establish the diagnosis, they are utilized. At this point it should be mentioned that in arriving at a diagnosis the negative findings observed in the course of the examination are just as important as the positive findings.

203

SUBJECTIVE CLINICAL MANIFESTATIONS

Pain

Broadly speaking, patients with lumbar disc lesions seek help because of pain. If given an opportunity to express themselves and with a little help from the examiner by the injection of a few pertinent questions, they will, as a rule, describe all the essential characteristics of their pain. It is helpful to have the patient point out the sites of pain; in most instances, they do this voluntarily. The localization of the pain is most essential and is the first step in determining the specific disc and nerve root affected.

During an acute attack, the pain is usually localized in the lumbar area, and radicular pain may or may not be present. The patient has difficulty in delineating back pain, but this is not true of leg pain if it is present. It should again be pointed out that there are two components of radiating pain: cutaneous or superficial pain and deep pain. The latter is the result of stimulation of the mesodermal tissues whose nerve supply is derived from the same embryonic level as the nerve root involved. For example, the L5-S1 disc derives its nerve supply from the same embryonic level as the S1 nerve root; likewise, the L4-L5 disc is related to the L5 nerve root, and the L3-L4 disc to the L4 nerve root, and so on. The intensity of this deep pain in the back and leg varies with the degree of disruption of the disc tissues and the amount of irritation of the nerve root.[22, 23, 25] The intensity of the leg pain is a good index as to the amount of tension and pressure that is being exerted on the root by sequestrated nuclear tissue. Characteristic of deep pain is its dull, aching nature; it is referred to the deeper structures of the leg, especially the muscles which are located in the scleratomes involved.[22, 23, 25] Therefore, the patient may indicate that he has a diffuse ache in the muscles of the inner or outer, or anterior or posterior, aspect of the leg but be unable to specify a definitive area in the leg.

In contrast to the nature of deep referred pain, superficial or cutaneous pain is clearly localized by the patients and the area depicted corresponds to the dermatome of the nerve root involved.[16, 25] It is sharp, lancinating and restricted to the dermatome of the affected nerve root. The spread of the radiation and the intensity is governed by the amount of tension and pressure that is being exerted on the sensitive root by the displaced nuclear tissue. Therefore, it may radiate no further than to the knee, calf or sole of the foot, or the entire dermatome may be involved. From time to time, this type of pain is sharply confined to one small area of the dermatome, such as the sole of the foot, the heel, the calf or the buttocks (Fig. 11-3). One type of radiation which may be confusing is sharp, superficial pain in the region of the iliac crests and in the groin. It should be remembered that these areas are supplied by branches from the posterior division of the nerve root and that these fibers in the root can be and occasionally are stimulated by displaced nuclear tissue.

Both the sclerotomes and dermatomes exhibit varying amounts of overlap. However, particularly in the case of the dermatomes, the pattern of distribution and spread of pain is specific enough to permit localization of the disc and nerve root involved. This is especially true of cutaneous pain in the lower leg. In fact, in the lower leg, the distribution of the pain is like a road sign pointing to the nerve root and the most likely disc to be involved. Pain in the sole of the foot, the heel and the calf points to the L5-S1 disc and the S1 nerve root. Pain on the anterolateral aspect of the lower leg and dorsum of the foot indicates the L4-L5 disc and the L5 nerve root, whereas pain on the anteromedial aspect points to the L3-L4 disc and the L4 nerve root (Figs. 11-6, 11-7 and 11-8).[15] Deep pain in the muscles of these areas, although less specific, also indicates the responsible roots and discs. Pain in the muscles of the calf specifies involvement of the L5-S1 disc and the S1 nerve root; pain in the anterior tibial compartment of muscles and the peroneal muscles shows involvement of the L4-L5 disc and the L5 nerve root; and pain in the anteromedial muscles points to the L3-L4 disc and the L4 nerve root (Figs. 11-6, 11-7 and 11-8). When one considers that the vast majority of disc lesions (95 per cent) are found at the L5-S1 and the L4-L5 levels, it becomes obvious that the margin of error in identifying the responsible nerve root is indeed small.

The clinical picture may be very confusing if the pain distribution is the result of implication of two nerve roots at one level. In this case, bilateral leg symptoms are present. Also, the pattern of pain may be caused by irritation of two contiguous roots on the same side. This results in considerable overlap of the pain patterns. On rare occasions, the following situation may occur: two discs at different levels with an unaffected disc between them may be responsible for the presenting pain distributions; this may produce a bizarre group of symptoms. However, if the examiner keeps in mind the possible combinations of nerve root involvement, the pain patterns become clear.

The pain patterns and the intensity of the pain may be influenced by other factors of which the patient is keenly aware. When the syndrome is acute, unguarded movements of the trunk and limbs produce a marked accentuation of the pain; in fact, the nerve roots may be so irritable that even insignificant movements are capable of severe aggravation of the pain. A sudden increase in intrathoracic and intra-abdominal pressure, such as occurs in coughing and sneezing, produces the same effects. The patient soon becomes aware that certain positions of the trunk and legs accentuate the pain, whereas others relieve it. He assumes certain postures of the trunk, which, by decreasing the tension and pressure of the nerve root, bring about some relief of pain. These postures will be discussed in more detail subsequently. The patient notes that any movement of the affected leg which necessitates increased flexion of the limb with the knee extended causes an aggravation of the pain. This mechanism will be considered more fully when the straight leg test is discussed. He learns that by decreasing vertical loading of the spine he can attain some relief of pain. This he achieves by lying on a firm bed or even on the floor, usually assuming the fetal position with hips and knees acutely flexed.

At this point, it must again be emphasized that the acute pain may be present in the leg only, without back pain. If the nerve root is very irritable and the leg pain is severe, it is not uncommon that a patient with no back pain exhibits severe muscle spasm of the lumbar spine with complete obliteration of the lumbar curve and, perhaps, even a tilt of the trunk to one or the other side. In such a patient, it is reasonable to assume that absence of pain is made possible by the vise-like grip that the muscles maintain on the spine, preventing even the slightest motion at the level of the involved motor unit. On the other hand, in less acute and in chronic syndromes in which there is little or no pain in the back, the patient may exhibit a remarkable range of motion in the lumbar spine. This is also true in some patients with an acutely painful spot localized to a small area in the distribution of the dermatome.

During the chronic stage of the syndrome when the acute symptoms have subsided, the patient may still complain of the same pain patterns described for the acute syndrome but the intensity of the pain is markedly reduced or may even disappear. Here too, the patient observes that certain factors may aggravate the pain or initiate an acute syndrome. Excessive activity, lifting objects from the floor with the trunk bent and long rides in an automobile all aggravate the existing pain or may evoke an acute attack.

Both in the acute and chronic syndrome, patients are encountered whose chief complaint in addition to pain may be a sense of instability in the leg or a diminished sense of awareness of the limb. This subjective complaint is readily explained by the fact that sensory nerves also contain proprioceptive fibers which may be affected along with sensory fibers. Lastly, the patient may exhibit all the sensory and motor deficits of a lumbar disc lesion and yet have no pain. The pain which was at one time relatively severe has either suddenly or gradually disappeared. This may not be an indication that the nerve root is free of any noxious agent but rather that severe tension or compression of the root resulted in total loss of function of the root. This is a serious complication which demands immediate investigation lest serious permanent dysfunction of the root ensues. The situation is comparable to a massive nuclear extrusion causing sudden compression of the cauda equina.

Sensory Disturbances

Sensory alterations in the dermatome of the involved nerve root are frequently observed in lesions of the lumbar disc. However, the patient is often not aware of these abnormalities until the lesion is far advanced. However, from time to time, a patient indicates a feeling of numbness or of "pins and needles" in an area of a dermatome distribution. It should be remembered that dermatome distributions vary from person to person and that in any one individual considerable overlap may exist; this is especially true of the L4, L5 and S1 nerve roots. This anatomic fact precludes positive identification of the nerve root involved on the basis of sensory alterations alone; this can only be done by correlation of the abnormal sensory findings with the site of referred pain and the presenting motor deficits.

Motor Deficits

Although abnormalities in motor function are more objective than subjective clinical manifestations, not infrequently one of the concerns of the patient is weakness or complete loss of function in a group of muscles. This is more likely to occur in disc lesions involving the L5 nerve root; in this instance, the patient may notice that he is unable to dorsiflex the foot or that he "slaps" the foot while walking. This alteration in gait is caused by weakness or paralysis of the anterior tibial, the extensors of the toes and the peroneal muscles. If the S1 root is affected there may be inability to stand on the toes because of motor dysfunction in the muscles of the calf. Loss of power may not be complete in any of these muscle groups because of the overlap of nerve supply; for example, the extensors of the foot derive their nerve supply from the L4 and L5 roots, the peroneal muscles from the L5 and S1 roots, and the calf muscles from the S1 and S2 roots. Massive extrusions of nuclear material compressing the cauda equina may produce partial or complete paralysis of both lower extremities, widespread sensory changes and loss of sphincter control.

OBJECTIVE CLINICAL MANIFESTATIONS

Many of the objective clinical features of lumbar disc lesions are so typical and so characteristic of the disorder that a diagnosis of the sites of the affected disc and the implicated nerve root can often be made without difficulty. An orderly scheme of examination of the patient should be followed; this ensures recognition of all the positive and negative findings and establishes a base of reference for comparision with the observations noted in subsequent examinations.

Gait

The gait of the patient during an acute attack of lumbar disc lesions is very striking and characteristic of the stage of the lesion. The trunk is bent forward and may also be tilted to one side. Every step is taken slowly and deliberately; the foot on the affected side is placed on the floor very gently. At all times the painful leg is held flexed at the hip and knee and the foot is plantar flexed, so that when the patient is walking only the ball of the foot touches the floor. The heel is never lowered to the floor. It appears as if the patient purposely avoids any movements of the trunk, which he holds rigid, and prevents any movements of the leg which might stretch the sciatic nerve.

The attack may be so severe that no form of ambulation is possible, and the patient is completely incapacitated and forced to lie down. These patients are in obvious pain and are very apprehensive; they refrain from the slightest movement of the trunk and hold both legs flexed at the hips and knees.

Posture in the Erect Position

During an acute attack the patient exhibits a distinctive posture: the lumbar spine is flattened due to a reduction of the normal lumbar curve; or, in some cases, the lumbar curve is actually reversed. The entire trunk is bent forward at the hips and the painful leg is flexed at the hip and knee so that only the ball of the foot rests on the floor (Fig. 12-1). When the involved nerve root is under severe tension, the patient develops a list of the trunk to one side or the other; this posture is referred to as "sciatic scoliosis" (Fig. 12-2). Postural or sciatic scoliosis is a variable clinical feature in that the trunk may shift from one side to the other side in the same patient. Tension in the nerve root is produced by extruded nuclear material, producing severe pain in the distribution of the dermatome of the affected root. In order to reduce the tension and decrease the intensity of the pain, the patient involuntarily shifts the trunk in the direction which tends to reduce nerve root tension. Depending on the relationship of the nuclear sequestrum to the nerve root the list of the trunk may be either toward the side of the irritated root or away from it. Should the relationship of the root to the nuclear extrusion change, the direction of the list of the trunk changes accordingly. Postural scoliosis may disappear suddenly if a rapid decrease in root tension occurs.

Not infrequently, the deviation of the trunk to one side is so insignificant that it may be almost imperceptible and unnoticed by the patient. However, lateral listing of the trunk is readily appreciated when the patient bends the trunk forward. Sciatic scoliosis may persist for short or long intervals. It is not uncommon for the abnormal posture to be present for many months, and we have observed it in some patients for several years.

Nature of Movements

Movement in the normal spine and especially in young people is a thing of beauty. The spine moves in any direction, forward or backward, from side to side or in a rotatory manner, with a smooth, uninterrupted rhythm. It bends, sways and twists like a pine in the breeze. Even in an older person the normal spine is capable of these free, unrestricted movements; however, the degree of flexibility of the spine varies from person to person. Broadly speaking, movements are freer and easier in the tall, lanky person than in the short, stout, muscular person.

In lumbar disc lesions, the movements of the spine with which we are particularly concerned are extension, flexion, lateral flexion and rotation. As a rule, in acute lesions, extension and flexion are seriously restricted while lateral flexion and rotation are relatively free. The degree of restriction of movements is governed by the phase and severity of the local pathologic process. During an acute attack, the striking feature of the spine is the complete loss of its inherent flexibility. The patient avoids motion in any direction; the spine is held rigid with the knees and hips slightly flexed; the normal lumbar curve is flattened or even reversed. Movements of the spine are best examined with the patient in the erect position with both feet together and the extended arms at the sides.

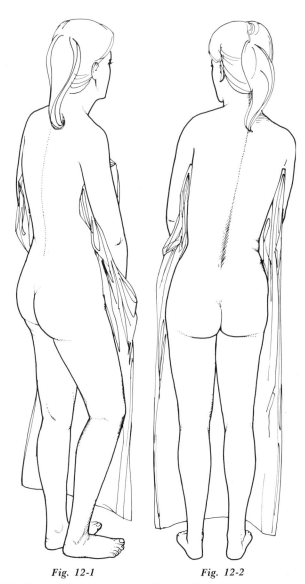

Fig. 12-1   *Fig. 12-2*

Figure 12-1   Posture frequently assumed by a patient with an acute attack of back pain with sciatica. The lumbar curve is diminished or even reversed; the trunk tends to tilt forward and the hip and knee are flexed.

Figure 12-2   Patient with a sciatic scoliosis; in this instance, the trunk lists toward the side of the sciatica.

EXTENSION AND FLEXION

The normal spine readily extends by increasing the lumbar lordosis. During an acute attack, as previously pointed out, the lumbar curve is flattened or reversed so that no extension of the lumbar spine is possible. Instead when the patient attempts to extend the lumbar spine he tends to lean the entire trunk backward and to hyperextend the cervical spine. If the examiner braces the lower lumbar spine with the palm of his hand and asks the patient to extend the lumbar spine against the resistance of his hand, severe pain may be elicited (Fig, 12-3).

During an acute attack, flexion of the lumbar spine is more seriously impaired than extension. The spine appears as a rigid structure and any attempt to flex it causes excruciating pain. Normally, the spine bends forward in a smooth arc and the degree of flexion is readily ascertained by measuring the distance from the fingertips to the floor. In an acute attack, little or no flexion occurs in the lumbar spine. Whatever forward bending the patient is able to perform occurs at the hip joints and in the dorsal and cervical spines (Fig. 12-4). If the patient's trunk is listed to one side in the erect position, the lateral shift of the trunk becomes even more obvious upon forward bending. Any attempt to force the lumbar spine into flexion causes severe pain. In less acute syndromes, some limited degree of flexion does occur in the lumbar spine; however, the movement lacks rhythm and smoothness; instead, it is irregular and jerky in nature. This same irregular movement is observed when the flexed spine returns to the erect position.

From time to time a patient exhibits all the spinal characteristics of an acute attack. The spine is held rigid, flexion and extension of the lumbar spine is not possible, and even a list of the trunk may be present, yet the patient has no pain. Forced maneuvers that attempt to flex or extend the spine evoke no discomfort or pain. In these patients, the spine is held as if in a vise by profound muscle spasm which is readily discernible; the grip on the spinal segments is so firm that not even the slightest motion in flexion or extension is permissible; hence, the patient has no pain.

In contrast to this manifestation of the acute lesion is the not infrequent occurrence of severe radicular pain without impairment of movements of the spine. In these cases, patients exhibit relatively free motion in all directions; however, their radicular pain is invariably accentuated when tension in nerve roots is increased as in the straight leg raising test (Fig. 12-15).

In less acute lumbar lesions in which muscle spasm is less pronounced, flexion and extension of the spine is affected accordingly. In fact, during the interval between attacks when muscle spasm is minimal or lacking, the spine may exhibit a free range of motion in all directions.

LATERAL FLEXION AND ROTATION

During an acute attack, lateral flexion and rotation of the spine show little or no impairment. The range of lateral motion can readily be determined by measuring the distance the extended fingers reach on the thigh.

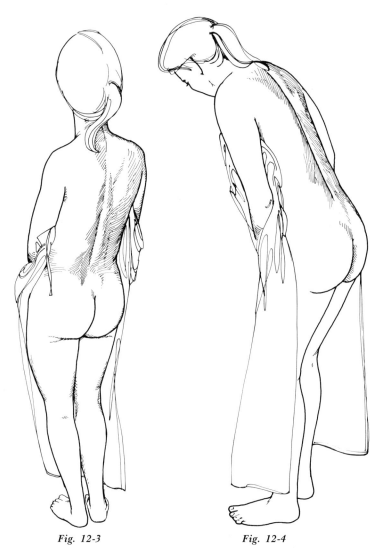

Fig. 12-3   *Fig. 12-4*

Figure 12-3 During an acute attack the lumbar spine may be held rigid. When the patient attempts to extend the spine he leans backward and extends the hips but not the lumbar spine.

Figure 12-4 During an acute attack the spine may be held rigid. Upon forward bending flexion occurs in the hips and dorsal and cervical spine but not in the lumbar spine.

Rotation of the spine is measured by having the patient turn the head and shoulders as far as possible in one direction and then in the other while the examiner steadies the pelvis with one hand on each of the iliac crests. Under normal conditions the arc of rotation of the shoulders is almost 90 degrees, but this varies slightly with the stature of the individual. As a rule, during an acute episode some restriction of lateral flexion is detectable and it may be more on one side than on the other; but severe impairment of lateral flexion rarely occurs. Rotation of the spine is less affected than lateral flexion (Fig. 12-5). However, if the patient is forced to move the trunk in lateral flexion or in rotation beyond the painless arc of motion, pain may be elicited.

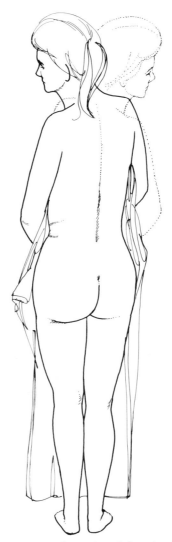

Figure 12-5 During an acute attack rotation of the spine is not seriously affected.

Muscle Spasm

Spasm of the paravertebral muscles in the lumbar spine is a consistent finding during an acute attack. It is a reflex protective mechanism over which the patient has no control. It is readily apparent to the expert examiner and it is always palpable. The muscles are tense and board-like to the touch and the spasm may be more pronounced on one side than on the other. This protective mechanism, holding the spine rigidly, is responsible for the flattening of the lumbar curve and the list of the trunk to one or the other side so frequently observed during an acute attack. Even when the patient is in the prone position the spasm persists. Spasm of muscles is best appreciated by gently palpating the paravertebral muscles with the pulp of the fingers; the muscles are tender to pressure. With experience, this simple method readily reveals the extent of the spasm when compared with unaffected muscle masses. Muscle spasm and pain is associated with derangement of the lumbar disc and may not be associated with nerve root irritation. It is not unusual to see a patient with severe spasm of the paravertebral muscles, a sciatic scoliosis and obliteration of the lumbar curve without leg pain. On the other hand, severe nerve root irritation due to extruded nuclear tissue may give rise to the same clinical picture, plus radicular pain. It was previously noted that muscle spasm and pain without leg pain is mostly due to entrapment of a sequestrum of nuclear tissue between the vertebral bodies.[2] Occasionally, with certain movements, the nuclear tissue slips back into the space between the bodies; this is often accompanied by the sudden relief of pain. Likewise, a nerve root suddenly relieved of pressure by extruded nuclear tissue results in diminution of the pain.[2]

Muscle tenderness may be associated with nerve root irritation; in an acute attack, tenderness of the buttock, the thigh and the calf on the affected side is often demonstrable.[21, 22] Referred pain of sclerogenic origin may also be accompanied by specific areas of local tenderness, usually at a distance from the site of irritation and usually at the insertion of tendon to bone, and also by aching in the muscles. When pain is localized to a specific area along the course of the sciatic nerve, careful regional examination is most essential in order to rule out local lesions irritating the sciatic nerve, such as abscess, neurofibroma, glomus tumor, lipoma or sterile abscess following injection of drugs to relieve the local pain.

Palpation and Percussion

These methods provide pertinent information providing the results are accurately interpreted. Palpation, light and deep pressure of the lumbar region, with the patient in either the erect or the prone position, may evoke tender areas in the midline at the level of the disc lesion and also in the paravertebral area on the side of a nuclear extrusion. It is not uncommon to be able to elicit tenderness along the iliac crest or even over the posterior aspect of the sacroiliac joint on the side of an irritated nerve root. It was previously pointed out that these areas are supplied by the posterior primary divisions of the lumbar roots and that these fibers may be stimulated by extruded nuclear material as are the fibers of the anterior division of the affected root. Tenderness is frequently noted when pressure is made over the sciatic notch on the affected side; this can readily be explained by the hypersensitivity of the fibers of an affected root comprising the sciatic nerve.

Percussion is less informative than palpation and light or deep pressure. It is true that in some instances of an acute attack even light fist percussion over the lumbar spine, in the midline, will produce such severe accentuation of the local and radiating pain that the patient's knees may buckle and he may show evidence of a vasovagal response. On the other hand, in some patients, particularly those with pronounced muscle spasm in which the lumbar spine is rigidly fixed, even forceful percussion may evoke no response. When the test is positive it gives a fair index of the sensitivity of the affected tissues and of the affected nerve root, but when it is negative it neither confirms nor eliminates the presence of a lumbar disc lesion.

Motor Dysfunction

Impaired motor function results in varying degrees of loss of muscle power and mass. It was previously pointed out that minor degrees of motor dysfunction are very often not recognized by the patient; however, in some cases it may be the presenting symptom. During an acute attack, leg and back pain may so dominate the clinical picture that what is obvious motor impairment to the examiner is not even noticed by the patient. However, some cases of long standing, associated with severe root compression, may exhibit advanced muscle dysfunction with little or no pain. This is due to total disruption of the nerve root function.

Although there is considerable overlap in the innervation of the muscle groups of the leg, the different groups derive their main nerve supply from specific nerve roots and are clinically identified with special movements of the joints they motorize. Therefore, impairment of certain movements of the toes, ankle, knee and hip indicates implication of specific muscle groups, which in turn points to involvement of a specific nerve root. This is especially true of movements of the toes and ankle.

Advanced muscle wasting is readily noted by both the patient and the examiner; however, minor or subtle changes in muscle bulk may be more difficult to identify. Often the state of the muscle mass can be ascertained visually and even minor degrees of flaccidity of the muscle group can be noted by light palpation. To ascertain the degree of muscle wasting or atrophy, both limbs should be compared one with the other. Differences in the circumferences of the thigh and calf of both legs are readily established by measurements made at the same level on both extremities. The circumference of the thigh is measured at a fixed distance above the superior pole of the patella; the calf is measured at a fixed distance from the superior aspect of the tibial tubercle. Measurements of the thigh and calf should be made when the muscles are completely relaxed, which is best induced when the patient is in the supine position with both legs extended.

Loss of muscle mass frequently occurs in the gluteal muscles. Here it is impossible to measure accurately the extent of muscle atrophy. However, when the patient is standing, any differences in the muscle masses of the affected and unaffected side readily become apparent by simple inspection and palpation of the two muscle groups.

Clinical assessment of the motor power in any group of muscles is best determined by having the particular group of muscles act against resistance. To determine the difference in power of the abductor muscles of the hips, the patient is examined in the supine position with both legs extended and together. The examiner grasps both ankles and tests the strength of the abductor muscles while the patient attempts to abduct the legs against resistance (Fig. 12-6). Next, adduction power is tested by having the patient adduct the legs from the abducted position against resistance (Fig. 12-7). Flexion power of the hips is also best determined with the patient in the supine position and the legs extended and together. The examiner makes firm pressure on the knees and determines the strength of the flexor muscles while the patient attempts to flex first one leg and then the other (Fig. 12-8).

Flexion and extension power of the knee joint is tested with the patient in the sitting position and with both feet free of the floor. The examiner grasps both ankles and notes the power of flexion and extension of the knee joint against resistance (Figs. 12-9 and 12-10).

Motor function of the ankles and toes is far more significant in localizing the nerve root involved than differences in power of the muscle groups activating the hip and knee. Motor dysfunction at the ankle and in the toes, in most instances, points to implication of either the L5 or S1 nerve root, the two roots which are involved in almost 95 per cent of all disc lesions in the lumbar spine. Because evidence of motor dysfunction in the group of muscles motorizing the ankle joint and the toes is so important in localizing the site of the lesion, the tests to determine the power in the muscle groups concerned should be performed with meticulous care. The power of the muscles should be noted against manual resistance and under weight bearing. The manual resistance test requires the patient to hold the foot in dorsiflexion while the examiner tries to force the foot into plantar flexion; this determines the strength of the dorsiflexors of the ankle (Fig. 12-11). To test the stength of the calf, the patient holds the foot in plantar flexion while the examiner tries to force the foot into dorsiflexion (Fig. 12-12). By these procedures, even minor differences in muscle power between the affected and the unaffected leg can be determined. More revealing is the action of these muscle groups under weight bearing. The group of calf muscles is tested by asking the patient to walk on his toes. A tendency to drop the heel to the floor is indicative of loss of power in the calf muscles, a phenomenon frequently associated with absence of the Achilles reflex. To test the dorsiflexors of the ankle, the patient is asked to walk briskly; if there is weakness of the dorsiflexors, the patient exhibits a slap foot gait on the affected side due to his inability to dorsiflex the foot completely. Weakness of the dorsiflexors of the foot can also be demonstrated by having the patient walk on his heels; because of the inability to dorsiflex the foot on the affected side, the patient reveals considerable difficulty in walking.

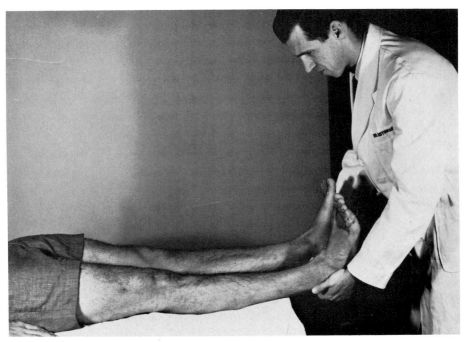

Figure 12-6   Test for the strength of the abductors of the hip; with the legs adducted the patient attempts to abduct the legs against resistance.

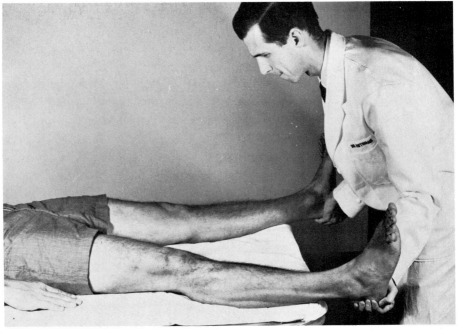

Figure 12-7   Test for the strength of the adductors of the hip; with the legs abducted the patient attempts to adduct the legs.

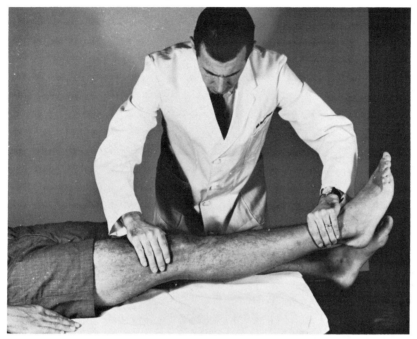

Figure 12-8   Test for the strength of the flexors of the hip; with the legs together and extended the patient attempts to flex the leg at the hip against resistance.

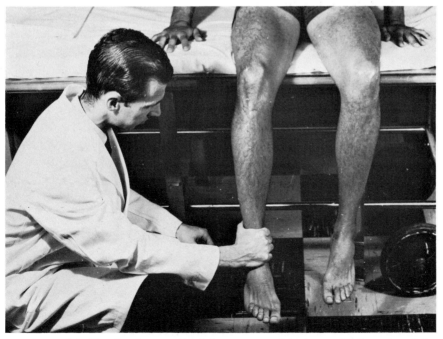

Figure 12-9   Test for the strength of the extensors of the knee; with the patient sitting and the legs free of the floor, the patient attempts to extend the knee against resistance.

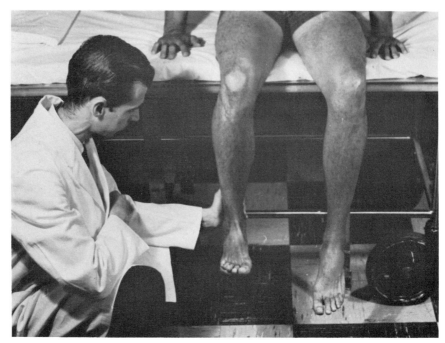

Figure 12-10　Test for the strength of the flexors of the knee; the patient attempts to flex the knee against resistance.

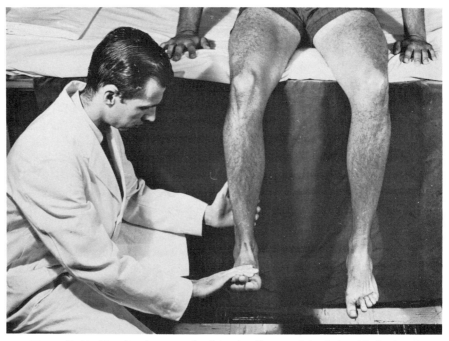

Figure 12-11　Test for the strength of the dorsiflexors of the foot; with the foot dorsiflexed, the patient attempts to hold this position while the examiner attempts to force the foot into plantar flexion.

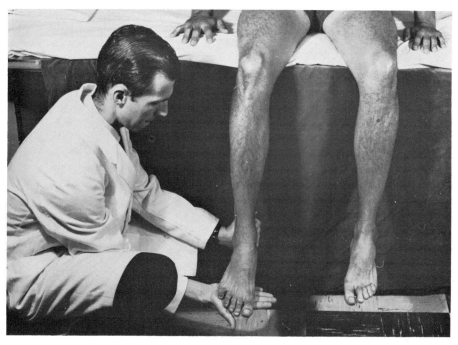

Figure 12-12 Test for the strength of the plantar flexors of the foot; the patient attempts to hold the foot in plantar flexion while the examiner tries to force the foot in dorsiflexion.

Weakness of the extensors of the toes is the most important test of muscle function in determining implication of the L5 nerve root. It is best performed with the patient in the standing position and asking him to dorsiflex both great toes against the resistance of the examiner (Fig. 12-13). Whereas weakness of the dorsiflexors of the ankle and toes is indicative of involvement of the fifth lumbar nerve root, loss of power in the calf muscles is positive evidence of implication of the first sacral nerve root. Both the fifth lumbar and first sacral nerve roots innervate the muscles of the buttock which produce abduction, extension and external rotation of the hip. However, from a functional viewpoint, involvement of the first sacral root has practically no effect on the above movements of the hip joint. Also both nerves supply the evertors of the foot and the flexors of the knee joint; however, functionally, the fifth lumbar root plays a far greater role in flexion of the knee and eversion of the foot than the first sacral nerve; in fact, the role of the first sacral nerve root is insignificant.

Motor dysfunction of the quadriceps femoris muscle, demonstrated by loss of muscle bulk and by diminished power of extension of the knee against resistance, indicates movement of the fourth lumbar nerve root. In addition to decreased power of extension of the knee, implication of this root may be associated with weakness of inversion of the foot. Like the fifth lumbar root, the fourth root also innervates the abductors, extensors and external rotators of the hip; but, whereas the fourth root innervates the extensors of the knee and the invertors of the foot, the fifth root supplies the flexors of the knee and the evertors of the foot (Figs. 12-14a and 12-

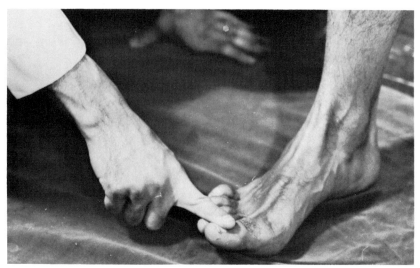

Figure 12-13   Test for the strength of the extensors of the toes; the patient attempts to extend the toes against resistance.

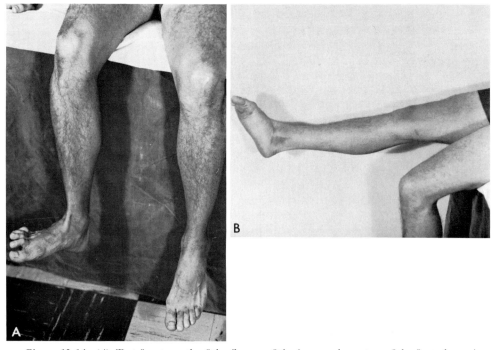

Figure 12-14   (*A*), Test for strength of the flexors of the knee and evertors of the foot; the patient forcefully flexes the knee and everts the foot. The main nerve supply to these muscles is from the L5 nerve root. (*B*), Test for the strength of the extensors of the knee and invertors of the foot; the patient forcefully extends the knee and inverts the foot. These muscles derive their main nerve supply from the L4 nerve root.

14b). It was previously noted that lesions of the fourth lumbar root are rare and, in the majority of cases, the source of irritation is nuclear material extruded from the L4-L5 disc which migrates cephalad.

Implication of the third lumbar root is even less common than involvement of the fourth root. When it does occur, the motor deficits are confined to the hip and knee. This root innervates the abductors, internal rotators and the flexors of the hip joint and the extensors of the knee joint. At this point it must be emphasized that impairment of function of a certain group of muscles does not always point to implication of a specific nerve root. Most muscles in the lower leg receive their nerve supply from more than one spinal nerve. Also, there is considerable overlap of the dermatomes of the lower leg. It becomes apparent, then, that the clinical picture is not always crystal clear as far as correct identification of the specific nerve root is concerned. However, in spite of these anatomical peculiarities, which vary from patient to patient, a careful study of the type of motor deficit found correlated with the sensory abnormalities present and the localization of the referred pain will, in most instances, identify the nerve root or roots affected.

Sudden, partial or complete paresis of all the roots of the cauda equina, associated with loss of function of the sphincter muscles, is indicative of severe compression of the cauda equina and may be produced by a massive extrusion of disc material from any of the lumbar discs, but it usually occurs at the L5, L4 or L3 interspace. Because all the roots are involved there is little difference in the clinical picture regardless of the site of nuclear extrusion. Usually there is profound muscle weakness and atrophy, and the patient is unable to walk because, except for the ability to flex the thighs and extend the knees, a flaccid paralysis involves all muscle groups of both extremities. When the lesion is at the L4 interspace, the patient has a bilateral foot drop in addition to other muscle involvement; when the lesion is at the L5 interspace there is paralysis of the plantar flexors of the feet; and when the lesion is at the L3 interspace there may be weak extension of the knees (Figs. 12-9, 12-11 and 12-12).

The clinical picture produced by massive extrusion of nuclear material from one of the lumbar discs is very similar to that produced by an intraspinal tumor located at the same interspace. Bilateral motor and sensory deficits are more commonly the result of intraspinal tumors, and such deficits have an insidious onset rather than the sudden onset so characteristic of massive nuclear extrusions.

This is one lesion of the lumbar discs that demands immediate surgical intervention. The cauda equina must be decompressed immediately; if not, the convalescence will be long and complete return of motor function will be most unlikely.

Sensory Manifestations

Abnormal objective sensory manifestations may or may not be associated with involvement of a nerve root in lumbar disc lesions. However, when present, because of the wide overlap of the dermatomes of the spinal nerves it may be difficult to identify the specific root involved. The overlap is not consistent from patient to patient; rather, it shows considerable variations. For this reason, the investigators concerned with this problem have evolved dermatome charts which exhibit little similarity. The abnormal sensory pattern noted in a patient is only of clinical significance in identifying the affected nerve root if it correlates with the pattern of referred pain and with the motor deficit presented by the patient. The sensory findings observed below the ankle are far more reliable than those occurring above the ankle and above the knee. It is generally conceded that the dermatome charting evolved by Foerster is the most reliable (Figs. 11-1 and 11-2).[15, 18, 23, 32]

Differences in sensation of two adjacent cutaneous areas are readily discernible by lightly circumscribing the leg with the sharp end of a pin. The patient will immediately give notice of any change in sensation at the point where it occurs. In the same fashion, by using first the blunt end of a pin and then the sharp end, any alterations in discrimination are readily noted.

Reflex Changes

An abnormal tendon reflex response at the knee or ankle is frequently observed in lumbar disc lesions when a specific nerve root is involved. Changes in the Achilles tendon reflex at the ankle joint are most significant; such a change invariably points to implication of the S1 nerve root. This reflex may also be altered by involvement of the S2 nerve root; but, since the S2 nerve root is rarely affected and the S1 root is frequently involved in lumbar disc lesions, it is safe to consider any alterations of the Achilles tendon reflex to be related to the S1 nerve root. However, it should be remembered that not all the patients with lumbar disc lesions at the L5-S1 level with leg pain have changes in the Achilles tendon reflex; in fact, almost 50 per cent of the patients show no alterations. Also, it should be remembered that 15 to 29 per cent of patients with lesions at the L4-L5 level exhibit a decreased or absent Achilles tendon reflex.[10]

The patellar tendon reflex at the knee joint is not affected by lesions implicating the L5 and S1 nerve roots except in very rare cases when it might be slightly diminished. In fact this reflex is never absent regardless of the level of the lesion, but it may be decreased in intensity by lesions involving the L3 or L4 nerve roots.

Another interesting observation should be recorded regarding tendon reflex responses at the knee and ankle; namely, that there is no correlation between the degree of tendon reflex changes and the impairment of muscular function. A patient with an absent Achilles tendon reflex may exhibit normal power in the muscles of the calf.

CLINICAL TESTS

Valsalva Maneuver

During an acute episode of backache, alone or associated with sciatica, mechanisms such as coughing, sneezing and straining may produce a sudden, sharp accentuation of the pain; both the low back pain and the leg pain may be affected. The cause of this sudden increase in pain is readily explained by the so-called Valsalva maneuver. Valsalva was an Italian anatomist who first described, in 1704, how secretions in the middle ear could be extruded through the external canal by blowing with the mouth and nose closed.[34] Today, Valsalva's maneuver is described as forced expiration against a closed glottis, a closed pharyngoesophageal orifice and a tightening of the sphincters of all the other body cavities. This maneuver is associated with marked contractions of the musculature of the thorax and abdomen, producing an increase in intrathoracic and intra-abdominal pressure. The mechanism is normally employed to expel material from these cavities. Also the increased intrathoracic and intra-abdominal pressures produced by this maneuver provide added support to the spinal column, particularly the lumbar spine, when the back is loaded in a position of forward bending. These pressures tend to straighten and elongate the spine and resist compression forces acting on the spinal column. Batson describes the maneuver as having two functions, visceral and muscular. Coughing and sneezing are visceral functions; whereas lifting a weight from the floor in front of the axis of the body is a muscular function.[5, 4, 12, 28]

Coughing is a normal use of the Valsalva maneuver; essentially, it consists of a sudden opening of the larynx following compression of air in the lungs. This act is followed by a sharp reduction of intrathoracic pressure, which tends to blow secretions or foreign material from the tracheobronchial tree and from the larynx. Sneezing is an act similar to coughing except that the air currents pass through the nose. Defecation and micturition are concerned with the abdominal functions of the maneuver; the act is effected by increasing the intra-abdominal pressure and concurrently relaxing the proper sphincter.

During the Valsalva maneuver venous blood does not flow into the cavities to return to the heart; in fact venous blood is actually forced out of the cavities. The question that naturally arises is, Where does the blood go? In 1940, Batson described a system of veins which are without valves, the vertebral vein system.[5] This system consists of all the veins of the head and neck, the veins of the body wall whose valves are competent where they join the cavity veins, the nonvalved veins of the extremities and the great longitudinal epidural plexus of veins. During the maneuver, the vertebral vein system fills with blood which cannot enter the cavities; it also accommodates the blood forced out of the cavities.

As a result of this retrograde flow of venous blood, several other phenomena occur. Some of the venous blood enters the cerebrospinal canal and, with a rise in the intrathoracic and intra-abdominal pressures, there is also an immediate rise in the intraspinal fluid pressure.[17] In addition, the epidural veins compress the dural sac and the dural sac increases in height and decreases in diameter.[31] These phenomena may explain the sudden accentuation of leg pain during a Valsalva maneuver; the increase in the pressure of the cerebrospinal fluid and the increase in length and decrease in diameter of the dural sac together may increase the tension of the nerve roots. This sudden increase in tension may have no effect on normal roots, but it may evoke marked accentuation of leg pain in a sensitive root already under abnormal tension.

Aggravation of the back pain during the Valsalva maneuver as noted on coughing and sneezing may be due to the sudden and abrupt reflex contraction of the erector spinae muscles and of the musculatures of the abdominal and thoracic cavities necessary to produce increased intra-abdominal and intrathoracic pressures; this mechanism tends to elongate the spine. The sensitive disrupted tissues associated with a lumbar disc lesion may be suddenly jarred and disturbed by this mechanism, thereby markedly accentuating the back pain. Also, the momentary increase in the venous pressure at the site of the disc and ligaments injured may play a role in aggravating the back pain. Coughing, sneezing and straining during defecation rarely produce accentuation of referred pain to the buttocks and posterior aspect of the thighs. This is in contrast to the radicular pain that these mechanisms produce by increasing the tension of a sensitive nerve root.

Leg Tests

There are several leg tests which point to implication of the lower lumbar nerve roots and, in a measure, to the severity of involvement. Before performing any of the tests, it is most essential to rule out the possibility of hip disease which may be responsible for referred pain to the thigh, especially in the region of the knee. It is not unusual to see a patient who has been under treatment for a lumbar disc lesion when the true site of pathology is in the hip; the converse is also true, particularly when the patient complains of pain in the buttocks. Diseases of the hip invariably produce restriction of motion; a free range of painless motion in the hip eliminates involvement of the joint. This is best demonstrated with the patient in the supine position and the legs extended at the *hips* and *knees*. Internal and external rotation are readily tested by rolling the limbs in either direction; also, these movements should be tested with the hips and knees flexed to 90 degrees. It should be mentioned that, during an acute episode, some patients hold the affected leg partially flexed at the hip and knee even in the supine position and are unable to extend the limb without accentuation of the pain. In these instances, movements of the hip are best tested by bringing the leg to a position of 90 degrees flexion at the hip and 90 degrees flexion of the knee.

STRAIGHT LEG RAISING

This test is frequently erroneously referred to as the Lasègue test. It is undoubtedly the most important of all the leg tests and is positive in all acute attacks and subacute attacks of lumbar disc lesions associated with nerve root irritation. The test is performed with the patient in the supine position with the legs extended at the hips and knees and the feet in the relaxed position of slight plantar flexion (Fig. 12-15). Next, the leg to be tested is flexed at the hip with the knee extended. Normally, the leg can be

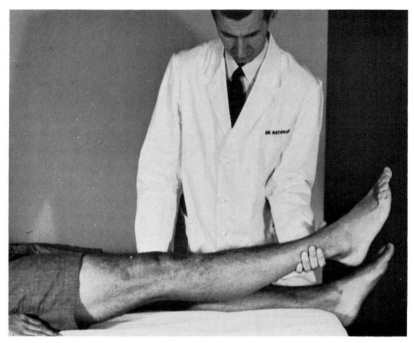

Figure 12-15 Demonstrating the straight leg test; normally the leg extended at the hip and knee and with the foot in plantar flexion can be raised 80 to 90 degrees.

raised to 80 or 90 degrees, depending on the tightness of the posterior musculature of the leg and the type of body build of the patient. Also, this maneuver stretches the sciatic nerve but no movement of the lower lumbar nerve roots occurs until 30 to 40 degrees of flexion are attained. Stretching of the sciatic nerve and movement of the nerve roots produce no pain under normal conditions. This is not true in the presence of a sensitive root already under normal tension by extruded nuclear material. Now the extent to which the leg can be raised is greatly diminished, and any attempt to raise the leg beyond this point produces excruciating pain in the leg or the back or both. In some instances, the leg cannot be raised from the table to any angle. In addition to the pain evoked in the leg and back when the leg is raised beyond the diminished angle, reflex spasm occurs in the muscles of the back and in the extremity, preventing further elevation of the leg. This maneuver does not cause compression of the affected nerve root because, as previously pointed out, direct compression of a nerve root is not associated with pain, but rather the stretching and increased tension of a sensitive root is responsible for the ensuing accentuation of pain.

As a rule, a positive straight leg raising test on the affected side is accompanied by some restriction of elevation of the unaffected leg; however, the angle to which the leg can be raised is greater on the unaffected side than on the side of the lesion. In addition, the straight leg raising maneuver on the uninvolved side may produce pain on the opposite side. The explanation for this phenomenon, previously recorded, is that raising the leg on one side normally causes the lower lumbar nerve roots on the opposite side, especially the L5 and S1 roots, to move slightly down-

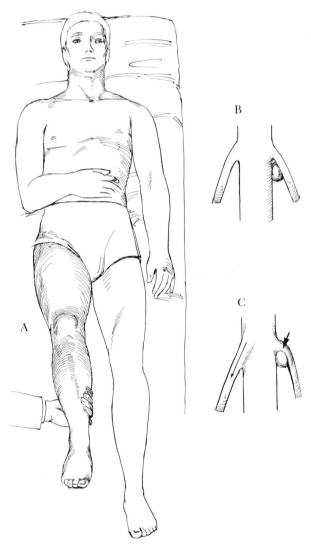

Figure 12-16 Movement of nerve roots when the leg on the opposite side is raised. (*A*), When the leg is raised on the unaffected side the roots on the opposite side slide slightly downward and toward the midline, (*B*). In the presence of a disc lesion this movement increases the root tension (*C*).

ward and toward the midline of the spinal canal.[37] In the presence of a disc lesion causing root irritation this minimal amount of movement of the roots is sufficient to further irritate the sensitive root and thereby accentuate the pain (Fig. 12-16).

The limit to which the leg on the affected side can be raised is a fairly good index of the degree of sensitivity of the nerve root. In fact, in some very severe, acute attacks, simple dorsiflexion of the foot with the leg extended at the hip and knee is sufficient to produce excruciating pain. This simple maneuver stretches the sciatic nerve and pulls it taut.

LASÈGUE TEST

Lasègue's test is frequently confused with the straight leg raising test and is often referred to as Kernig's test. It is performed with the patient in the supine position with the legs extended at the hips and knees and the feet in plantar flexion. First the knee is flexed and then the thigh is flexed to 90 degrees; next the knee is extended. Normally the knee can be extended to 180 degrees without causing pain, except for a sensation of tightness of the posterior leg muscles and in the back (Fig. 12-17). In the presence of a disc lesion causing nerve root irritation the limit to which the knee can be extended is diminished; beyond this point, pain is produced in the leg or back or both. Pain can also be reproduced by extending the knee to the position of tolerance and then sharply dorsiflexing the foot; this maneuver also stretches the sciatic nerve and increases the tension on the nerve root.[26]

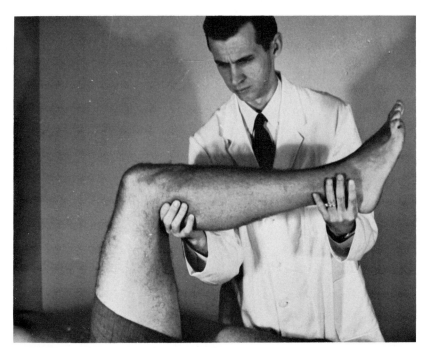

Figure 12-17 Demonstrating Lasègue's test; first the knee and then the thigh is flexed to 90 degrees; next the knee is extended. Normally the knee can be extended to 180 degrees without pain.

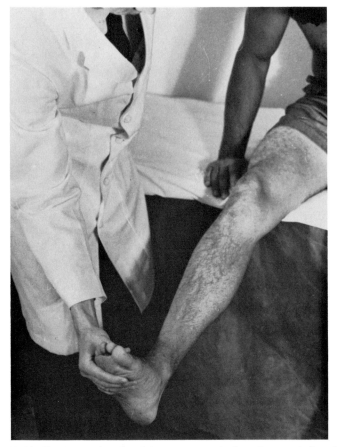

Figure 12-18   Demonstrating the sitting root test; the knee is extended to the point of resistance, then the cervical spine is suddenly flexed. In the presence of a sensitive nerve root, this maneuver evokes severe pain along its distribution.

SITTING ROOT TEST

This test is performed with the patient in the sitting position with the legs hanging free. First, the knee is extended to the point of resistance; next, the examiner places one hand behind the head over the occipital region and then sharply flexes the cervical spine. The sudden increase in tension of a sensitive nerve root caused by flexion of the cervical spine evokes severe pain along the distribution of the root (Fig. 12-18).

FORWARD BENDING WITH THE KNEES EXTENDED

Essentially this test is a modification of the straight leg raising test. By forward bending of the trunk with the knees extended, the sciatic nerve is stretched. In the presence of a sensitive root with increased tension, this test produces accentuation of the radicular pain. During an acute attack in which there is radicular pain, the patient will bend forward only a few degrees and then will stop because of the pain and reflex spasm of the muscles of the back and the extremity which are initiated by this maneuver. In patients with no sciatic radiation there is a surprisingly free range of forward motion of the trunk. However, little or no flexion takes place in the lumbar spine; most of the forward motion occurs at the hip joints, whereas the trunk is held rigid by the severe spasm of the paravertebral muscles.

Peripheral Vascular Examination

Examination of the vessels of the lower extremities must never be overlooked. Symptoms produced by diseases of the peripheral vessels may simulate lesions of the lumbar discs. The pain of intermittent claudication is usually localized in the buttocks, the hamstring muscles and the calves. Characteristically, the pain appears with activity, such as walking, or even with standing; it is relieved by a short period of rest but reappears upon resumption of activity. Careful examination of the character of the pulse of the femoral artery, of the popliteal artery and of the posterior tibial and dorsalis pedis arteries should be made in every case in which a lumbar disc lesion is suspected.

Jugular Compression Test

This is another test revealing the effect of increased tension on a sensitive nerve root. By compression of the jugular veins, a rise in the pressure of the intraspinal fluid occurs; this in turn produces stretching of the dura and its extensions covering the nerve roots. The resulting increased tension on a sensitive root already under abnormal tension is sufficient to cause sharp pain along the distribution of the root.

The test is best performed with the patient in the sitting position. Firm digital pressure is made simultaneously over both the internal and external jugular veins for at least two minutes. If the test is positive, the patient experiences pain along the distribution of the involved nerve root beginning in the back, then in the buttock, in the thigh and finally in the leg. If positive, the test confirms the existing evidence of nerve root irritation; if it is negative, it does not rule out nerve root implication.

Abdominal and Rectal Examination

No examination of the back is complete without inquiry into any change in the patient's bowel and bladder habits and an abdominal, pelvic and rectal examination. Primary and metastatic tumors of the spine and retroperitoneal, lumbar and pelvic malignancies may mimic lesions of the lumbar discs. These lesions will be considered more fully in the discussion concerned with differential diagnosis. Nevertheless, the abdomen and pelvis should be carefully palpated for the evidence of tumors and areas of tenderness, and a digital examination of the prostate and rectum should be made to exclude the presence of tumors in these regions. One patient in our series presented signs of a lumbar disc lesion with sciatic radiation; however, at surgery the bulging mass under the L5 nerve root proved to be a metastatic lesion from a renal tumor. In two others, the cause was a retroperitoneal tumor. It should be remembered that aortic aneurysms produce back pain; however, evidence that the pain is of mechanical origin is lacking.

SPECIAL DIAGNOSTIC TESTS

Examination of the Cerebrospinal Fluid

Usually examination of the cerebrospinal fluid is not necessary to establish a diagnosis of a lumbar disc lesion. If it should be performed, its only significance is in the negative findings. The flow of the cerebrospinal fluid in the subarachnoid space is not obstructed when sequestra of nuclear material are extruded from the disc, except when there is a massive extrusion which fills completely the spinal canal and compresses the cauda equina. In the usual case, the amount of the total protein of the fluid is not significantly increased, ranging from 60 to 80 mg. per 100 mls. Less than ten per cent of the disc lesions have elevated total protein. This finding is in contrast to that occurring when the flow of the fluid is completely or almost completely obstructed. Now, the protein content of the fluid distal to the obstruction may be as high as 200 to 400 mg. per 100 mls. and is a consistent finding in space occupying lesions of the spinal canal such as tumors. When the diagnosis of a lumbar disc lesion is not clear, the cerebrospinal fluid should be examined. For the test to be significant, the fluid must be drawn from the subarachnoid space distal to the obstructing lesion; this may be difficult in cases of a lesion at the L4-L5 level and impossible if the obstruction is at the L5-S1 level.

Lumbar puncture is not an innocuous procedure; a nerve root may be traumatized, puncture of a vein may be followed by hemorrhage into the subarachnoid space and, finally, the introduction of pyogenic organisms into the subarachnoid space is not a far-fetched possibility. The procedure should be performed under strict aseptic technique and done only when the clinical picture of a disc lesion is not clear and where there is evidence that some other lesion may be responsible for the symptom complex.

Electromyography

This test is of no significant value in the diagnosis and localization of a lumbar disc lesion. In our experience the findings recorded by this test have never established the diagnosis or influenced our decision as to the management of the patient. It is a valueless exercise for both the patient and the surgeon.

Radiographic Examination

Radiographic study of the lumbar spine is mandatory in the evaluation of a person presenting the clinical manifestations of a lumbar disc lesion. Certain radiographic features indicate a definite pathologic process in a disc; however, these characteristic findings may be observed in lumbar discs which do not give rise to symptoms. It becomes obvious that specific radiographic findings can only be used to re-enforce the clinical diagnosis of a lumbar disc lesion. We have confined our discussion here to lesions of the lower lumbar discs which relate to the posterior elements of the spine and to the lumbar or sacral nerve roots, but a pathologic disc may also implicate the lateral and anterior aspects of the spine. These latter lesions are not associated with radicular pain, but they may give rise to local and referred pain. Their recognition, therefore, is most important; and careful radiographic study will help not only in establishing the diagnosis but also in determining the type and stage of the pathologic process in the affected disc.[29, 32]

The radiographs should be of good quality and should be taken with careful attention to all the details of an established technique. The study should include anteroposterior, lateral and oblique views. In addition, in some cases, tomograms may be necessary to disclose the disc pathology. Plain radiography may point to involvement of the disc by the following features: (1) narrowing of the intervertebral space, (2) osteophyte formation along the peripheries of the adjacent vertebral bodies, (3) sclerosis or condensation of the subchondral bone of the vertebral bodies above and below the affected disc, (4) relative posterior displacement of the proximal vertebral body, (5) sacralization of the fifth lumbar vertebra, (6) calcification in the nucleus pulposus or in the annulus fibrosus and (7) the "vacuum or pneumatization phenomena."

NARROWING OF THE INTERVERTEBRAL SPACE

With or without extrusion of nuclear material the pathologic condition may exist in the disc without any appreciable diminution of the disc space. Also, the decrease in height of the space may be so subtle that it may be difficult to determine whether true diminution exists or whether the alteration is the result of faulty radiographic technique. Although varying degrees of narrowing is the most valuable single radiographic finding in localizing the disc involved, it is a very changeable observation and discernible only in approximately one-third of the cases (Fig. 12-19). It should be remembered that narrowing of the disc space is not peculiar to degeneration of the nucleus pulposus as encountered in the lumbar disc lesions, but may also occur as the result of other pathologic processes affecting the spine, such as pyogenic infections, tuberculosis and primary or metastatic malignancies.

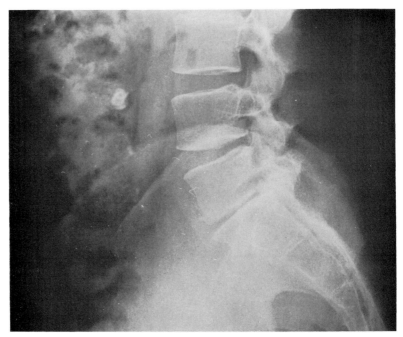

Figure 12-19 Observe the marked thinning of the disc between L5 and S1. There is no radiographic evidence of secondary changes in the vertebral bodies or the posterior joints. At operation, a large extrusion of disc material was found at the L5-S1 level.

ARTHROSIS OF THE INTERVERTEBRAL JOINT

The radiographic features characteristic of this process are narrowing of the intervertebral space, formation of osteophytes along the peripheries of the vertebra above and below the involved disc, and sclerosis and condensation of the subchondral bone of the two opposing vertebral bodies. In the presence of a clear clinical picture of a lumbar disc lesion the above findings are most significant in localizing the site of pathology, provided that no other motor unit is similarly affected. When these alterations are common to several motor units it is difficult to select the level responsible for the patient's symptoms on these changes alone (Fig. 12-20).

In elderly persons the above alterations may implicate many motor units of the lumbar spine and yet not give rise to symptoms. This is also true during the period of middle age when one, two or more units may be affected. The alterations represent the terminal stage of the pathologic process in the discs of the motor units involved.

RELATIVE POSTERIOR DISPLACEMENT OF THE VERTEBRAL BODY

With degeneration of the disc and collapse of the intervertebral space, secondary alterations occur in the posterior articular joints, and there may be some change in the alignment of the proximal vertebra to the distal vertebra of the motor unit affected. The change in alignment is essentially a relative retrodisplacement of the upper vertebra in relation to the lower

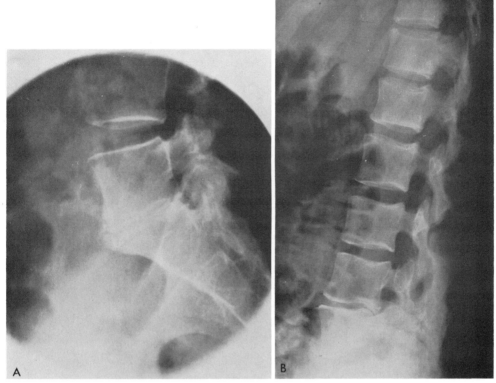

Figure 12-20 (*A*), This is the terminal stage of the degenerative process affecting the L5-S1 disc. The disc is completely collapsed; osteophyte formation along the peripheries of the L5 and S1 vertebral bodies is clearly evident; some calcification has occurred in the anterior longitudinal ligament and in the remnants of the L5 disc; some subchondral sclerosis is present in the posterior articular joints. This lesion was asymptomatic. (*B*), Terminal stage of disc degeneration at the L4-L5 level. Observe the narrowed disc space and subchondral sclerosis of the adjacent surfaces of L4 and L5. The fourth vertebra is displaced backward. This lesion was symptomatic and required excision of disc material and fusion.

vertebra. This occurs when the posterior facets are in an oblique downward and forward plane allowing the upper vertebra to settle in a slightly posterior position in relation to the lower vertebra (Fig. 12-21). This does not occur if the articular facets lie in a vertical plane.[14] Usually, backward displacement of the proximal vertebra occurs at the L5-S1 level; however, it may be encountered at the L4-L5 and L3-L4 levels. Relative posterior displacement of the centrum may also be explained by the anatomical fact that the lower surface of the fifth vertebra is in many cases wider than the articular surface of the sacrum so that, as the fifth vertebra settles down, its posterior surface is in a slightly backward position to that of the sacrum.[36] However, in cases with an acute lumbosacral angle, especially when the sacrum is almost in the horizontal plane, even vertical facets of the sacrum assume a downward and backward inclination as related to the horizontal. When the disc collapses, this configuration at the lumbosacral joint allows, in many instances, the fifth lumbar vertebra to attain a backward position in relation to the sacrum (Fig. 12-22).

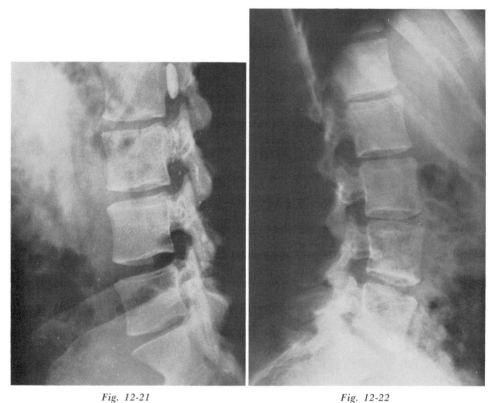

Fig. 12-21   Fig. 12-22

Figure 12-21 The L5 disc has collapsed and the L5 vertebra is displaced slightly backward. This retrodisplacement occurs when the posterior facets are in an oblique downward plane.

Figure 12-22 Observe the exaggerated lumbosacral angle; the sacrum is almost in a horizontal plane. With collapse of the disc, the L5 vertebral body is displaced slightly backward.

SACRALIZATION OF FIFTH LUMBAR VERTEBRA
(CONGENITAL THIN DISC)

Among the many congenital abnormalities of the lumbosacral region, partial or complete sacralization of the last lumbar vertebra and partial or complete lumbarization of the first sacral vertebra are most frequently associated with a thin disc (Fig. 12-23). Rarely is this thin disc the site of a pathologic alteration comparable to that which occurs in the discs proximal to it. However, degenerative changes can and do occur in the congenital thin disc, but this depends on the amount of motion present at the abnormal interspace. In a patient with a classic lumbar disc lesion, the responsible disc is, as a rule, at the first intervertebral space proximal to the congenital thin disc. The abnormal motion at this level and the secondary alterations that ensue may be the sources of back pain. If a lumbar disc lesion occurs above the abnormal disc and if the patient comes to surgery, a spinal fusion should be done extending from the vertebra proximal to the site of the lumbar disc lesion to the sacrum. By obliterating motion at the site of the congenital disc the patient is protected from future disability that might arise from the thin disc.

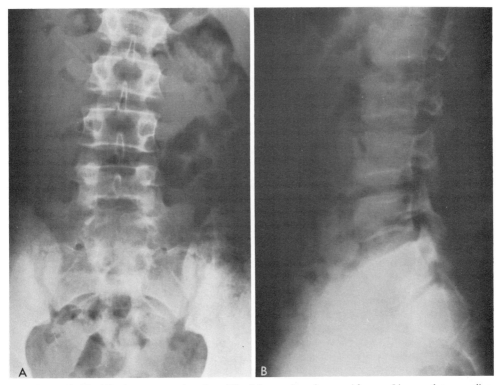

Figure 12-23 (*A*), Anteroposterior view. The L5 vertebra shows evidence of incomplete sacralization. (*B*), Lateral view. Observe the congenital thin disc between the partially sacralized vertebra and the first true sacral segment. This is rarely the site of degenerative disc disease.

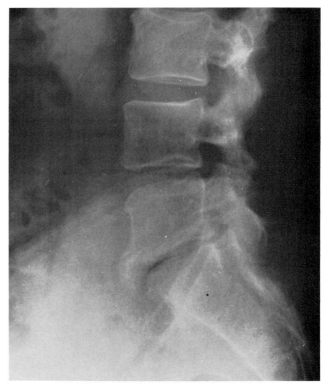

Figure 12-24 Advanced arthrosis of the L5-S1 intervertebral joint. Observe the thin L5 disc and the calcification and bone formation in the anterior longitudinal ligament.

CALCIFICATION OF THE DISC

Calcification of the nucleus pulposus of the lower lumbar disc rarely occurs in the classic pathologic process of lumbar disc lesions. This cannot be said of calcification of necrotic areas in the annulus, particularly its anterior portion. It is not uncommon to encounter varying degrees of calcification or even bone formation in the anterior portion of the annulus in persons with advanced pathologic changes which are now comparable to the changes of intervertebral arthrosis (Fig. 12-24). Ratheke found calcification in the annulus fibrosus in 71 per cent of all the spines examined (post mortem specimens) and only 6.5 per cent showed calcium deposits in the nucleus pulposus.[30]

VACUUM OR PNEUMATIZATION PHENOMENA

Magnusson (1937) first described the "vacuum phenomena" observed by radiography in the nucleus pulposus of the lumbar disc.[27] Vacuoles or "air bubbles" are discernible in the nucleus pulposus. The method which produces these defects is not clear. Some workers presume that while the spine is subjected to longitudinal forces which tend to separate the vertebrae and elongate the spine (such as in hyperextension of the spine), the gases in solution in the nuclear material are liberated and may be observed lying within the nucleus. The gases disappear when the tension is removed.[19, 20] Because this phenomenon is not observed constantly, in fact it is rarely demonstrable, and because its mechanism is still not clear, very little clinical significance is attached to it.

OTHER FORMS OF LUMBAR DISC LESIONS

It is true that in most disc lesions that produce back pain or leg pain or both, the posterior elements are primarily involved; namely, the posterior portion of the annulus fibrosus, the posterior longitudinal ligament and the nerve roots. However, the same pathologic process responsible for implication of these structures can also involve the anterior and lateral structures, and the superior and inferior cartilaginous plates. In many of these cases, the nature of the involvement is discernible in the radiographs (Fig. 12-25).

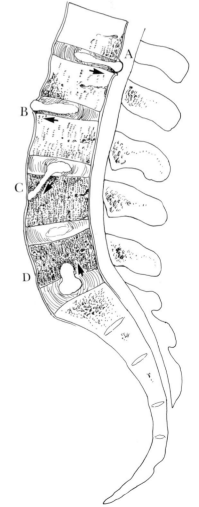

Figure 12-25 Directions the degenerated disc may take: (*A*), It has ruptured the annulus and the posterior longitudinal ligament and now lies in the spinal canal. (*B*), It has penetrated the annulus and now lies under the taut anterior longitudinal ligament. (*C*), It has traversed the annulus and lies under the epiphyseal plate. (*D*), It has pierced the annulus and the articular plate and now lies in the centrum.

ANTERIOR PROTRUSIONS AND EXTRUSIONS OF THE NUCLEUS PULPOSUS

During the course of degeneration of the nucleus pulposus some nuclear material may follow the radial fissures in the annulus which pursue an anterior direction. The nuclear tissue may eventually displace or penetrate the anterior fibers of the annulus and come to lie immediately beneath the tough anterior longitudinal ligament which deflects its course. In this position the nuclear sequestrum is compressed firmly against the anterior margin of the vertebral body, producing an erosion of the centrum at this site (Fig. 12-26). The size of the anterior extrusion varies; when associated with skeletal disorders such as dyschondroplasia, it may reach enormous proportions. On lateral radiographs the erosion of the anterosuperior border of the centrum is readily seen. In older lesions, peripheral osteophytes form where the fibers of the annulus have been detached from the border of the vertebral body. These alterations are also demonstrable in radiographs.

Anterior displacement of nuclear material is commoner than generally appreciated. Batts records an incidence of six per cent of 50 spinal columns he studied.[6] Many of these are asymptomatic, whereas others may cause deep seated local pain and also referred pain.

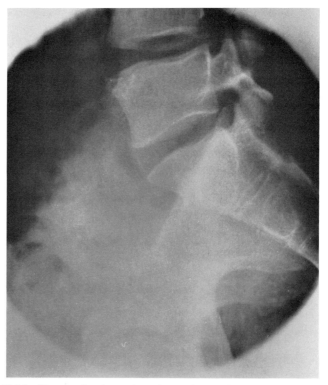

Figure 12-26   Observe the absorption of a portion of the anterosuperior portion of the L4 vertebra. The most likely cause of this alteration is extrusion of disc material under the tough anterior longitudinal ligament.

EXTRUSIONS OF NUCLEAR MATERIAL
BENEATH THE EPIPHYSEAL RING

Degenerated nuclear material may penetrate the articular plate at its junction with the epiphyseal ring.[32] The displaced nuclear material may force a crescentic segment of bone to separate from the vertebral body; the detached fragment of bone remains attached anteriorly to the anterior longitudinal ligament. By this same mechanism, pieces of the centrum may be detached from its inferior margin and, in rare instances, from its posterior margins. These lesions have been erroneously called "persistent epiphyses." They are encountered in adults and in children; in the former, the lower lumbar vertebrae are more frequently involved, whereas in the latter, the upper lumbar vertebrae are more often affected. Occasionally, considerable reactive bone forms at the site of the lesion. Healing may occur between the centrum and the detached fragment, leaving only the sequestrated nuclear material within the substance of the body.

These lesions may produce local backache and even referred pain to the lower abdomen and the renal region. They are frequently mistaken for other disorders such as tuberculosis of the spine, or considered as part of an overall degenerative process of the spine.

EXTRUSIONS OF NUCLEAR MATERIAL INTO
THE VERTEBRAL BODY

Schmorl was the first to describe extrusions of nuclear material into the spongiosa of the vertebral bodies. Usually, the nuclear tissue penetrates the defective cartilage plate just behind its center and is extruded into the substance of the vertebral body. However, the nuclear material may penetrate more peripheral areas of the body; the size of the nodes vary considerably. The nuclear material initiates a reactive process in the spongiosa characterized by the formation of a thin layer of dense bone around the displaced material. This encompassing shell of thin bone makes the lesion discernible in plain radiographs; at times tomograms may be necessary to locate the lesion (Fig. 12-27).

These lesions are frequently encountered in association with Scheuermann's disease, which affects adolescents. The herniations of nuclear material into the vertebral bodies may be the primary cause, and the disturbance of growth at the epiphyseal ring a secondary manifestation, in the pathogenesis of this disorder. The vertebrae of the lower thoracic and upper lumbar spine are frequently involved. Retardation of growth occurs in the anterior portion of the body because of involvement of the epiphyseal rings in this area; this together with some collapse of the anterior portion of the body produces the typical wedge-shaped vertebrae of Scheuermann's disease. The typical Schmorl's nodes may be seen in all the vertebrae affected; it may be necessary to employ tomography in order to visualize some of the lesions (Fig. 12-28).

Similar lesions may occur in later life and are usually associated with degenerative changes occurring in a motor unit. They may give rise to no symptoms; however, occasionally they do cause pain at the site of involvement and also referred pain to the lower thoracic and upper abdominal regions.

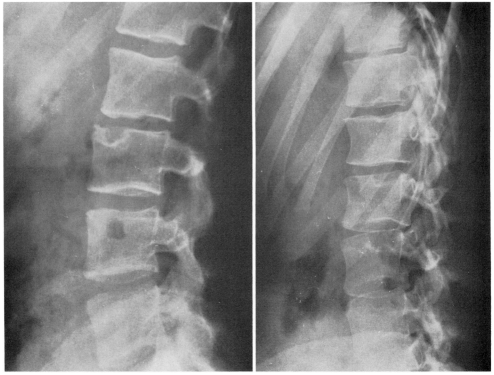

Fig. 12-27   *Fig. 12-28*

Figure 12-27 Radiographic appearance of a Schmorl's node. Observe the defect in the superior articular plate of the affected vertebral body; also note the thin line of dense reactive bone surrounding the displaced nuclear material in the spongiosa of the vertebral body.

Figure 12-28 This is the radiographic appearance of Scheuermann's disease. Some of the vertebrae of the lower thoracic and upper lumbar spine are wedge-shaped, caused by interference of the normal growth of the anterior portion of the bodies because of implication of the epiphyseal rings. Typical small Schmorl's nodes are discernible in many of the affected vertebrae.

NARROWING OF THE INTERVERTEBRAL FORAMINA

Plain radiography may disclose constriction of the intervertebral foramina, especially when the cause of the constriction is the formation of bony spurs at the posterior margins of the vertebrae or at the apophyseal joints. The abnormalities are best seen in lateral and oblique views of the lumbar spine. These alterations may give rise to no symptoms; however, if the findings correlate with the clinical picture, then they are of real significance, particularly if surgery is contemplated.

This point is illustrated by a male patient, 52 years old, who presented symptoms and signs indicating the L5 nerve root. The disc at the L4-L5 level was explored, and a degenerated disc was excised; this was followed by a spinal fusion from L4 to the sacrum. In spite of the fact that the fusion became solid, the patient's symptoms were never relieved. One year later, a study of the radiographs taken before the surgery revealed definite constriction of the intervertebral foramen transversed by the L5 nerve root. A

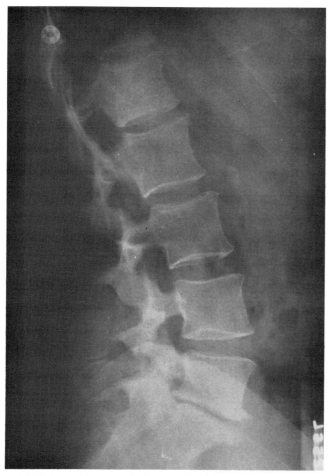

Figure 12-29 Encroachment on the intervertebral foramen. The foramen is narrowed considerably by collapse of the disc and osteophytes on the rims of L5 and S1 vertebrae, particularly in the region of the anterior boundary of the foramen.

foraminotomy at this level on the affected side relieved the patient's symptoms (Fig. 12-29).

Myelography

In the recent past, many well-documented communications have appeared in the literature which emphasize that: (1) routine myelography should not be performed in cases of lumbar disc lesions; (2) the accurate diagnosis of this symptom complex should and can be made on the presenting signs and symptoms; (3) myelography should be reserved for those cases in which the clinical picture is not clear, or in which some other space-occupying lesion is suspected, or if the disc lesions are suspected at multiple levels. With these concepts we are in full accord. But, in spite of these warnings, there are many surgeons who still employ myelography as a

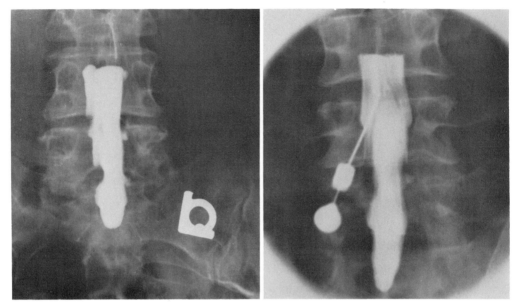

Fig. 12-30   *Fig. 12-31*

Figure 12-30   Myelogram showing the typical lateral defect in the column of dye caused by nuclear material extruded laterally. The size of the defect is not indicative of the amount of nuclear material extruded. In this instance, the nuclear material was extruded from the L5-S1 disc; however, evidence of a degenerative process is also present in the L4-L5 disc. Observe the thinning of the disc and the secondary osteochondral changes at the peripheries of the bodies of L4 and L5 vertebrae.

Figure 12-31   Myelogram showing a symmetrical constriction of the column of dye caused by a large midline protrusion of disc material. The dural sac is almost completely obliterated except for a small open column in the midline.

routine diagnostic tool, and more regrettably, some surgeons justify its routine use to re-enforce their clinical diagnosis in case legal implications should arise.

Myelography is not an innocuous procedure as some physicians write and it does carry a certain amount of risk to the patient. Some patients are subjected to considerable pain both during and after the test. There is, as yet, no assurance that the radio-opaque materials currently used are non-irritating in all cases; certainly this was not true of some of the materials used in the past, as attested by the many cases of arachnoiditis reported after their use. Complete removal of the radio-opaque material is not achieved in many instances, and it may be seen in the subarachnoid space years after the test is performed. Faulty technique may result in placing the dye outside the subarachnoid space, and its recovery becomes impossible. The nerve roots of the cauda equina may be traumatized and impairment of normal sphincter control may occur.

Even when the technique is accurately performed, the incidence of error ranges from 20 to 30 per cent. The investigation may fail to reveal the presence of extruded material if it is small in size, and lies far laterally in the lateral recess of the canal, and has no contact with the dural sac. On the other hand, the defect made by large extrusions bearing on the dural sac is readily seen. The test may be positive when, in fact, no lesion exists.

This may be attributed either to artifacts resulting from faulty technique, such as the leakage of radio-opaque material from the puncture hole in the subarachnoid membrane into the subdural space, or to congenital or acquired abnormalities of the subarachnoid space itself.[3, 13, 24]

Myelography should be done by one who is expert in its technique and who is able to attain the necessary exposures in different planes and to interpret them accurately. The different filling defects disclosed by myelography can be grouped into four categories.

1. A lateral defect or indentation in the column of dye as noted on anteroposterior projections. This type of defect is produced by nuclear material extruded laterally, but which is still in contact with the dural sac. The size of the indentation in the column of dye is not indicative of the true size of the nuclear mass (Fig. 12-30). Lateral defects are not always located at the level of the disc interspace. Occasionally, the extruded material may migrate up or down from its site of extrusion, so that the defect produced in the column is at the level of a vertebral body.

2. A more or less symmetrical constriction of the column of dye producing an hour-glass deformity. The defect indicates that the dural sac is almost completely obliterated except for a small open column in the midline. It is the type of defect seen in large midline protrusion of disc material (Fig. 12-31).

3. Defects depicting alterations in the normal anatomy of the nerve roots. These appear as: failure of the dye to fill the nerve root sheath, asymmetrical filling of the sheath, and elevation and distortion of the sheath. These lesions are often difficult to decipher accurately and are frequently overlooked (Fig. 12-32).

4. The so called "block defect" is indicative of a massive extrusion of nuclear material which almost completely seals off the dural sac. The defect is usually seen at the level of the interspace but may also be seen at the level of a vertebral body. Characteristic of this lesion is its irregular, shaggy outline at the level of the block (Figs. 12-33, 12-34 and 12-35).

INTERMITTENT PROLAPSE

Some mention must be made of the so called "intermittent prolapse" of nuclear material. Attention was first called to this type of lesion by Dandy (1941) who designated it the "concealed disc." Degenerated nuclear material still within the confines of the annulus (which may be weakened by the degenerative process but which is still intact) may bulge beyond its normal limits when the spine is subjected to certain stresses. According to the stresses, the prolapse appears and then disappears. Extension and hyperextension of the spine favor the prolapse which, by myelography, can be seen producing a defect in the anterior aspect of the column of dye. When the spine is relieved of stress, such as when the patient is lying relaxed in the prone position, the defect in the column disappears. Prolapse of nuclear material will not be evident at the time of surgery when the patient is completely relaxed. Such a lesion should be kept in mind when at operation no disc lesion is demonstrable in a patient presenting a typical clinical picture of a lumbar disc lesion.

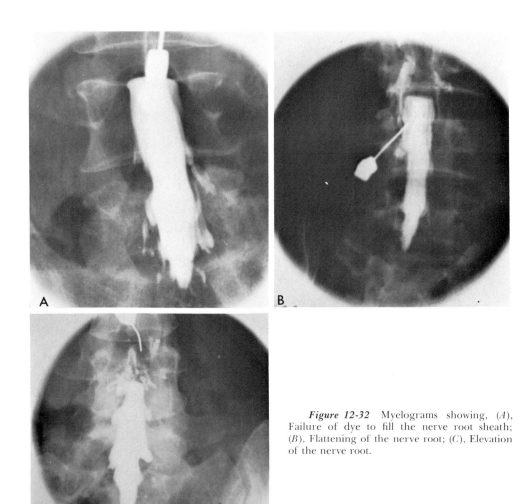

Figure 12-32 Myelograms showing, (*A*), Failure of dye to fill the nerve root sheath; (*B*), Flattening of the nerve root; (*C*), Elevation of the nerve root.

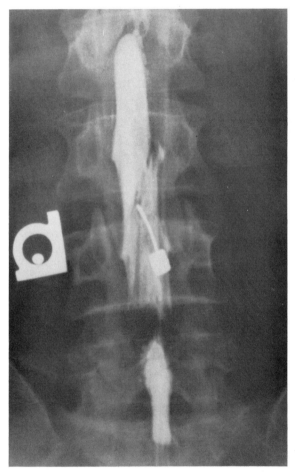

Figure 12-33 Myelogram showing "block defect" caused by a massive extrusion of nuclear material that permits some leakage of the dye past the obstruction. Observe the irregular shaggy outline at the level of the block.

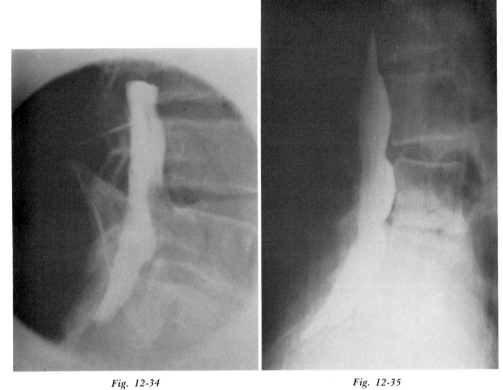

Fig. 12-34   ***Fig. 12-35***

Figure 12-34   Myelogram (lateral view) showing massive extrusion of nuclear material at the L4-L5 level. Observe that the lower portion of the defect lies opposite the vertebral body of L5, indicating downward migration of the extruded material.

Figure 12-35   Myelogram (lateral view) showing a defect in the column of dye caused by bone formed along the posterior superior rim of the fifth lumbar vertebra. This finding was confirmed at operation.

Many factors produce false readings of myelograms. Among these are: injection of the dye in the extra subarachnoid space, artifacts produced by the needle, abnormal configurations of the subarachnoid space, hypertrophy of the ligamentum flavum, osteophytes at the posterior margins of the vertebral bodies, adhesions of the arachnoid membrane and adhesions inside and outside the nerve root sheath. Likewise false negative readings may be made when the extrusion occupies an extreme lateral position and is not in contact with the dural sac; negative readings are abnormalities of the dural sac, such as short cul-de-sac, and faulty technique.

In summary, our position is simply this: myelography should not be done routinely to establish the diagnosis and the level of the lumbar disc lesion; the clinical picture in all but exceptional cases, is sufficiently clear to make the diagnosis. Myelography is not an innocuous procedure and should be reserved for those cases in which the clinical picture is not clear and when there is evidence suggesting the possibility of some other lesion. It should never be performed just to satisfy inquiries which might arise from medico-legal action. There are many factors which may produce a false positive or a false negative reading. Finally, if the investigation is to be done, it should be performed by one who is expert in the technique and competent to read the radiographs accurately.

Discography

We have never been convinced that discography is justified to establish the site of the pathology in lesions of the lumbar discs. What has been expressed concerning myelography is also true of discography; that is, that the diagnosis of lumbar disc lesions in the majority of the patients can be made on the clinical manifestations alone and that routine discography is not necessary.

Although the procedure is often referred to as a simple, harmless test, it must be admitted that this is far from the truth. Long term observations relating to the fate of lumbar discs following puncture of the annulus and injecting a foreign material in the naturally chemically unstable nucleus pulposus have never been reported. Such a study should include the late observations on normal and degenerated discs. In practice, more than one disc is usually injected with the radio-opaque substance, so that many normal discs are punctured needlessly. In our experience, in several cases, simply puncturing asymptomatic discs in the cervical region has produced spontaneous fusion of the adjacent vertebrae with obliteration of the intervening disc. In these instances, saline was injected into the nucleus pulposus and distended. (This is the so called distension test which we employ to isolate the symptomatic cervical disc. See page 90). Whether further insult was added to an already degenerated nucleus pulposus or whether the puncture and distension initiated a pathologic process terminating in destruction of a normal disc is not clear. This sequel was noted in cervical discs and it is reasonable to assume that it may also occur in lumbar discs subjected to the same test.

There is no doubt that discography has provided many answers related to the pathologic process that occurs in lumbar and cervical disc lesions, but it is very doubtful that it is selective enough to justify its routine use. Also, in our study of the cervical spine after anterior fusion was performed, many patients exhibited rapid degeneration of the disc above or below the fused segment. Was this degenerative process initiated or accentuated by the distension test, or did the increased stress at these sites following fusion of a segment of the cervical spine evoke the pathological process?

REFERENCES

1. Aird, R. B. and Noffziger, J. C.: Prolonged jugular compression; New diagnostic test of neurologic value. Proc. Amer. Neurol Assoc. 66:45-49, 1940.
2. Armstrong, J. R.: Lumbar disc lesions. Baltimore, Williams & Wilkins, 1965.
3. Aronson, H. A. et al.: Herniated upper lumbar discs. J. Bone Joint Surg. 45-A:311-317, 1963.
4. Bartelink, D. L.: The role of abdominal pressure in relieving the pressure on the lumbar intervertebral discs, J. Bone Joint Surg. 39-B:718-725, 1957.

5. Batson, O. V.: The Valsalva maneuver and the vertebral vein system. Angiology 11:443-447, 1960.
6. Batts, M., Jr.: Rupture of nucleus pulposus: Anatomical study. J. Bone Joint Surg. 21:121-126, 1939.
7. Begg, A. C. et al.: Myelography in lumbar intervertebral disk lesions: A correlation with operative findings. Brit. J. Surg. 34:141-157, 1946.
8. Begg, A. C. and Falconer, M. A.: Plain radiography in intraspinal protrusion of lumbar intervertebral disks: Correlation with operative findings. Brit. J. Surg. 36:225-239, 1949.
9. Begg, A. C.: Nuclear herniations of the intervertebral disc. Their radiological manifestations and significance. J. Bone Joint Surg. 36-B:180-193, 1954.
10. Brown, H. A. and Pont, M. E.: Disease of lumbar discs: Ten years of surgical treatment. J. Neurosurg. 20:410-417, 1963.
11. Dandy, W. E.: Concealed ruptured intervertebral disks: A plea for elimination of contrast mediums in diagnosis. J.A.M.A. 117:821-823, 1941.
12. Eie, N. et al.: Measurements of the intra-abdominal pressure in relation to weight bearing of the lumbosacral spine. J. Oslo City Hosp. 12:205-217, 1962.
13. Falconer, M. A., McGeorge, M. and Begg, A. C.: Observations on cause and mechanism of symptom-production in sciatica and low-back pain. J. Neurol. Neurosurg. and Psychiat. 11:13-26, 1948.
14. Fletcher, G. H.: Backward displacement of fifth lumbar vertebra in degenerative disc disease: Significance of difference in antero-posterior diameters of fifth lumbar and first sacral vertebrae. J. Bone Joint Surg. 29:1019-1026, 1947.
15. Foerster, O.: The dermatomes in man. Brain 56:1-39, 1933.
16. Gasser, H. S.: Pain-producing impulses in peripheral nerves. A. Research Nerv. and Ment. Dis. 23:44-62, 1943.
17. Hamilton, W. F. et al.: Physiologic relationships between intra-thoracic, intra-spinal and arterial pressures. J.A.M.A. 107:853-856, Sept. 12, 1936.
18. Head, H.: Studies in neurology. London, Oxford University Press, 1920.
19. Hendry, N. G. C.: The hydration of the nucleus pulposus and its relation to intervertebral disc derangement. J. Bone Joint Surg. 40-B:132-144, 1958.
20. Höffken: Der röntgenologische Nochweis von Spaltbildungen un Zwischenwirbelscheiben. Zbl. Chir. 716, 1951.
21. Inman, V. T. and Saunders, J. B. de C. M.: Referred pain from skeletal structures. J. Nerv. and Ment. Dis. 99:660-667, 1944.
22. Inman, V. T. and Saunders, J. B. de C. M: Anatomico-physiological aspects of injuries to intervertebral disc. J. Bone Joint Surg. 29:461-475, 1947.
23. Keegan, J. J.: Dermatome hypalgesia associated with herniation of intervertebral disk. Arch. Neurol. and Psychiat. 50:67-83, July, 1943.
24. Lansche, W. E. et al.: Correlation of the myelogram with clinical and operative findings in lumbar disc lesions. J. Bone Joint Surg. 42-A:193-206, 1960.
25. Lewis, T.: Pain. New York, Macmillan, 1942.
26. Lasègue, C.: Considérations sur la sciatique. Arch. Gén. de Méil 2 (Série 6, Tome 4):558-580,1864.
27. Magnusson, W.: Über die Bedingungen des Hervortretens der wirklichen Gelenkspalte auf dem Röntgenbilde. Acta. Radiol. (Stockh.) 18:733-741, 1937.
28. Morris, J. M. et al.: Role of the trunk in stability of the spine. J. Bone Joint Surg. 43-A:327-351, 1961.
29. Neidner, F.: Zur kenntnis der normalen und pathologischen anatomie der wirbelkörper-randleisten. Fortschr. Röntgenstr. 46:628, 1932.
30. Ratheke, L.: Über kalkablagerungen in den Zwischenwirbelscheiben. Fortschr. Röntgenstr. 45, 1932.
31. Reitan, H.: On movements of fluid inside the cerebrospinal space. Acta Radiol. 22:762-779, 1941.
32. Schmorl, G. and Junghanns, H.: The human spine in health and disease. New York, Grune & Stratton, 1959.
33. Sherrington, C. S.: Experiments in examination of the peripheral distribution of the fibers of the posterior roots of some spinal nerves. Phila. Trans., Roy. Soc. Lond. 184-B:641-763, 1893.
34. Valsalva, A. M.: De Ame Humana Tractatus. Bologna, 1704.
35. Viets, H. R.: Two new signs suggestive of cauda equina tumor. New Eng. J. Med. 198:671-674, 1928.
36. Willis, T. A.: Lumbosacral anomalies. J. Bone Joint Surg. 41-A:935-938, 1959.
37. Woodhall, B. et al.: The well-leg-raising test of Fajerstajn in the diagnosis of ruptured lumbar intervertebral disc. J. Bone Joint Surg. 32-A:786-792, 1950.

Chapter 13

CONGENITAL AND ACQUIRED ABNORMALITIES OF THE LUMBAR SPINE
(Their Relation to Back or Back and Leg Pain)

Mechanical dysfunction in the lumbosacral region is undoubtedly the commonest cause of low back pain. The impairment of function resulting from disintegration of the lower lumbar discs is responsible for back pain or back pain with sciatica in the majority of the patients. This truth must not close our eyes and minds to the fact that there are other sources of mechanical dysfunction in the lower lumbar spine and that if each source is critically analyzed and understood, appropriate therapeutic measures can be instituted to relieve the patient of his symptoms. Too often, the primary mechanical disorder and the structures involved are not clear to the physician or surgeon; hence, the intensity and even the veracity of the complaints are too often underestimated. The suffering patient is treated in a casual manner by half-way measures, producing the inevitable results: discouragement and disillusionment for the patient, and pessimism for the attending physician.

Man's intense desire to stand on his hind legs in order to free his upper limbs for prehensile purposes has been fulfilled at a price; the greatest portion of which has been assumed by the lower lumbar and lumbosacral regions. Even under the most ideal conditions, these regions are made to meet functional demands which are beyond their capacity. It is for this

6. Spina bifida with a long spinous process of the fifth lumbar vertebra
7. Abnormalities of the spinal canal
8. Rotational deformities of the lower lumbar vertebrae
9. Tropism of the articular facets

Spondylolysis

Spondylolysis is a relatively common abnormality; one or both of the neural arches may be affected. Essentially it is characterized by a defect in the neural arch midway between the superior and inferior articular facets. It differs from spondylolisthesis in that there is no forward displacement of the vertebral body of the affected neural arches (Fig. 13-1). Some believe that the defect is developmental in origin while others favor the concept that the zone of dissolution through the neural arch is the result of excessive stress comparable to fatigue fractures.[5, 13, 16] The authors have seen and reported one case in which dissolution of both neural arches occurred in a vertebra (L3) proximal to a fusion mass;[3] radiographs taken before the operation showed the arches to be intact. The defect is readily seen in good

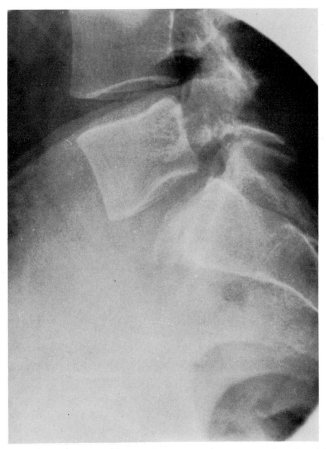

Figure 13-1 Spondylolysis. Observe the defect in the neural arch of L5 midway between the superior and inferior articular facets. The L5 disc is thin and there is some irregular sclerosis of the bone on either side of the defect in the neural arch.

oblique views of the lumbar spine. In long standing cases, the line of the defect is irregular and the adjacent bone is dense and sclerotic.

Many of these defects are found accidentally; they cause no symptoms. When they are symptomatic, the patient usually experiences mild deep-seated pain in the lumbar region; occasionally, in an acute episode, the pain (scleratogenous pain) may be referred to the gluteal areas and even to the posterior aspect of the thighs. This referred pain is never the dominant complaint. In uncomplicated cases, radicular pain is never a feature of the clinical picture and the patient is rarely completely incapacitated. The symptoms are usually aggravated by activity and relieved by rest.

The physical examination is not revealing. Generally, there is a free range of motion in the spine; there may be some pain at the extremes of extension; mild muscle spasm may be present and there are no associated motor, sensory or reflex changes.

This lesion, however, may co-exist with a degenerative disc of the same motor unit (Fig. 13-1). In such a case, if the disc lesion is symptomatic, the patient exhibits all the clinical manifestations of a lumbar disc lesion. What relationship the spondylitic defect has to the degenerative lesion of the disc is not clear; but it is reasonable to assume that the instability of the abnormal motor unit may add considerable abnormal stress to the disc, thereby enhancing the pathologic process.

Spondylolisthesis

Of all the congenital variations encountered in the lumbar spine, spondylolisthesis is most frequently associated with pain in the lumbosacral region and it is frequently associated with sciatica. The main features are: dissolution of both neural arches between the superior and inferior articular facets and forward migration of the vertebral body on the lower vertebra (Fig. 13-2). In most instances, the defect occurs in the fifth lumbar vertebra, but it may occur in the fourth and, in rare cases, in the third. Although not common, it also may occur in two contiguous vertebrae. Much has been written on the etiology of this lesion without agreement among most of the investigators. What is clear, however, is that heredity plays a role in many instances. The authors' files contain several incidents of both father and son showing identical lesions.[7, 12, 13]

This lesion exhibits several characteristic features; the forward displacement of the vertebral bone is easily recognized in lateral views of the spine. The degree of forward slipping varies from patient to patient; there may be only minimal displacement or the body may be completely displaced in relation to the vertebral body below (Figs. 13-3 and 13-4).

In some individuals, the forward displacement of the body reaches a certain point on the lower body and stops; in others, the migration continues until the vertebra is in front of the lower vertebra. This latter phenomenon was seen in two cases in our series and the progressive displacement was easily demonstrable in serial radiographs taken at six-month intervals.

If the fifth lumbar vertebra is involved, as the vertebral body proceeds

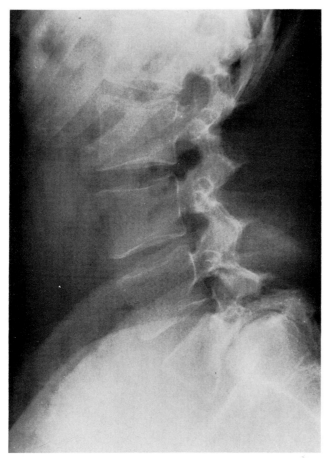

Figure 13-2 Spondylolisthesis with marked forward displacement of the fifth lumbar vertebra on the sacrum. There is severe degeneration of the intervertebral disc between L5 and S1. The defects in the neural arches of L5 are clearly seen.

forward the configuration of the lumbar spine at the affected level is markedly altered. The features characteristic of the displacement vary in severity depending on the degree of slippage. The posterior elements of L5 (those lying posterior to the neural arch defects) maintain their normal anatomic relation to the posterior elements of the sacrum below, while the anterior elements move forward with the spinal column. Now the anterior aspect of the spinal canal is markedly distorted and compromised by the ledge formed by the upper and posterior margins of the sacrum. In later life, the formation of osteophytes along this ledge increase its size considerably. The intervertebral foramen at the L5-S1 level are widened in their anteroposterior diameters. A similar deformation occurs in the dural sac; and to this must be added the indentation on the posterior wall of the dura made by the lamina of the fourth lumbar vertebra as the entire spinal column moves forward (Fig. 13-5).

It becomes apparent from the description of the abnormality that we are dealing with a very unstable motor unit, which is often the site of advanced degenerative alterations frequently noted in middle-aged and elderly patients. This instability undoubtedly has a pernicious effect on the

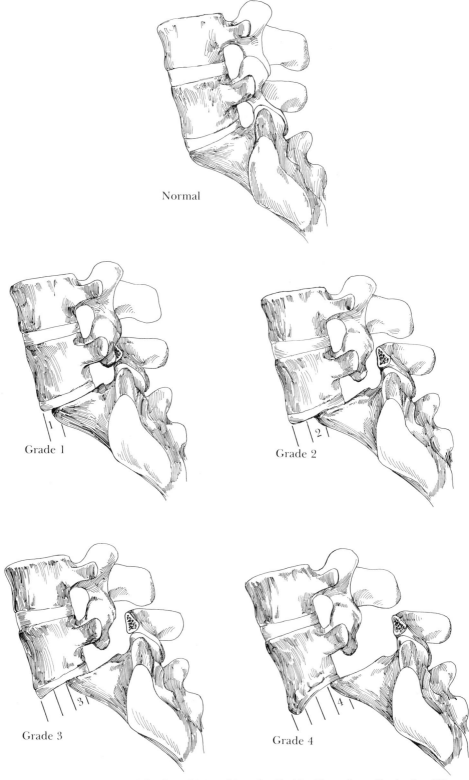

Figure 13-3   Degrees of slipping of L5 on S1 as classified by Meyerding—Grades I to IV.

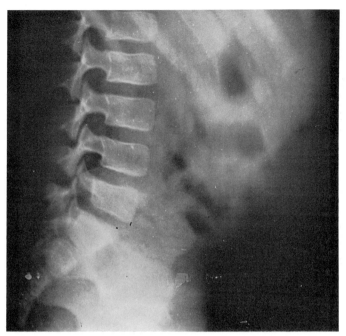

Figure 13-4 Spondylolisthesis at the L5-S1 level in a child 6 years old. There is only minimal forward displacement of L5 on S1. The defects in the posterior neural arches of L5 are clearly seen.

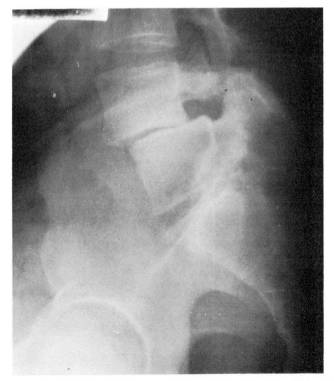

Figure 13-5 Spondylolisthesis. Observe the forward displacement of L4 on L5, thinning of the L4-L5 disc, sclerosis of the vertebral bodies of L4 and L5, and distortion of the spinal canal anteriorly by the upper and posterior margin of L5 and posteriorly by the laminae of L3.

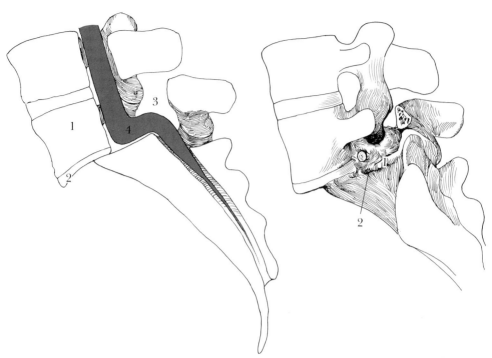

Figure 13-6 Pathologic changes that occur in an established spondylolisthesis: *A.*, (1) Forward displacement of L5 on S1. (2) Thinning of the L5 disc. (3) Widening of the anteroposterior diameter of the intervertebral foramen. (4) Deformation of the spinal canal. *B.*, (1) Formation and accumulation of fibrocartilaginous tissue within the foramen. (2) The nerve root is enmeshed in fibrous tissue.

disc immediately below the displaced vertebra. The disc often undergoes rapid and severe degeneration. This instability also is responsible for advanced proliferative soft tissue changes which produce large irregular masses of fibrous tissue, fibrocartilaginous and even osteocartilaginous tissue, all of which crowd the site of the defect in the pars interarticularis and spill over into the intervertebral foramina. In the latter position, the nerve roots become emmeshed in and pressed by the reactive tissue. In addition, posterior protrusion of nuclear material may further compromise the spinal canal and the intervertebral foramina (Fig. 13-6). An interesting variation of this deformity is spondylolisthesis associated with an exaggerated lumbosacral angle. In these cases, the posterior elements, the spinous process, the laminae and the inferior articular processes form a tight band of osseous tissue across the posterior aspect of the dural sac which indents the dura. When the posterior elements are removed, the dura actually bulges through the defect in the posterior spinal column.

The types and sources of pain now should be clear. The markedly disrupted and unstable motor unit alone is capable of producing deep-seated low back pain and referred pain to the posterior aspect of the thighs and gluteal regions. Encroachment of the nerve roots by tough, dense, fibrous tissue in and about the intervertebral foramina may occur, producing radicular pain.[1, 4] Rarely are both roots involved. This is due to rotation of the vertebra as it slips forward so that one or the other root may be spared. The roots traversing the foramina are affected, that is, the L4 roots in the L4-L5 foramina and the L5 roots in the L5-S1 foramina. The nerve roots may also be implicated before they enter the foramina. It was pointed out that in spondylolisthesis the spinal canal is compromised by the ledge formed by the posterior rim of the caudal vertebra as the cephalic vertebra migrates forward. If the displacement is severe, the posterior ledge may exert considerable pressure on the nerve roots as they pursue their course to their respective foramina. Lesions involving the fourth lumbar vertebra implicate the fifth lumbar roots; and those involving the fifth lumbar vertebra, the first sacral root.

The clinical manifestations of spondylolisthesis are fairly typical of a mechanical disorder. Once the symptoms are initiated, the patient has some constant back discomfort which is aggravated by activity and relieved by rest. These are periods in which the pain is more intense than others, but, unless the picture is complicated by a severe bout of sciatica, total incapacitation is rare. The patients are seldom aware of any sensory or motor deficits; however, the presenting complaint of one patient in our series was difficulty in function of the bladder and rectal sphincters. The bouts of pain tend to increase in intensity and duration with the passage of time. At this point it should be pointed out that in some persons even severe displacement gives rise to no disability. It is not uncommon to see a middle-aged or elderly person with spondylolisthesis who, except for some occasional mild discomfort, was never aware of any back disorder (Fig. 13-7). On the other hand, we have yet to see the individual who, once the back

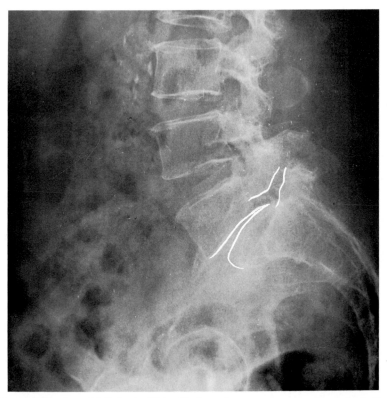

Figure 13-7 Spondylolisthesis. This elderly patient was unaware of any back disorder except for occasional mild discomfort. The disc is completely replaced by fibrous tissue or perphaps even bone that is stabilizing this motor unit.

really becomes symptomatic, was ever completely free of some discomfort and disability. Although symptomatic spondylolisthesis is usually encountered in adults, not infrequently patients in their teens (and we have seen three cases under ten years of age) have symptoms of such severity that their routine daily activities are curtailed.

The objective features of this syndrome are fairly characteristic of the lesion. In the absence of any radicular pain the patient exhibits no postural scoliosis, but there is always present an exaggeration of the lumbar curve and a visible "step-off" or dimple in the midline at the site of the abnormality.

Occasionally mild muscle spasm is demonstrable and, in most instances, some tenderness can be elicited by making firm pressure directly over the lesion. Movements in all directions are usually freely executed except that on hyperextension of the spine mild pain is evoked in most of the cases. In many, forward bending is limited and appears to be caused by shortening of the posterior structures of the legs.

In the presence of unilateral or bilateral sciatica of the nonradicular type the clinical picture is that of a typical lumbar disc lesion with implication of a nerve root.

Radiographs, particularly the lateral views, confirm the diagnosis. Even the slightest amount of forward slipping of the body of the affected vertebra is readily discernible, and the oblique views disclose the dissolution of both neural arches between the superior and inferior articular facets (Fig. 13-8).

Exaggerated Lumbosacral Angle

Accentuation of the lordotic curve is a relatively common abnormality. In some such lumbar spines, the sacrum lies almost in a horizontal position (Fig. 13-9). It was previously noted that the lumbosacral region is anatomically and phylogenetically poorly adapted to meet the functional demands of the upright position which man has assumed. An increase in the lumbar curve increases the stresses applied to the lumbosacral spine, the greatest stress falling on the posterior articulations between L4 and L5 and L5 and S1. Also, the intervertebral discs at these levels are subjected to unusually abnormal stresses and, in many instances, show evidence of rapid degeneration. In the uncomplicated cases the patients experience a deepseated discomfort or even moderate to severe pain in the lumbar region. The pain is due to the abnormal stresses acting on the posterior elements of the last two lumbar vertebrae. A contributing factor in the production of the pain may be degeneration of one or both of the last two lumbar discs. It is not uncommon for a typical lumbar disc lesion to develop in these spines. When this occurs, the patient exhibits clinical manifestations of a lumbar disc lesion with or without monoradicular pain. In our experience, this abnormality is more prevalent in women.

The clinical picture is characterized by a constant discomfort in the lower back which may progress to mild or even severe pain when the spine performs strenuous activity. Walking and standing tend to aggravate the

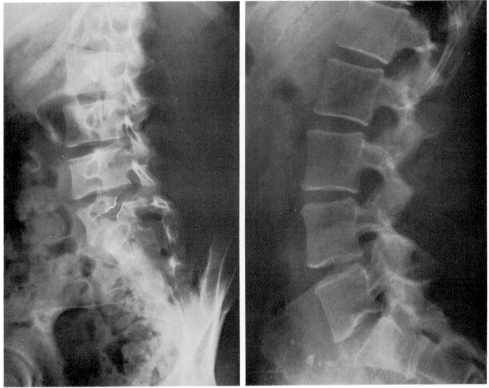

Fig. 13-8   *Fig. 13-9*

Figure 13-8   Spondylolisthesis, oblique view. The defects in the neural arches of L5 are clearly seen; note the wide separation between superior and inferior facets of L5.

Figure 13-9   Lumbar spine with an exaggerated lumbosacral angle. The posterior articulations between L4 and L5, and L5 and S1 are subjected to abnormal shearing stresses.

pain, and rest tends to relieve it. Occasionally the pain is referred to the gluteal areas and at times to the posterior aspect of the thighs; rarely does it extend below the knees.

Examination reveals the obvious increase in the lumbar curve; mild muscle spasm may be present. Movements of the spine are relatively free, except that there is usually some limitation of forward motion due to shortening of the soft tissue structures of the lower back and lower extremities. At the extreme of extension some pain is generally felt. Pressure over the spinous processes of L4 and L5 invariably elicits tenderness. There are no motor, sensory or reflex abnormalities.

In the event that the situation is complicated by a lumbar disc lesion, then the patient shows all the typical features of this lesion, especially if one of the lower nerve roots is involved (Fig. 13-10).

Radiographic study clearly demonstrates the accentuated lumbar curve, and if a lesion of one or both of the discs is present there may be narrowing of the affected vertebral interspace and reactive changes in the adjacent vertebrae. In long standing cases, there may be varying degrees of

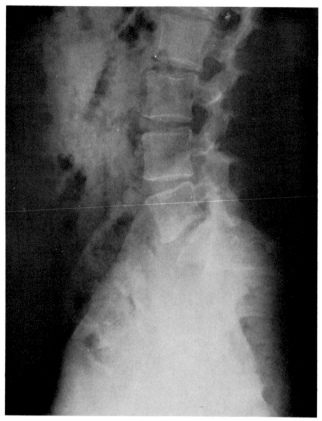

Figure 13-10   Lumbar spine with an exaggerated lumbosacral angle. Note the narrowing of the L4 and L5 discs; this is indicative of degeneration of the nucleus pulposus at both levels.

subluxation of the posterior articular facets of the involved motor unit and evidence of arthritic changes in the posterior articulations.

In severe forms of this abnormality, we are of the opinion that one source of pain is the firm pressure that the posterior elements of the fifth vertebra make on the dural sac. At operation the posterior elements resemble a bony band constricting the dural sac, much like a tight collar around a thick neck. The effect of this constriction is two-fold: it irritates the sensory nerve endings in the dura, and it narrows the anteroposterior diameter of the spinal canal. Should even a small nuclear extrusion appear at this level the nerve root would most likely be compressed against the anterior surface of the lamina.

Increase or Decrease in the Number of Free Lumbar Vertebrae

Variations in the number of free lumbar vertebrae are relatively common. They arise either from lumbarization of the first sacral vertebra, or from sacralization of the last lumbar vertebra, or by a reduction or increase

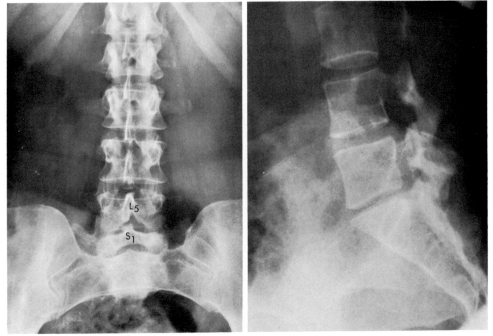

Fig. 13-11   *Fig. 13-12*

Figure 13-11   Lumbar spine showing six free vertebrae. The last vertebra is transitional; it has neither the pure characteristics of a lumbar or a sacral vertebra.

Figure 13-12   Lateral view of the lumbar spine depicted in Fig. 13-11. The disc between the last free vertebra and the sacrum is symmetrically narrowed; this is a congenital development that may undergo degeneration.

in the number of thoracic vertebrae. It is very doubtful that these abnormalities per se play a primary role in the production of low back pain. However, implication of one of the lower lumbar discs is a common finding associated with these variations. Whether or not the mechanics of the lower spine is altered sufficiently to predispose this region to degeneration of lumbar discs is not clear. Radiological examination clearly reveals the presence of four or six lumbar vertebrae. In order to determine accurately the number of lumbar vertebrae present, the radiographs should visualize the thoracolumbar region (Figs. 13-11 and 13-12).

Sacralization (Partial or Complete) of the L5 Vertebra and Lumbarization (Partial or Complete) of the S1 Vertebra

These are common abnormalities, and their frequency and variations emphasize the transitional state of development in the lumbosacral region. It appears as if nature is trying all combinations in an attempt to find an arrangement that will be stable and yet meet the functional demands of the erect position. The transverse processes of the fifth lumbar vertebra show considerable variation in size. They may completely fuse with the sacrum or form a false joint with it; this partial or complete sacralization may be unilateral or bilateral. The vertebra may be seated deep in the pelvis and its

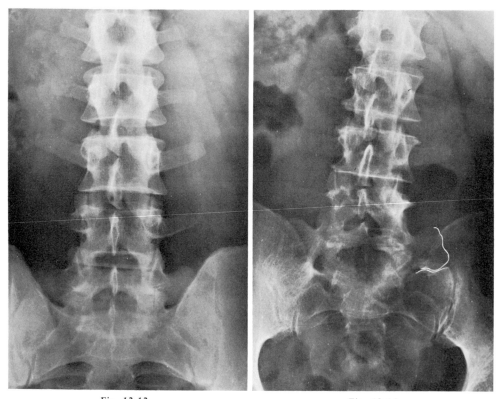

Fig. 13-13   *Fig. 13-14*

Figure 13-13   Incomplete sacralization of the fifth lumbar vertebra. The tranverse processes are larger than normal, but they are free and make no contact with the sacrum.

Figure 13-14   Incomplete sacralization of the fifth lumbar vertebra. The large massive transverse process on the left is incorporated into the body of the sacrum, whereas the one on the right forms a false joint with the sacrum.

large transverse process may fail to make contact with the sacrum (Figs. 13-13 and 13-14).

What has been recorded for the fifth lumbar vertebra in relation to the sacrum is also true of the first sacral vertebra in relation to the ilium. As a rule, the disc between the transitional vertebra and the main body of the sacrum is vestigial and may be completely devoid of any nuclear material. However, this rudimentary disc may undergo degenerative changes which may produce symptoms. If a lumbar disc lesion should develop, the affected disc is proximal to the rudimentary disc (Figs. 13-15 and 13-16).

The abnormalities per se may be the source of low back pain and in some incidences of radicular pain. Pain may arise from arthritic changes in the pseudo joint between the enlarged transverse processes and the sides of the pelvis; it may be evoked by degenerative changes in the vestigial disc; and finally, the altered mechanics, when the transitional vertebra is settled deep in the pelvis, may be the source of pain. It was previously noted that radicular pain may also be associated with some of these abnormalities. This is achieved by irritation of a nerve root whose downward course in the

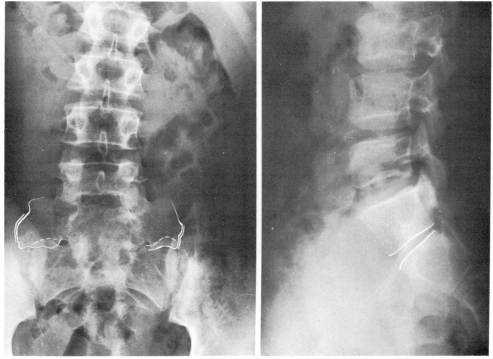

Fig. 13-15   Fig. 13-16

Figure 13-15   The transitional vertebra is the first sacral vertebra. Its lateral masses (designed to be transverse processes) form false joints with the body of the sacrum.

Figure 13-16   The lateral view of the lumbar spine depicted in Fig. 13-15 reveals the vestigial nature of the disc between the transitional vertebra and the main body of the sacrum.

pelvis happens to be in the vicinity of the anterior surface of a pseudo joint undergoing degenerative changes. The nerve roots involved are either the fourth or the fifth; the first sacral root passes too far below the site of the false joint to be implicated. The fourth root is involved when the transverse process of the fifth lumbar vertebra participates in the formation of the false joint, and the fifth lumbar root when the first sacral vertebra is the participant (Fig. 13-17).

Radiological examination clearly reveals the characteristic features of the abnormalities. Degenerative changes at the pseudarthrosis are made evident by irregularity of the opposed joint surfaces, subchondral sclerosis on one or both sides of the joint line and, in advanced lesions, hypertrophic bone formation at the margins of the joint (Fig. 13-17). The vestigial disc is narrower than the normal discs and, if degeneration has occurred, the characteristic features of an arthritic joint are discernible. The interspace may be further collapsed, spurring at the margins of the vertebrae and condensation of subchondral bone.

Clinically, the patient presents the picture of a mechanical back disorder. Pain is localized at the site of the false joint and pressure over this area

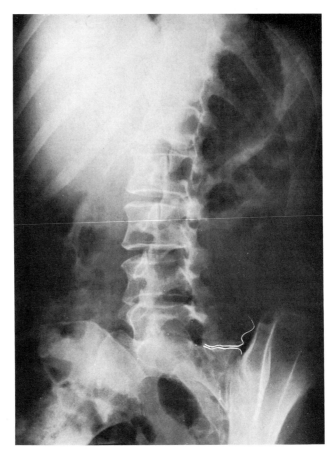

Figure 13-17 The right transverse process of the fifth lumbar vertebra forms a false joint with the sacrum. The joint shows evidence of degeneration. In this instance, the patient presented evidence of implication of the fourth lumbar root.

elicits tenderness. Some muscle spasm may be present, usually on the side of the lesion. Movements of the spine are somewhat limited, especially extension and lateral flexion. A dull back pain is always present and is accentuated by certain movements and by activity; it is relieved by rest. Motor, sensory and reflex deficits are absent.

If the fifth or the fourth lumbar root is irritated or if a lumbar disc lesion above the transitional vertebra is affected and is associated with nerve root irritation, then all the clinical manifestations of a lumbar disc lesion are present. When considering the differential diagnosis between back pain with nonradicular pain arising from a true disc lesion and root irritation associated with degenerative changes in a false joint, it should be remembered that the syndrome produced by the latter mechanism is relatively rare, whereas that evoked by the former is common. Also, the clinical manifestations characteristic of involvement of a certain nerve root should correspond to the root most likely to be affected by the false joint; for example, the fifth root, if the first sacral vertebra forms the false joint.

Spina Bifida With Long Spinous Process of L5 Vertebra

Failure of fusion of the posterior bony elements in the midline of the fifth lumbar or first sacral vertebrae produces a posterior defect in the neural arches known as spina bifida. The abnormality is common and we doubt that it, per se, is cause for back pain. Many of these deformations are associated with true lumbar disc lesions; but there is no evidence that the presence of the defect renders the lower lumbar discs more vulnerable.

There is one exception: a spina bifida of the first sacral vertebra may co-exist with an abnormally long spinous process of the fifth lumbar vertebra. Low back pain may be initiated by pressure of the long spinous process on the soft tissues covering the posterior defect in the first sacral vertebra when the spine is extended. This is particularly true if the lordosis of the lumbar spine is congenitally accentuated. The patients complain of a dull constant ache directly in the midline, and extension of the spine aggravates the pain.

Radiographs show the midline defect in the fifth lumbar or first sacral vertebra and also the elongation of the spinous process of the fifth lumbar vertebra. The close proximity of the spinous process to the defect is more fully appreciated when this region is exposed surgically.

Abnormalities of the Spinal Canal

A rare developmental anomaly is congenital narrowing of the lumbar or lumbosacral spinal canal. In some instances, it is responsible for a symptom complex markedly different from that of lumbar disc lesions. Plain radiography does not give enough information to make the diagnosis because all the osseous elements appear to be of normal proportions; however, myelography readily discloses the abnormal configuration of the spinal canal.[9, 10, 12]

The clinical picture is characterized by low back pain and evidence of multiple nerve root involvement as noted by the diffuse motor, sensory and reflex changes. One distinguishing feature is the appearance of the symptoms when the patient is in the erect position, such as standing and walking, and the relief of symptoms when the patient lies down.[11] Awareness of this congenital anomaly is most important in establishing the diagnosis.

Other abnormalities which may compromise the spinal canal in the lumbosacral region are: spondylolisthesis, severe exaggeration of the lumbosacral angle and spina bifida of the first sacral vertebra associated with a long spinous process of the fifth lumbar vertebra which dips into the defect. These variations have already been discussed.

Rotational Deformities of the Lower Lumbar Vertebrae

Not infrequently developmental rotational deformities of the lower lumbar vertebrae are encountered. The fourth and fifth lumbar vertebrae or the fifth alone are most commonly involved. This rotational deformity is independent of the rotation of lumbar vertebrae associated with idiopathic scoliosis or scoliosis due to multiple congenital malformations of the vertebrae such as hemivertebrae. The abnormality may be accompanied by other developmental defects that occur in this region.

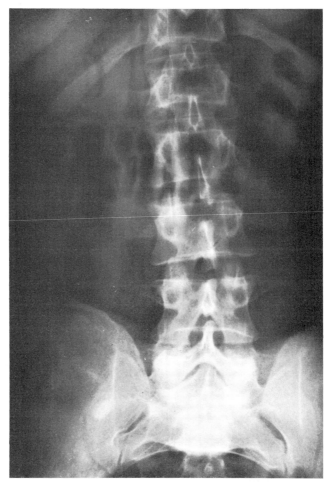

Figure 13-18   Rotational deformity. There is a mild rotational deformity of the last three lumbar vertebrae. Lesions of the discs and degenerative changes both of the discs and the posterior intervertebral joints may complete this abnormality.

The abnormal mechanics of the lumbosacral spine produced by the rotational deformity plays a major role in the early development of degenerative changes both in the intervertebral joint and in the posterior intervertebral joints. Before the development of degenerative changes, there may be mild back pain which is aggravated by activity and relieved by rest; later when degenerative changes are well advanced, the clinical manifestations become more pronounced and continuous. Radicular pain is absent and there are no motor, sensory or reflex changes. However, there may be deep-seated referred pain to the gluteal regions and to the posterior aspect of the thighs.

At any time these abnormalities may be complicated by a true lumbar disc lesion. In the event that this occurs, the patient shows the typical clinical manifestations of this lesion.

Radiological examination shows the nature of the deformity; later, when the degenerative changes are established, these also are readily identified (Fig. 13-18).

Asymmetric Posterior Intervertebral Joints

Much has been written on tropism of the posterior articulations, especially those at the lumbosacral level. At one time, many observers were of the opinion that this asymmetry was responsible in a large measure for chronic low back pain and also that this arrangement made the lumbosacral articulations vulnerable to even minor stresses.[12, 13]

Anatomic studies of the lumbosacral region reveal that asymmetry of the planes of the joints at the lumbosacral level is very common; in fact, it is more prevalent than the symmetrical arrangement. It is our opinion that tropism of the lumbosacral articulations alone cannot be considered as a causative factor in the production of low back pain (Fig. 13-19).

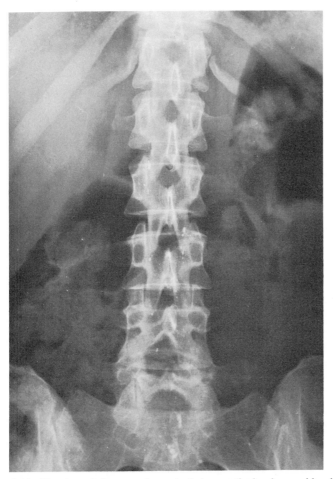

Figure 13-19 Tropism of the posterior articulations at the lumbosacral level. Note that the articular surface of the left articulation is in the sagittal plane, whereas that on the right is in the coronal plane.

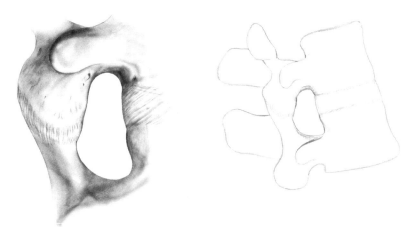

Figure 13-20   Boundaries of the intervertebral foramina. These comprise: anteriorly, the posterior and lateral aspects of the vertebral bodies and the disc; and posteriorly, the posterior intervertebral joint.

ACQUIRED ABNORMALITIES OF THE LUMBOSACRAL REGION

At this juncture we are primarily concerned with the pathologic processes capable of compromising the lower lumbar canal and the intervertebral foramina. Those disease processes which produce gross and obvious destruction and disfiguration of the motor units will not be discussed but just mentioned. Essentially these are such diseases as: osteomyelitis, tuberculosis, syphilis, fractures and fracture-dislocations of the lumbar spine. It should be remembered that some anatomic features of the lower lumbar canal and foramina render them receptive to distortion and narrowing.

There is considerable variation in the size and shape of the lumbar canal. It was previously recorded that the average anteroposterior depth of the canal is 17.4 mm. and its average width is 23.4 mm. However, these dimensions vary from person to person, and in some persons there is actually a constriction of the canal with all the osseous elements uniformly reduced in size. The configuration of the canal also varies considerably; it may be ovoid, triangular or trefoil.[1] The trefoil-shaped canal has long lateral recesses which render the lumbar roots particularly vulnerable to compression against the anterior surfaces of the laminae.

The intervertebral foramina are intimately related to the discs and the posterior articulations. The anterior boundary of a foramen is formed by the posterior and lateral aspect of the vertebral body and disc; the posterior boundary is formed by the posterior intervertebral articulations (Fig. 13-20). The lumbar foramina are, in essence, elongated canals which are five or six times the size of the lumbar roots traversing them. However, the width of the canals decreases from above downward, and the diameter of the roots increases. It becomes obvious that the last two lumbar roots have less room in their respective canals than the upper lumbar roots and are more likely to be compressed by space-occupying lesions.

Arthrosis of the Intervertebral and Posterior Intervertebral Joints

The lumbar spinal canal may be distorted and compromised by the formation of osteophytes on the posterior and posterolateral rims of the vertebral bodies. At autopsy these are common findings in elderly persons. Some nuclear material may extrude posteriorly, augmenting the size of the mass protruding into the spinal canal. In most instances, these lesions, if they should cause symptoms and do not directly irritate any nerve roots, produce a syndrome typical of osteoarthritis of the lumbar spine (Fig. 13-21).

Degenerative changes are usually encountered in middle life and in the elderly. The patients complain of a deep seated ache and stiffness in the lumbar spine which is aggravated by activity, relieved by rest and influenced by changes in weather. Periods of inactivity such as sitting or lying

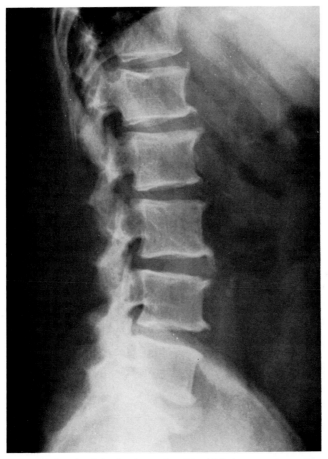

Figure 13-21   Arthrosis of the lumbar spine. Note (*A*) the posterior and anterior osteophytes; the former reduce the size of the intervertebral foramina; (*B*) the narrow discs and subchondral sclerosis of the adjacent vertebrae. This patient had backache but no radicular pain.

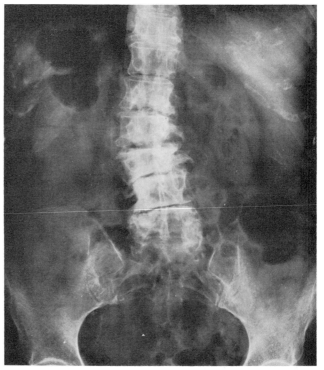

Figure 13-22   A spine with advanced degeneration of all the discs of the lumbar spine in an elderly patient. Observe the thinning of the discs, sclerosis of the vertebrae and marked bone proliferation along the peripheries of the vertebral bodies. This patient had radicular pain caused by irritation of the L4 and L5 nerve roots, bilaterally.

also aggravate the symptoms. Patients frequently volunteer the information that they "can't get started in the mornings" or that they "have to loosen up" before they experience some relief. Some poorly localized pain may be referred to the buttocks and the posterior aspect of the thighs; it is not of the radicular type. There are bouts of exacerbation of the pain but it is rarely so severe that the patient is incapacitated.

The objective clinical manifestations are never outstanding. Postural deformities are, as a rule, lacking although there may be some flattening of the lumbar spine. All movements are somewhat curtailed, muscle spasm is never severe and pressure over the spine may elicit only mild tenderness. There is no evidence of motor, sensory or reflex abnormalities. The characteristic feature observed by radiological examination readily establishes the diagnosis.

On the other hand, the posterior osteophytes may be of sufficient size to actually irritate some nerve roots before they leave the dura, producing a unilateral or bilateral sciatica. Now the clinical picture changes completely, and manifestations of nerve root irritation become evident. The patient may exhibit a postural scoliosis; the lumbar spine assumes a flattened configuration; movements are more restricted, especially extension and forward bending; the straight leg test is positive, usually on both sides.

Motor, sensory and reflex abnormalities may exist and correspond to the specific root or roots involved, either the fourth or fifth lumbar roots. In the presence of true radicular pain the symptoms due to degeneration of the spine become insignificant. It should be remembered that the possibility of extrusion of nuclear material, as occurs in uncomplicated lumbar disc lesions, does occur in the presence of arthrosis of the lumbar spine (Fig. 13-22).

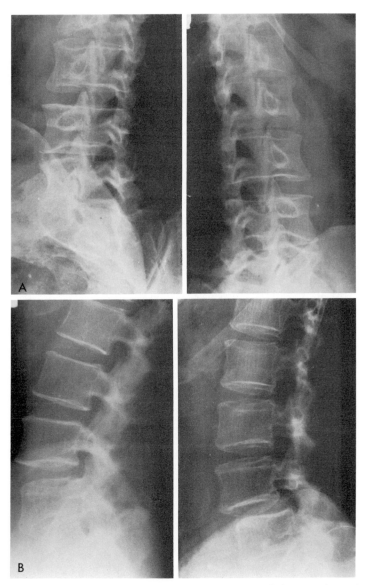

Figure 13-23 Arthrosis of intervertebral joint (L4-L5) and the posterior articulations with forward displacement of L4 on L5 in a 67-year-old patient. (*A*), Oblique views of the lumbar spine taken in 1961, showing normal alignment of the posterior articulations and no forward displacement of L4. (*B*), Radiographs taken in 1969 show marked displacement of L4 on L5.

The posterior boundary of the intervertebral foramina is formed by the posterior intervertebral joints. These joints are always involved to some degree in arthrosis of a motor unit. Spurring and osteophyte formation at the margins of the joints reduce the size of the foramina. When such a lesion co-exists with similar changes on the posterior rims of the vertebral bodies, the foramina may be profoundly compromised. The posterior articular joints are synovial joints; arthrosis involving the joints is associated with a proliferative reaction in the synovial membranes and capsule. Swelling and edema of these structures reduce the dimensions of the foramina.

Occasionally, as the result of degeneration of both the intervertebral and posterior intervertebral joints and of laxity of the ligamentous structures, marked instability of the motor unit occurs and the proximal vertebra tends to slide forward. This forward displacement of the body and the posterior osseous elements reduces the size and distorts the configuration of both the spinal canal and the foramina. It should be noted that when narrowing of the spinal canal and the foramina by the degenerative alterations just described occurs, a myelogram may depict a defect in the opaque column consistent with an extruded disc when no extrusion really exists (Fig. 13-23).

Another interesting factor producing narrowing of the canal is related to the shape of the spinal canal and the position of the articular facets. Articular facets are found at varying distances from the midline, depending upon the shape of the canal. Large osteophytes located on the margins of laterally situated facets are more likely to cause root pressure than medially placed facets. There are two other entities which are capable of compromising the spinal canal and the foramina. These are: Paget's disease and ankylosing spondylitis.

Paget's Disease (Osteitis Deformans)

The spine may be affected as a part of the generalized process in Paget's disease; the pelvis and lumbar spine may show more involvement than other parts of the skeletal system. Characteristic of this disease, the subperiosteal proliferation of bone produces a marked increase in the size of the affected bones in all dimensions. When the vertebrae are involved, both the body and the posterior elements become sclerotic and markedly thickened. Thickening of the pedicles and the laminae may encroach on the lumen of the spinal canal. Although this is true, we have never seen a patient with Paget's disease whose spinal column was so reduced in size that pressure of the cauda equina occurred; this is not true of the intervertebral foramina. Thickening of the bony elements forming the boundaries of the foramina produces a decided reduction in the size of the foramina. The roots may be irritated and even compressed. The phenomenon may implicate more than one foramen. It becomes apparent that all the clinical manifestations of nerve root irritation or compression may be superimposed on the clinical picture produced by Paget's disease. Many of these patients have profound involvement of the bones of the hip joint which causes not only pain in the

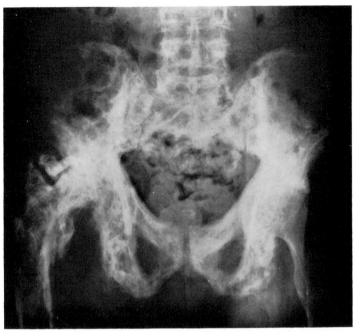

Figure 13-24 Generalized Paget's disease involving the entire skeleton. There is complete degeneration of both hips. This patient had true radicular pain caused by compression of the L5 nerve root. Thickening of the bony elements comprising the intervertebral foramen produced a reduction in the size of the foramen and compression of the nerve root.

region of the joint but also referred pain into the leg as far as the knee on the affected side. This must not be confused with radicular pain. Simple examination of the movements of the hip which are restricted and painful will establish the true source of the pain (Fig. 13-24).

Paget's disease of the lumbar spine, as elsewhere in the skeletal system, produces deep-seated pain in the low back; occasionally there may be diffuse poorly localized pain in the buttocks and the posterior aspects of the thighs. The pain is more or less constant but from time to time may become more intense. It does not have the characteristics of pain due to mechanical impairment; activity or rest influences its intensity very little. With implication of one or more roots the patient shows the signs and symptoms of nerve root irritation. There may be motor, sensory and reflex abnormalities, the nature of which depends on the roots affected. When nerve roots are involved in Paget's disease the radiating pain may be unrelenting and responds to no therapeutic measure short of decompression of the foramina. This differs from the pain caused by extruded nuclear material which after a reasonable period of time will reduce in size from shrinkage or will change its position in relation to the root so that tension in the root is lessened, thereby relieving the pain.

The diagnosis is easily established by the typical features seen in radiographs. Oblique views show the narrowing of the intervertebral foramina and the thickening of the boundaries of the foramina.

Ankylosing Spondylitis

This disorder is frequently seen in young adults, usually males. It is characterized by an inflammatory process involving primarily the soft tissue elements of the spine. The synovial membranes, capsules and ligaments of the joints of the spine become swollen, edematous and thickened; this is followed by calcification and eventually by ossification. The end result is bony ankylosis of all the affected joints. In ankylosing spondylitis the pathologic process is confined to the intervertebral joints, the posterior articular joints, the sacroiliac joints and the surrounding ligaments. The peripheral joints of the extremities are spared.

The proliferative process in the soft tissues in and about the intervertebral foramina (the capsules of the posterior joints, the ligamentum flavum and the posterior longitudinal ligament) narrows the outlets and may press and irritate the nerve roots traversing the bony canals. In addition, the sheaths of the nerves are involved so that the roots essentially are enmeshed and fixed in a mass of fibrous tissue. It becomes apparent that body movements tending to stretch the roots, such as flexing the leg when extended at the knee, will accentuate the pain in the back and leg.

Low back pain and sciatica are common complaints in all stages of this disorder, the incidence of sciatica being greater than generally realized. In the early stages, radiological examination is not informative, making the diagnosis very difficult. At this time the clinical picture may mimic that of a lumbar disc lesion. The authors have seen several patients, in the early stages of ankylosing spondylitis, in whom an erroneous diagnosis was made and who were subjected to exploration of the lower back. The early clinical picture does not unequivocally simulate that of a lumbar disc lesion. The low back pain is the first manifestation; the area of involvement is not localized to the lumbosacral region but spreads to the regions of the sacroiliac joints. Pain may be referred to the buttocks and the posterior aspects of the thighs. The syndrome is punctuated by remissions; the pain is not of a mechanical nature and is influenced by weather changes. The patient experiences considerable stiffness in the dorsal region and in the thoracic cage. Later, sciatica in one or both legs appears. All movements of the spine are restricted, especially forward bending. As time goes on, the lumbar spine is flattened, the patient begins to stoop forward, the cervical curve tends to be exaggerated and flexion contractures of the hips develop. Now the picture of ankylosing spondylitis is clearly evident and can be confirmed by radiological study, which reveals the characteristic changes in the posterior articulations and the sacroiliac joints.

At all times some muscle spasm of the entire dorsal and lumbar spines can be demonstrated. Some tenderness can be elicited over the spinous processes and a little to each side of the midline. As the process progresses, the excursions of the thorax become smaller and smaller until the thoracic cage becomes completely rigid and fixed. Throughout the active stages of the disease, the sedimentation rate is always elevated and is a good index to the activity of the process, but the serologic test for rheumatoid arthritis is frequently negative (Fig. 13-25).

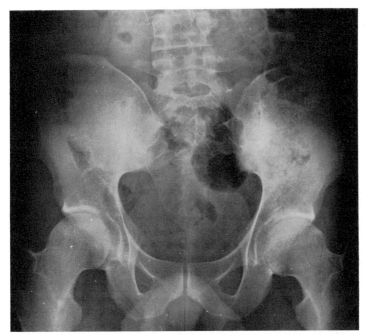

Figure 13-25 Ankylosing spondylitis. Both sacroiliac joints are fused. The same process is evident in the posterior articulations of the lumbar spine. Because of radiation of pain into both lower extremities, this patient had been treated for lumbar disc disease.

ABNORMALITIES OF THE NERVE ROOTS

Although rare, congenital malformations of the nerve roots and the sheaths may initiate a syndrome not unlike that of lumbar disc lesions. It may be impossible to distinguish one entity from the other on clinical or radiographic grounds. The true nature of the symptom complex can only be resolved by visualization of the nerve roots. Essentially the anomalies comprise preformations of the lumbosacral plexus in the spinal canal. The superadded nerve roots pursue abnormal directions. This peculiarity of the nerve roots poses considerable difficulty at operation, making it almost impossible to retract the roots in the usual manner in order to expose a pathologic disc. Adequate exposure of the spinal canal is necessary in order to visualize these anatomic variations.

The possibility of the existence of a prefixed or postfixed lumbosacral plexus must also be kept in mind. These variations are more common than generally realized, especially in association with variations in the number of free lumbar vertebrae. This possibility should be considered when determining the root affected in a lumbar spine with an increase or decrease in the number of lumbar vertebrae.

REFERENCES

1. Adkins, E.: Spondylolisthesis, J. Bone Joint Surg. 37-B:48-62, 1955.
2. Cozen, L.: The developmental origin of spondylolisthesis. Two case reports. J. Bone Joint Surg. 43-A:180-184, 1961.

3. DePalma, A. F. and Marone, P.: Spondylolysis following spinal fusion. Report of a case. Clin. Orthop. 15:208-211, 1959.
4. Gill, G. G. et al.: Surgical treatment of spondylolisthesis without fusion. Excision of the loose lamina with decompression of the nerve roots. J. Bone Joint Surg. 37-A:493-518, 1955.
5. Harris, R. I. and Wiley, S. S.: Acquired spondylolysis as a sequel to spine fusion. J. Bone Joint Surg. 45-A:1159-1170, 1963.
6. Hilel, N.: Spondylolysis; its anatomy and mechanism of development. J. Bone Joint Surg. 41-A:303-320, 1959.
7. Meyerding, H. W.: Spondylolisthesis. J. Bone Joint Surg. 13:39-48, 1931.
8. Meyerding, H. W.: Spondylolisthesis: As an etiologic factor in backache. J.A.M.A. 111:1971-1976, 1938.
9. Sarpyener, M. A.: Congenital stricture of spinal canal. J. Bone Joint Surg. 27:70-79, 1945.
10. Sarpyener, M. A.: Spina bifida aperta and congenital stricture of spinal canal. J. Bone Joint Surg. 29:817-821, 1947.
11. Verbiest, H.: A radicular syndrome from developmental narrowing of the lumbar vertebral canal. J. Bone Joint Surg. 36-B:230-237, 1954.
12. Willis, T. A.: An analysis of vertebral anomalies. Am. J. Surg. 6:163-168, 1929.
13. Wiltse, L. L.: The etiology of spondylolisthesis. J. Bone Joint Surg. 44-A:539-560, 1962.

Chapter 14

THE CONSERVATIVE THERAPY OF LUMBAR DISC DISEASE

The aims of nonoperative therapy of lumbar disc disease are threefold: relief of pain, increase of the functional capacity of the patient and slowing the progression of the disease. Reports on the efficacy of various types of conservative therapy vary tremendously. The most optimistic of these reports claims that of a total of 400 patients with acute disc lesions, only two required operative intervention after conservative therapy.[1] Our own experience has led us to become more cautious in responding to inquiries about the possible failure of conservative therapy and the necessity for operative intervention, which patients make when they have been assigned a diagnosis of acute disc herniation. It is our feeling that approximately 20 per cent of patients with a diagnosis of an acute disc lesion will ultimately require surgery when followed over a period of years.

The question of efficacy of various types of conservative therapy for this disorder is complex. It will depend upon the willingness of patients to accept not only various levels of chronic and acute pain but also an altered functional capacity. It must be kept in mind that disc degeneration is not a lethal disease. If the patient is willing to live with his pain, it is his prerogative to persist with a course of conservative therapy despite the treating physician's feeling that it has failed and operative intervention is required. On the other hand, patients with a bona fide disc lesion who do not respond to conservative therapy in a reasonable length of time should be granted the benefit of surgical intervention to allow them a more comfortable and active life.

The course of conservative therapy that will be presented here has evolved over a period of years and was found to be effective in a large patient population. The reasons for its efficacy are somewhat hypothetical, but it has been shown on an empiric basis to be the most efficient approach to the problem of acute and chronic disc lesions.

BED REST

The most important element of therapy in acute disc lesions is an adequate period of bed rest. In most instances this can be accomplished most effectively at home where the patient is in comfortable and familiar surroundings and cared for by his family. Should he lack adequate facilities for good home care, he should be admitted to the hospital for this treatment. It is expected that the patient remain at complete bed rest, with the exception of bathroom privileges for bowel movements once or twice a day, either with the use of a bedside commode or a nearby toilet facility. The short period of ambulation necessary to reach the bathroom is frequently less stressful than the acrobatics required to utilize a bedpan. If a firm mattress is available, we feel that bed boards are not necessary and in many instances will actually increase the level of discomfort noted by the patient.

While in bed, the patient should be placed in a position such that his hips and knees are flexed to a moderate degree. This has been found to be particularly necessary in disc herniations at the L4-5 level. The patient is cautioned against sleeping in a prone position which will result in hyperextension of the lumbar spine.

Patients with sensitive skin will find additional comfort in the use of a natural or synthetic "sheepskin" when placed at prolonged periods of bed rest.

The duration of this period of bed rest is of prime importance. Too frequently patients are mobilized and allowed to return to work before the inflammatory reaction to a disc herniation has subsided. The patient is informed that after an acute disc herniation a minimum of two weeks is required at complete bed rest whether at home or in the hospital. Subsequent to this, a week to ten days of gradual mobilization is instituted if he has had substantial relief of pain and is free of list and paravertebral muscle spasm. It should be mentioned parenthetically that any patient with a profound neurologic deficit or with a progressive neurologic deficit should undergo operative intervention; he is not a candidate for conservative therapy. It is unrealistic to expect a patient with a frank disc herniation to return to full activities in less than one month. Compromise on this point is frequently sought by the patient but in the long run will not be to his benefit. It should be pointed out to the patient that operative intervention, in itself, requires a prolonged period of rehabilitation and that strict adherence to a conservative program may preclude the necessity of operative intervention.

Based on present-day knowledge of the pathophysiology of disc degeneration, it is the authors' feeling that the modality of bed rest is important so that the secondary inflammatory reaction to disc degeneration may subside; bed rest is not instituted with the expectation that an extruded fragment will return to its original place within the annulus. Once extruded into the annulus or beneath the posterior longitudinal ligament, a fragment of nuclear material does not return to its original location. In many instances, however, if the edema and hyperemia of the soft tissues and nerve root surrounding the extruded fragment are allowed to subside, the patient will become free of his acute back pain and sciatica. This relief may or may not be permanent. The work of Nachemson has shown that it is only in the horizontal position that the disc is freed of significant stress.[2] The sitting position places a substantial burden upon the lumbar disc and patients must be informed that sitting at a desk or in an armchair does not provide adequate relief for the lumbar spine.

DRUG THERAPY

The intelligent use of drug therapy is an important modality in the treatment of lumbar disc disease. Three categories of pharmacologic agents are utilized: muscle relaxants, anti-inflammatory drugs, and analgesics.

If resolution of inflammation about a degenerated disc is the prime goal of conservative therapy, then anti-inflammatory drugs might be expected to be of importance in the treatment of these disorders. This is indeed the case. Most effective of these drugs is phenylbutazone (Butazolidin). In an acute disc herniation, patients are started on phenylbutazone at a level of 100 mg. four times daily with food or milk. The side effects of this drug are well known and include gastric irritation, fluid retention and blood dyscrasia. Buffering the stomach with food or milk is effective in preventing gastric irritation. Blood counts should be repeated at periodic intervals, and the patient cautioned about the appearance of ulceration in the mouth or other manifestations of blood dyscrasia. In those individuals who have a gastrointestinal intolerance to phenylbutazone, a less irritating analogue, oxyphenbutazone (Tandearil), may be utilized in an equivalent dosage scale.

It has been the authors' experience that certain patients who fail to show a response to phenylbutazone may get dramatic relief from the use of a short course of systemic steroids.[3] They should be utilized only in patients who are hospitalized and can be observed for the many potentially hazardous side effects of systemic steroids. Dexamethasone has been utilized in a dosage of 0.75 mg. four times daily which is tapered over a one-week period of time.

As patients resolve their acute disc herniations, they may have residual chronic symptomatology of low back pain which will require anti-inflammatory drugs, usually in lower dosages than those utilized for the acute lesion. A common dosage level for outpatient treatment is phenylbutazone 100 mg. twice daily. Periodic blood counts are obtained when this drug is utilized on an outpatient basis. If this drug has not shown itself to be effective in alleviating the symptomatology of a particular patient within a two-week period, it should be discontinued as it will probably not prove to be effective.

The use of muscle relaxants is effective in acute disc lesions in which muscle spasm shows itself as a prominent finding. Methocarbamol (Robaxin) and carisoprodal (Soma) are the drugs most commonly used for this purpose. The former is less likely to cause drowsiness. Soma is utilized in a dosage of 350 mg. three times daily, and Robaxin in a dosage of 1.5 Gm. four times daily. Occasionally, in an extremely acute problem with marked paravertebral muscle spasm, therapy will be initiated with the use of 10 ml. of intravenous Robaxin which is then continued with the oral form of the drug. This will frequently produce striking relief of both pain and limitation of motion. Muscle relaxants are rarely used in the chronic or subacute phase of disc degeneration where muscle spasm is a less prominent feature. Their major importance is during the acute phase of the disease process.

The judicious use of analgesics is of extreme importance during the acute phase of disc disease. It is our feeling that if the pain is of such a severe nature that parenteral narcotics are required, then morphine sulfate is the drug of choice. The dosage should be adequate to insure substantial relief of the patient's symptoms. Patients must be reassured that pain medication is available for their use and that a stoic attitude is therefore not essential. Many times during the early phases of treatment, the narcotics will be ordered on a regular rather than a p.r.n. basis. This alleviates the patient of the burden of summoning and waiting for nurses to obtain pain medication. Many of the opiates have constipation as an untoward side effect, and a stool softener should be added to the regimen if prolonged use of narcotics is required. As pain subsides, oral codeine or non-narcotic analgesics may be substituted for the more potent drugs.

It has often been found of value to add a sedative or mild tranquillizer to the patient's regime to alleviate anxiety and make the prolonged periods of bed rest more tolerable. Phenobarbital in doses of 15 to 30 mg. four times daily will accomplish this goal.

FLEXION EXERCISES

Lumbar flexion exercises become important in the subacute and chronic phases of lumbar disc degeneration (Fig. 14-1). The use of lumbar flexion exercises is based on the theory expounded by Williams.[4] The overall aim of lumbar flexion exercises is to reduce the lumbar lordosis. This reversal of the lumbar curve and full flexion of the lumbosacral joint will accomplish four goals. Subluxed or overriding facets of the apophyseal joints are placed in a position where they no longer overlap. Secondly, the spine is placed in a position of greater stability where the shearing strains are minimized at the lower lumbar disc levels. Third, the intervertebral foramina are widened, allowing for maximum room for exit of the nerve roots. A fourth goal of lumbar flexion exercises is strengthening of the abdominal musculature and flexors of the spine. Both of these muscle groups have been shown to be important in supporting the spine and alleviating stress of the intervertebral disc. All of these goals and reasons for the effectiveness of a lumbar flexion exercise program are theoretical and open to question. Their efficacy, however, on an empiric and clinical basis has been clearly shown.

Figure 14-1 Lumbar spine exercises.

Two exercise sessions every day: (Morning and night *OR* afternoon and night).

Start with two (2) of each and gradually increase to ten (10) of each (twice a day), over a period of 10 days to two weeks.

1. Stand with back against wall and heels flat on the floor. Flatten "small" of back against wall by rotating pelvis up and forward.

   NOTE: No space between small of back and wall.

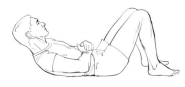

2. Lie on back with knees bent and feet flat on floor. Place hands on abdomen. Raise head and upper part of spinal column while contracting abdominal muscles.

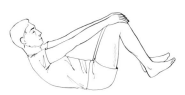

3. Lie on back. Separate legs. Bend knees and hips, and draw knees up toward axillae by clasping them with hands. *NOT TO BE DONE BY POSTOPERATIVE SPINE FUSION PATIENTS.*

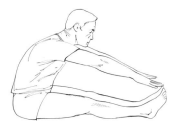

4. Sit on floor with legs outstretched. Touch toes without bending knees. When able to touch toes, stretch beyond toes. "Spring."

5. Lie flat on back. Without bending knees, lift one leg straight up, bending at hip; then the other; then both together.

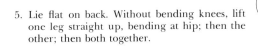

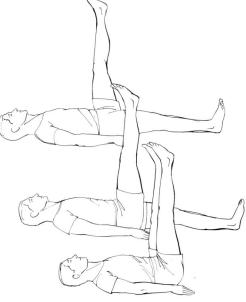

281

Lumbar flexion exercises should not be instituted in acute disc herniations until the patient's symptoms have subsided to the point where list and paravertebral muscle spasm are no longer noted and the major part of his acute symptomatology has subsided. This will usually be two to three weeks after the initiation of conservative therapy. Exercises are then started in a very gentle manner and are immediately discontinued if a flare-up of the patient's symptomatology appears. They may be reinstituted at a later date when the patient's tolerance for them has increased. It is not necessary, however, to wait until the patient is completely asymptomatic before instituting this program of exercises.

GENERAL MEASURES OF BACK HYGIENE

Along with a program of lumbar flexion exercises the patient with lumbar disc degeneration should be educated in certain measures of back hygiene which are in accord with the flexion management of these disorders.

He should be instructed to sleep on his side or back with his knees and hips in a position of flexion. He should be cautioned against the prone position which hyperextends the lumbar spine. If a patient is in a hospital bed, the Fowler's position should be utilized.

When sitting in a chair, he should sit with the buttocks well forward and his spine in a flexed position. This position is sometimes referred to as "slumping" and is regarded with a sense of horror by many physical therapists. It is our feeling, however, that people will habitually assume this position because of the comfort it provides. Crossing the legs while seated will add further flexion to this position and is also desirable.

Lifting heavy loads above the waist should be prohibited, particularly those in which the patient is forced to rock back into a position of hyperextension. When picking up a load from the floor the patient must be cautioned to utilize the musculature of his legs and bend from the knees and hips rather than the thoracic and lumbar spine.

PHYSICAL THERAPY

The most frequently used modalities of physical therapy are the application of heat and the use of light massage on the lower lumbar spine during the acute phases of disc herniation. Manipulation with or without anesthesia is not indicated in the treatment of lumbar disc disease. In many instances this will intensify rather than ameliorate the patient's symptomatology. The number of cases reported in the literature where a profound neurologic deficit has occurred, secondary to manipulation of the spine, are too great in number to justify the use of manipulation of the spine. It is particularly true when relief can be obtained by more judicious means.

The use of pelvic traction has not been found desirable or necessary by the authors in the treatment of lumbar disc disease. It is a cumbersome apparatus which makes bed rest less comfortable. Its therapeutic value is highly dubious and probably nonexistent except for enforcing a program of bed rest.

THE USE OF BRACES AND CORSETS

Rigid immobilization of the lumbar spine will rapidly lead to soft tissue contracture and muscle atrophy. For this reason the use of a rigid lumbar brace is seldom recommended. The young patient with degenerative disc disease is more advantageously treated with a program designed to increase his range of motion and strengthen his musculature rather than one based upon immobilization.

There are, however, certain instances in which external supports play a useful role.

The obese patient with poor abdominal musculature is frequently fitted with a firm corset with flexible metallic stays (Fig. 14-2). This corset will serve the function of reinforcing his abdominal musculature and thereby increases his efficiency in utilizing the thoracic and abdominal cavities to support the spine. The mechanism whereby the thoracic and abdominal cavities act as extensor of the spine is discussed in the chapter on the anatomy of the spine. It would, of course, be preferable to train these patients to develop their abdominal musculature and shed their body of unneeded adipose tissue.

A second category of individuals for whom braces are utilized are the elderly individuals with advanced multi-level degenerative spondylosis.

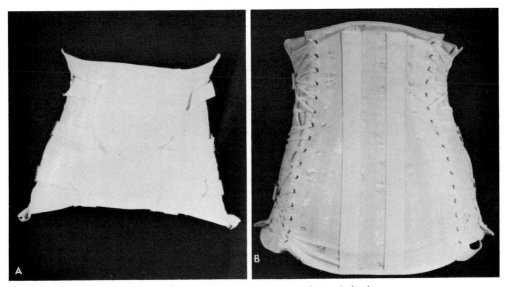

Figure 14-2 Lumbosacral corset; *A*, front, *B*, back.

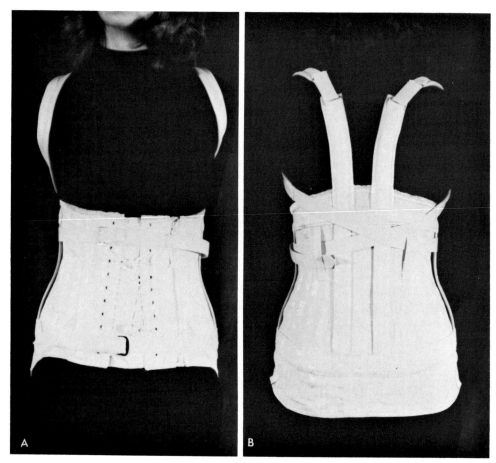

Figure 14-3   Knight-Taylor brace; *A*, front, *B*, back.

These patients will not tolerate an exercise program and, indeed, their symptomatology is frequently intensified by a program of mobilization. Depending upon the extent of their disease, a Knight-Taylor brace with shoulder straps or possibly a shorter lumbosacral brace with rigid metal stays is utilized to partially immobilize the spine and place these arthritic joints at rest (Figs. 14-3 and 14-4). Marked relief of pain is rapidly achieved in these individuals with bracing. It is frequently possible to wean these people from their support and this should be attempted if possible after their acute symptoms subside. This is to prevent further loss of muscle tone and stiffness in an already weakened spine.

A third use for bracing in the management of lumbar disc disease is in the postoperative management of patients who have undergone spine fusion (Fig. 14-4). Since the advent of the lateral fusion, the postoperative use of braces has declined. The authors currently use postoperative bracing only when more than one disc space has been fused. A typical lumbosacral fusion, that has been achieved with a lateral fusion technique, is mobilized without the use of any bracing or support whatsoever. This plan is also being considered in multi-level fusions but as yet has not been evaluated.

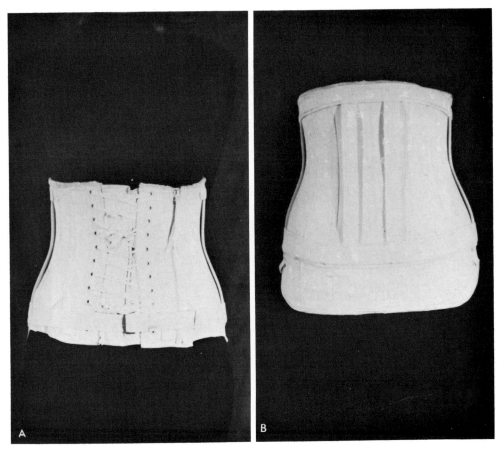

Figure 14-4 Lumbosacral brace; *A*, front, *B*, back.

PREGNANCY AND LUMBAR DISC DISEASE

One of the most challenging problems confronting the orthopedic surgeon is the pregnant patient presenting with symptoms of disc degeneration. It is our feeling that the intervertebral disc is placed under excessive stress during pregnancy for two reasons. The first of these is the obvious extra burden of carrying the fetus and the second is the unusual ligamentous laxity found during pregnancy. This is caused by the maternal production of relaxin or relaxin-like hormones. Relaxin is a hormone found in many mammals which produces the necessary ligamentous laxity about the pelvis which allows for the birth of offspring which may be larger than the bony pelvic outlet. It is possible that a similar hormone produced near term in humans may be an important cause of congenital hip dysplasia and can certainly be of importance in producing relaxation of the important ligamentous supporting structures of the spine.

The therapeutic modalities available are somewhat limited during pregnancy and for the most part one must depend upon bed rest and the use of a supporting corset. One hesitates to prescribe potent and potentially teratogenic drugs during pregnancy. Diagnosis is also somewhat hampered by the limited use of x-ray. Surgery, of course, is a court of last resort during pregnancy and is only indicated in the presence of serious neurologic findings. It is often necessary to prescribe long periods of bed rest for a pregnant patient in order to obtain any measure of pain relief. Use of a firm flexible corset is of great help in alleviating the spine of excessive stress.

REFERENCES

1. Marshall, L. L.: Conservative management of low back pain: A review of 700 cases. Med. J. Aust. 1:266-267, 1967.
2. Nachemson, A. et al.: In vivo measurements of intradiscal pressure. Discometry: A method for the determination of pressure in the lower lumbar discs. J. Bone Joint Surg. 46-A:1077-1092, 1964.
3. Naylor, A. and Turner, R. L.: ACTH in treatment of lumbar disc prolapse. Proc. Roy. Soc. Med. 54:14-16, 1961.
4. Williams, P. C.: Examination and conservative treatment for disk lesions of the lower spine. Clin. Orthop. 5:28-36, 1955.

Chapter 15

OPERATIVE TREATMENT OF
LUMBAR DISC DISEASE

Excision of one of the lower lumbar discs for the relief of sciatica is now an established procedure which no longer needs to be defended. Removal of the disc for back pain is still on equivocal ground and as yet there is no agreement as to whether a spine should or should not be fused following the excision of a pathologic lumbar disc. Relief of sciatica by excision of a lumbar disc can be expected in over 90 per cent of the patients; however, this high incidence of cures depends upon the accuracy of the selection of patients. Careful evaluation of all the features presented by the patients is the most important prerequisite of surgical intervention. If this is adhered to conscientiously, no procedure is more gratifying in terms of good results to both the surgeon and the patient. The converse is also true: with poor selectivity, no procedure is fraught with more disappointment, disillusionment, pessimism and psychic turbulence. No particular operation, no unusual surgical skill or dexterity will negate this fact.

In the selection of patients for surgery, the whole patient and his individual characteristics and traits must be considered. This includes not only the objective and subjective manifestations of the disease, but also the patient's occupation, social status, emotional response and psychic build. First and foremost let us not forget that other disorders may produce sciatica and back pain. Also, it should be remembered that we are not dealing with a specific treatment for a certain disorder but rather a specific treatment to be applied to a *patient* with a certain disorder. Don't let us put on the robe of the cultist who subscribes to the concept that only one causative agent can be responsible for a certain symptom complex. It is the moral obligation of every physician and surgeon to evaluate the whole patient and his disease; never to violate the patient's trust and confidence; and to dispel fear, apprehension and anxiety, all of which may augment pain and intensify the physician's objective findings.

Unfortunately, there are too many inept surgeons whose enthusiasm for surgical intervention in all patients presenting the features of lumbar disc lesions instills fear and augments the patient's anxiety, and in so doing lays down the foundation for the development of an intractable psychic phenomenon which will be a stumbling block to any form of treatment.

Many patients will have gone through the surgical mill once or several times and still the pain and the disability persist. Most of these patients present a pathetic picture of disappointment whose constant pain makes them apprehensive, suspicious and emotionally unstable; yet, they continue to seek some relief. Many can be helped by restoring their confidence, giving them hope and, after thorough evaluation and study, even restoring them to a useful and active life. What really happens in many instances is the complete opposite. Being unwilling to assume the responsibility or convinced that the patient is beyond the point of salvage, too many surgeons refer the patient to someone else. The patient makes the rounds of many consultants and clinics until he is depleted of funds and reason. With the proper approach to the problem, many forsaken patients with backache and sciatica can be salvaged to the point of living a comfortable and productive life, and it is the physician's responsibility to provide that approach.

In the same vein, too many patients whose symptoms are related with a compensable injury are looked upon with suspicion. This attitude has led to many injustices; the patient's objective and subjective manifestations should be thoroughly investigated and evaluated with an open mind before any judgment is made. In many instances, the complaints are honest claims and are often confirmed by the objective findings. On the other hand, we should always be attuned to the possibility that a patient motivated by financial gain may make fictitious claims unsupportable by the objective findings and other facts of the case.

The surgeon should have complete knowledge of the normal and variational anatomy of the lumbosacral region and should be able to cope with any anatomic situation he may encounter. He should be knowledgeable of the typical and atypical features of lumbar disc lesions and should keep a constant vigilance for atypical observations suggesting some other lesion. Having gathered all the facts of the presenting clinical picture, the surgeon should attempt to correlate the data with the nature of the pathologic process in the lumbar disc and in the surrounding structures, always keeping in mind that the disc pathology is progressive and that the relationship of the nerve root to the extruded nuclear material and the size of the extruded sequestra are subject to constant change. This changing pattern is also applicable to the surrounding tissues. Of particular importance is the effect of the inflammatory process on the neural elements. Fibrous tissue may implicate both the perineural and intraneural elements and the intensity of the involvement changes constantly. Some individual nerve fibers may be compressed and yet recover completely after the compression is removed; others undergo axonal degeneration producing permanent loss of function.

INDICATIONS FOR SURGERY

MASSIVE NUCLEAR EXTRUSION PRODUCING CAUDA EQUINA SYNDROME

Compression of the cauda equina by a massive posterior extrusion of nuclear material is the only condition requiring immediate surgery. This is a rare condition, but when it occurs, prompt recognition of the lesion and immediate decompression of the cauda equina is imperative. There must be no delay on the part of the surgeon in making a decision to operate. Myelography prior to surgery may be helpful in determining the level of the lesion, but myelography should not be performed unless a decision is made to follow through with exploration of the pathologic disc. A delay of several hours may make the difference between total recovery and serious muscular impairment and permanent dysfunction of the bladder and rectal sphincters.

UNRELENTING SYMPTOMS

Occasionally an acute attack of back pain and sciatica fail to respond to any form of conservative treatment. No patient with an acute syndrome, regardless of its intensity and without evidence of any significant motor involvement, should be subjected to surgery without a fair trial of conservative treatment, the essential feature of which should be complete bed rest. It should be remembered that approximately 30 per cent of patients experiencing the first acute attack will recover spontaneously and many of these patients will have no further symptoms for a long period of time. Colonna's study of a series of conservatively treated patients with proven disc lesions is revealing in that 29 per cent of the patients were symptom free at the end result study, 71 per cent had some residual disability and 57 per cent were intermittently completely disabled.[5]

In spite of the above statistics, some patients do not respond to conservative treatment and unrelenting symptoms persist even when narcotics are administered to relieve the pain. If the diagnosis is clear, a period of three to five weeks, in our estimation, should be allowed for conservative therapy; if there is no response, surgical intervention is justified.

RECURRENT ATTACKS

In spite of adequate conservative treatment some patients have recurrences of severe, incapacitating pain. Even between attacks, the overall activities must be curtailed because of the fear of initiating another attack. It is apparent that the pathologic process in the affected disc is such that bits of nuclear material are being repeatedly extruded and the healing process has as yet failed to seal off the defects in the annulus in order to prevent further extrusions. If the symptoms and signs are clearly indicative of a lumbar disc lesion the patient should be relieved by surgical intervention.

Recurrent episodes in another group of patients are less disabling and the intensity of the symptoms are well within the patient's tolerance and endurance. However, the attacks may occur frequently enough to interfere with the activities of normal living and with steady employment. Surgery in this group is indicated, especially in men and women who are otherwise healthy, sound and emotionally stable.

In this same category are patients with recurrent attacks which are relatively mild and rather infrequent. Some of these patients make a mental adjustment to their problem and are satisfied to carry on without surgical inteference. Conservative measures should be continued and the patient is urged to live within the capacity of his back. Some other patients that fit in this group are less tolerant, are unwilling to live a restricted life and become very apprehensive. If no contraindications to surgery exist, operative intervention is justifiable. It becomes obvious that each patient responds differently to the same situation and that the patient is not fitted to a surgical procedure; rather, surgery is considered only one tool in the surgeon's armamentarium to be used in a specific situation.

Finally, some patients have recurrences which increase in frequency and intensity with the passing of time. The patient's tolerance and work capacity become less with each attack and his emotional status begins to deteriorate. Surgery should be seriously considered in these patients provided the surgeon is convinced that all other methods will be ineffective.

MOTOR DEFICIT

Weakness or paralysis of a group of muscles is indicative of interference with normal root function caused by compression of a nerve root. The characteristic features of this situation are demonstrable motor, sensory and reflex changes while pain is absent or insignificant in intensity. Decompression should be performed when paralysis of a group of muscles suddenly appears and no improvement is discernible within several days. The amount of compression is expressed in the degree of motor dysfunction, which may vary from slight weakness and mild atrophy of the affected muscles to complete paralysis and profound muscle wasting. Immediate operation should be performed in all cases showing a progression of the motor deficit. Failure to decompress the affected nerve root may result in varying degrees of permanent root dysfunction. When the amount of root dysfunction is minimal, conservative measures should be continued as long as there is evidence of improvement; if the dysfunction shows no improvement or shows progression, exploration of the affected root should be carried out.

Indications for Surgery in Patients With Previous Operations

These patients are often very difficult to assess adequately; yet a thorough investigation is most essential before contemplating further surgery. In these patients, we see the most pathetic tragedies of disc surgery. Many exhibit much apprehension, emotional instability and complete loss of confidence. The functional overlay may completely dominate the clinical picture; yet in many, the psychosomatic state is the direct sequel of months or years of pain, restricted activity and invalidism. The study and evaluation of these patients should leave no stone unturned and all diagnostic aids available should be employed which could lead to the true cause of the pain and disability. Don't forsake these patients, because, as will be shown subsequently, many can be salvaged and restored to a useful existence. For the purpose of discussion, they can be grouped into specific categories:

1. Patients who, having a clear picture of a lumbar disc lesion preoperatively and complete relief of symptoms postoperatively, experience after varying intervals of time the reappearance of some or all of the clinical manifestations. In those patients who had a disc excision alone, for relief of back and leg pain, it must be assumed that all of the nuclear tissue was not removed, that the pathologic process in the affected disc continued to progress, and that eventually another extrusion occurred producing symptoms similar to those present before the operation. If these patients fail to respond to a fair trial of conservative treatment, exploration of the disc should be done. It is our belief that in addition to removal of the disc tissue, a spinal fusion should also be performed. This is based on the assumption that the instability of the motor unit after the first operation could very well contribute to extrusion of nuclear material. Also, we are of the opinion that the same line of reasoning is applicable to cases in which back pain alone or sciatica alone was the presenting symptom before operation. These, too, should be treated by the combined operation.

A number of patients in this category may have had the combined procedure performed at the first operation. Development of a pseudarthrosis in the bony fusion mass may be responsible for the return of symptoms. Although some pseudarthroses are asymptomatic, when they do become painful and disabling repair of the fusion and exploration of the affected disc becomes necessary.

2. Patients whose original symptoms were never relieved by the operative procedure. If the original symptom was primarily backache and excision of the disc failed to bring relief, the natural assumptions are that the backache was due not to derangement of the nucleus pulposus but rather to instability of the motor unit affected or that the wrong disc was excised. In these cases, stabilization of the motor unit involved by spine fusion is mandatory.

If the patient's original complaint was leg pain and the pain still persisted, it is apparent that either the wrong disc was explored or the nuclear sequestrum responsible for the sciatica was not found. Re-exploration of the affected disc must be performed in order to relieve the sciatica and the spine should be fused. Fusion assures the patient against developing backache due to the instability of the affected segment of the spine following a second exploratory operation.

3. Patients previously subjected to surgery who develop back pain, leg pain or both after an interval of time during which they were asymptomatic. However, the clinical manifestations are not the same as those before the operation was performed. Study reveals that the clinical features indicate implication of a disc at a different level. It should be remembered that four to six per cent of patients operated for lumbar disc lesions develop recurrent attacks due to extrusion of nuclear sequestra at the same or at a different level. Management should be similar to that in patients suffering a first attack; if conservative treatment fails, exploration of the affected disc is indicated.

4. Patients who have been subjected to numerous operations—six, seven, eight, nine and even ten procedures. Invariably, the patient was worse following each operation. The functional overlay which most of these unfortunate persons develop undoubtedly plays a major role in exaggerating the symptoms. It is interesting to note that in many of these patients the complaints prior to the first operation are not clearly consistent with lumbar disc lesions and, in many, multiple discs are excised at the first operation. Also many technical errors are obvious, such as: complete removal of all of the posterior bony elements of several segments, thereby destroying the stability of the lumbar spine; evidence of exploration of multiple levels and excision of multiple discs; and inadequate and poorly executed fusion when spine fusion was attempted. In our file are records of eight patients in whom an attempt to fuse the lower lumbar spine was made by simply transfixing the facets of the posterior articular joints with screws. As a rule, at least three sets of posterior joints were transfixed in each case.

It becomes apparent that these cases present many diverse problems ranging from erroneous diagnoses to poor surgical judgment and technique. The problems are compounded by the profound emotional instability developed over the period of months and, in some instances, years of suffering. No operative procedure will restore these patients to physical and mental normalcy. Each case must be thoroughly studied on its own merits over a long period of time in order to determine the organic basis of the complaints. The objective manifestations must be meticulously analyzed and an attempt made to correlate them with the existing pathology. It should be remembered that after repeated surgical trauma the muscles, fasciae and ligaments of the spine are profoundly changed by dense, inelastic fibrous tissue which is adherent to the posterior dura following a wide laminectomy. Also, there may be great loss of bone substance including the posterior articular facets. Myelography may provide little or no information because the contour of the subarachnoid space may be distorted by adhesions. The importance of arachnoid adhesions in the production of radicular pain has been overestimated. Many patients who have had previous surgery with recurrence of pain will show distortion of the opaque column presumably due to arachnoid adhesions; yet exploration of the right level often reveals the presence of extruded nuclear material making pressure on the nerve root responsible for the symptoms. All these factors must be taken into consideration if further surgery is considered.

In spite of all this, if those cases in which the functional element is the dominant factor are excluded, many of the remaining patients can and should be restored to a tolerable existence and even a gainful life by properly thought out and executed surgical procedures and postoperative management. These patients, as a group, will be discussed in more detail subsequently.

What has been said of the patient with multiple operations is also true of the patient who is being considered for surgery for the first time. A long drawn-out period of invalidism and pain demoralizes a patient and reduces his tolerance and confidence. Many show obvious evidence of emotional instability. These patients should be handled with great care and caution. Careful and critical analysis must be made of the objective features the patient presents. If sufficient evidence is found to justify the complaints on an organic basis, then surgery can be performed with reasonable assurance that the patient will be benefited. As for the remaining patients, whose functional overlay overshadows and dominates the clinical picture and whose objective manifestations cannot be justified on an organic basis, it would be foolhardy to subject them to surgery. Surgical intervention would only compound the neurotic problems and push the patient still further from realism.

CONTRAINDICATIONS TO SURGERY

THE COOPERATIVE PATIENT

Many patients with lumbar disc lesions are able to adjust their lives in such a fashion that the disorder is not an insurmountable situation. These patients should be carried on an adequate conservative program until the pathologic process in the disc has expended itself and a painless, stable motor unit evolves. If such a patient understands the problem and is willing to bide his time and to cooperate in a conservative program of treatment, surgery is contraindicated.

On the other hand, many cooperative patients with uncomplicated lumbar disc lesions fail to respond to conservative treatment because the prescribed program is inadequate or has not been pursued for a sufficient period of time. If these patients do not show significant motor deficits, an adequate, closely supervised program of therapy should be instituted; surgery at this time is contraindicated.

WHEN THE CLINICAL PICTURE IS AT VARIANCE WITH THE DIAGNOSIS OF A LUMBAR DISC LESION

Surgical intervention should never be considered when the presenting clinical picture is vague and even at variance with that of the typical lumbar disc lesion. Most of the surgical tragedies following surgery on the lumbar spine are the result of failure to adhere to this principle. When the clinical manifestations are not well-defined it behooves the surgeon to study the case carefully, to weigh all the possibilities capable of producing the presenting picture and to consider surgery only after a diagnosis is established with reasonable certainty. It is true that in cases of back pain without sciatica, the level of involvement may be difficult to determine and, in these instances, myelography and radiological examination may provide no confirmatory evidence. It is also true that in some cases the disc affected can only be found by exploration of several interspaces. However, the exploration should not be undertaken until the surgeon, as the result of his studies, is reasonably certain that the causative agent of the symptoms is a pathologic disc and not some other lesion.

It should be remembered that chronic backache is not synonymous with disc pathology and may be due to mechanical instability of a motor unit. Excision of one or more discs in such a situation as this is doomed to failure.

Double disc lesions may confuse the picture. Although these occur, we are convinced that their presence is overestimated. A symptom complex exhibiting involvement of more than one nerve root must be regarded with great suspicion, and the possibility of a tumor of the cauda equina seriously considered. In such cases, surgery must not be undertaken before all diagnostic aids are used and carefully analyzed in order to establish the diagnosis.

OBJECTIVES OF SURGICAL INTERVENTION

The surgeon's objectives (and, incidentally, the patient's hopes) are: (1) to relieve the patient's current pain, (2) to insure the patient of no further recurrences of the syndrome and (3) to provide a stable lumbar spine capable of meeting all of the functional demands that may be required of it. To say the least, these are truly idealistic aims, particularly when weighed against the statistics of some reliable long-term end result studies. Nevertheless, these should be our goals; and, although at the present time many of us fall short of this high level of achievement, there is reason to hope that with a better understanding of the causes of low back and radicular pain and with the evolution of better surgical techniques these goals may in the near future be achieved. How best to achieve them cannot be dictated to any surgeon concerned with lumbar disc lesion. The philosophy of treatment, the methods to solve the problems and the technical skills to execute these methods must come from within himself; his ultimate crystallized approach will be a product of much thought, critical analysis of his cases, open-mindedness to new ideas and a perfection of the surgical techniques he is best able to perform. To the uninitiated, the great variance in the statistical analyses of series of cases from many reputable sources is confusing and even baffling. To the experienced surgeon it is understandable, for he realizes that some surgeons with their own methods are capable of doing what is almost an impossibility for other surgeons using the same methods and techniques. These human variables in the thinking process (and even intuition), in the mental and manual dexterity and in the drive for perfection cannot be passed from one individual to another by reading a communication or a book. Or, it can be said the way the tough Marine sergeant put it when he was evaluating his men after a strenuous period of basic training in a boot camp. He looked down on a pathetic little Marine, who in eight weeks never executed a perfect maneuver, and, shaking his head, said, "Cheer up, Joe, some guys got it and some don't."

To Fuse or Not to Fuse

Over the past 30 years, the question of whether to fuse or not to fuse a segment of the lumbar spine following excision of an intervertebral disc has concerned us greatly. If we compare the long-term end results of recognized, competent surgeons we soon come face to face with the fact that there is a definite difference in the incidence of satisfactory results between the cases treated by disc excision alone and those treated by the combined operation, disc excision and primary spine fusion, but the difference is not too great. The significant observation is that those who do not fuse the spine claim the difference in their favor, whereas those who fuse the spine routinely claim it to their favor. Young et al. presented the end result studies of two groups of consecutive patients who were followed for a minimum of six years and a maximum of ten years since operation.[13] In one group, the patients were treated by disc excision alone and, in the other, by excision of the protruded disc and primary fusion of the lumbar spine. Statistically it was shown that the chances of obtaining a long-term good result were about 20 per cent greater after the combined operation than after disc excision alone; and that the rate of failure was ten per cent less after the combined operation than after removal of the disc without spine fusion. Raaf reported the end result studies in 430 patients who had excision of the disc alone; excellent and good results were obtained in 91 per cent of the patients.[10] A second group of 147 patients in the same study had the combined operation; excellent and good results were obtained in 79 per cent of them. Discrepancies such as these appear in the literature many times. On the other hand, the discrepancies in other reported series varies from as low as 50 per cent to 97.6 per cent satisfactory results. Certainly the validity of these reports must not be challenged. Then, what makes the difference in opinions and reported statistics?

The answer to this question is not simple. In our opinion, the determining factors, which lie within the surgeon himself, are: selectivity — the ability to select the patient that has an excellent chance of obtaining a good result by the operative procedure the surgeon intends to employ; experience — the experience of the surgeon in regard to knowledge in depth of the pathologic process acting in the lumbar spine, surgical skill and dexterity, and familiarity of the normal and variational anatomy of the lumbar region, and the conviction that his decision is based on solid ground. However, what may be the solid ground of conviction for one surgeon may not be so for another. It is this divergence of opinion that stimulates and motivates minds to delve more deeply into a problem in the hope that the true answer to all differences will eventually be found.

We are of the opinion that all abnormal motor units which have been further deranged by excision of the nucleus pulposus should be stabilized by fusion unless there are definite contraindications to do so. In our hands, the patient has a better chance of attaining a good result if we perform the combined operation. This belief is based on a wide experience of disorders of the spine and has evolved over a period of many years; it was not a sudden acquisition. Years back (1953), when our present conviction was not as yet firmly grounded, the senior author performed 100 consecutive operations in which the disc alone was excised.[6] All of these cases had a disc protrusion demonstrable at the time of surgery. After the completion of the series in 1955, a period of five years was allowed to expire; then the cases were critically evaluated by an independent investigator. Of the 100 patients, 83 were available for study with a postoperative period ranging from five to seven years. Briefly, the end result study disclosed the following statistics: 58 per cent were rated excellent or good, 22 per cent fair and 20 per cent poor. In other words, 58 per cent were considered satisfactory and 42 per cent unsatisfactory. The unsatisfactory results were too high and were not acceptable. At this point, it is interesting to note that many of the patients who at the end of the study were considered as having satisfactory results have since that time developed recurrent pain sufficiently severe to warrant an arthrodesis of the affected motor unit. Had these patients decompensated sooner, the number of satisfactory results would have dropped precipitously. This observation also points up the fact that it is difficult to designate a fixed time period for end result studies. We are certain that if our cases had been evaluated at the end of a three-year period the end result figures would have been considerably better than 58 per cent.

Justification for Spine Fusion After Excision of the Disc

Under normal conditions, the lower lumbar spine functions at a disadvantage because of its anatomic arrangement; it is vulnerable to excessive stresses. The degenerative process, which afflicts the nucleus pulposus as early as the third decade, renders the spine even more vulnerable. Surgical insult, by removing the nucleus pulposus and thereby destroying the disc upon which depends the stability of the motor unit, renders the spine very unstable. It is hoped that by excision of the disc, a reparative process is evoked which will terminate in fibrous ankylosis of the affected segment of the spine. It is generally acknowledged that fibrous ankylosis of any of the peripheral joints is invariably synonymous with a painful joint and that such a joint is very irritable and responds unfavorably to even minor abnormal stresses. It is reasonable to assume that the same situation is applicable to an intervertebral joint, except that the normal range of motion in the intervertebral joints as compared to the peripheral joints is considerably less, and therefore stability is more readily achieved by a tough, fibrous ankylosis. Nevertheless, these joints are not completely stable, and many are prone to decompensate when subjected to excessive stresses.

If the above analogy is made to osteosynthesis of the peripheral and vertebral joints, it is an accepted fact that osteosynthesis is tantamount to a painless joint. It is argued that bone is a living structure with sufficient elasticity to allow some movement at points of maximum stress and, if this premise is applied to the spine, the motion may give rise to pain.[8] In practice, the amount of movement possible within an area of osteosynthesis produces no pain. This is a natural physiological phenomenon; a fused joint is a painless joint.

It becomes apparent that, in theory at least, arthrodesis of a spinal segment is the most favorable situation following excision of a pathologic disc; it not only eliminates pain but also provides stability sufficient to meet the demands of a normal active life. It has been suggested that arthrodesis should be reserved for only certain situations; among these is failure to achieve a firm, painless fibrous ankylosis either by conservative methods or after surgical excision of the disc. In our opinion, in these instances, the patient and the surgeon have performed an unnecessary exercise. Conservative management of a lumbar disc lesion which is associated with recurrent episodes of back and leg pain and considerable disability requires a period of many months and even years before the desired end point is reached. The end point, which is a stable fibrous ankylosis, may never be attained. Much time is saved, and the patient is spared much pain and great financial loss by an arthrodesis of the affected segment of the spine.

It should be mentioned at this time that the statement, often made, that "the entire nucleus is removed through a posterior approach" is a fantasy. In very few instances is the surgeon capable of removing the entire nucleus through a hole in the annulus. At best, this is a blind-and-touch procedure, and much nuclear material is inaccessible and remains in situ. This is attested to by the amount of nuclear tissue that is removed at second operations and also by the fact that extrusion of nuclear sequestra following a so-called "excision of the disc" is not an infrequent occurrence. Moreover, following removal of a disc, the postoperative period of convalescence is long and tedious before fibrous ankylosis, if achieved at all, is attained. By the current methods of securing an arthrodesis and the postoperative management, the patient is returned to normal activity in a much shorter period of time.

Arthrodesis

Arthrodesis of the spine, when indicated, is an accepted surgical procedure that needs no defense. In our opinion, for the reasons previously enunciated, it should be performed whenever an intervertebral disc is removed except in the few specific instances where it is contraindicated. In the hands of one experienced in surgery of the spine, the techniques (and there are many) to achieve a solid bony ankylosis should pose no problems either for the surgeon or for the patient. The one great objection to osteosynthesis of the spine has been the high incidence of failure to attain a bony ankylosis. In the past, and even today in the hands of many surgeons, the high rate of failure and the subsequent problems that arise have forced some surgeons to look at the procedure in an unfavorable light and to seek alternate methods to solve the problems raised by an unstable motor unit, whether it is the result of a lumbar disc lesion or some other etiologic factor. The formidability of the procedure is compounded when it is intended to bridge more than one interspace by bone; the greater the number of vertebrae fused the higher the rate of failure.

Fortunately, methods of arthrodesis have been evolved which, if properly executed, overcome all the objections previously registered against arthrodesis of the spine. The incidence of failure has been reduced to insignificant proportions, less than three per cent; this includes single level and multi-level fusions. The convalescent period is no longer a protracted one; the patients are out of bed within the first week after operation. In single level fusions, no bracing is needed; in multi-level fusions, a light corset brace is worn for three to four months. Sedentary occupations can be resumed within four to six weeks and full activity in four to six months. This postoperative program measures well with any program instituted when the disc alone is removed and better than most. When successful, the incidence of recurrent protrusions of nuclear material at the same level is markedly reduced. In addition, the patient is assured of a stable, painless back capable of meeting the stresses of a normal life.

There are certain anatomic variations, either congenital or acquired, which make arthrodesis mandatory when complicated by a lumbar disc lesion. The excessive amount of instability common to these lesions requires bony stabilization if a good result is to be anticipated. These are: spondylolysis, spondylolisthesis, congenital neural arch anomalies, increase in the number of free lumbar vertebrae, exaggerated lumbosacral angle, partial sacralization of the fifth lumbar vertebra, partial lumbarization of the first sacral vertebra, arthrosis of a motor unit and an excessively mobile unit, a condition which is indicated by a long history of backache aggravated by activity and relieved by rest and which may or may not be associated with a narrowed disc space as demonstrated by radiographs.

The few contraindications to arthrodesis are: the elderly patient with a lumbar disc lesion in which the dominant feature is sciatica, the elderly person with generalized arthrosis of the lumbar spine and patients with medical problems which preclude any extensive surgical procedure.

PERTINENT ANATOMIC FEATURES RELATED TO LUMBAR DISC LESIONS

Comprehension of the normal and abnormal anatomic features of the lower lumbar spine is most essential in the exploration of the spinal canal. Many of the osseous configurations are discernible by radiological examination, such as: spondylolysis, spondylolisthesis, spina bifida of the fifth lumbar or first sacral vertebra, partial or complete lumbarization of the first sacral vertebra, partial or complete sacralization of the fifth lumbar vertebra, increase or decrease in the number of free lumbar vertebrae, exaggeration of the lumbosacral angle, narrowing of one of the lower lumbar discs and advanced arthrosis of one of the intervertebral joints.

Knowledge of these abnormalities and consideration of them in the planning of the operation facilitates the execution of the surgical procedure. However, it should be remembered that in determining the level of the affected disc, radiological observations may be misleading and should only be considered meritorious if they confirm the clinical impression.

Some abnormalities are less discernible or are not revealed in the radiological examinations; yet, awareness of these changes is necessary in order to expose the spinal canal with the least structural damage and still obtain an adequate exposure to visualize fully the local pathology.

CONGENITAL NARROWING OF THE LUMBAR SPINAL CANAL

It was previously mentioned that congenital narrowing of the spinal canal may occur. This anomaly is not often recognized on plain radiographs; however, myelography does reveal the abnormal configuration of the canal.[11] When encountered, a more extensive exposure may be necessary than would normally be made in order to adequately explore the contents of the spinal canal. A small canal is to be expected in small persons.

VARIATIONS IN THE CONFIGURATION OF THE SPINAL CANAL

As previously recorded, the configuration of the spinal canal varies considerably from person to person. The flat trefoil canal is most likely to cause the most difficulty in discovering a nuclear protrusion which may lie deeply in the flat lateral gutter of the canal.[1] A wide exposure extending far laterally will facilitate mobilizing the root and extracting the protrusion.

VARIATIONS IN THE SIZE OF THE LAMINAE

Not infrequently the distance between the midline and the facets is markedly diminished. Reduction in the width of the laminae may offer some difficulty in exposing the spinal canal. Because of the smallness of the bony parts, the fenestration through the laminae and the interlaminar space must be performed with great care in order to avoid traumatizing the contents of the canal.

NARROW INTERLAMINAR SPACE

The interval between the laminae of the cephalic and caudal vertebrae of the affected motor unit may be markedly reduced. Here again, great care must be taken in approaching the spinal canal.

TROPISM OF THE ARTICULAR FACETS

As will be noted in a later section, the spine is partly prepared for a primary fusion before the spinal canal is explored. In doing so, a portion of the inferior facets of the cephalic vertebra is removed. Asymmetry of the facets of the lower lumbar vertebrae is a frequent, if not a common, finding; awareness of this fact aids in localization of the plane of the posterior articular joints.

INCREASE OR DECREASE IN THE NUMBER OF FREE LUMBAR VERTEBRAE

When these variations, which are readily demonstrable in plain radiographs, are present, they should be utilized in the localization of the lower lumbar nerve roots. It was previously noted that in the presence of these abnormalities the relationship of the roots to the intervertebral discs changes. When there are six lumbar vertebrae the S1 nerve root is in relation to the L5-L6 disc, the S2 root to the L6-S1 disc, and the L5 root to the L4-L5 disc (Fig. 15-1). When there are four lumbar vertebrae, the L5 nerve root relates to the L4-S1 disc and the L4 root to the L3-L4 disc; the S1 root does not relate to any disc. It should be understood that these anatomic relationships are valid provided the lumbar plexus is normal. A prefixed or postfixed plexus will nullify the disc-root relationship.

ANOMALIES OF THE LUMBAR NERVE ROOTS

Although anomalies of the nerve roots are relatively rare, they occur more frequently than generally realized. Awareness of these variations is

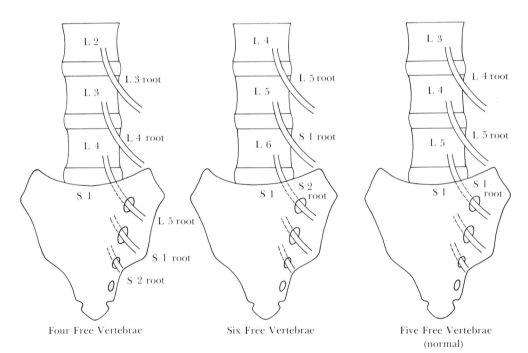

Four Free Vertebrae   Six Free Vertebrae   Five Free Vertebrae
                                                      (normal)

Figure 15-1   Site of exit of the nerve roots when there are four free vertebrae and six free vertebrae. Four vertebrae: The L5 nerve root is in relation to the L4-S1 disc. Six vertebrae: The S1 nerve root is in relation to the L5-L6 disc and the S2 root relates to the L6-S1 disc.

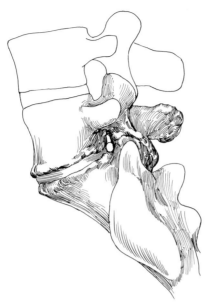

Figure 15-2 Narrowing of intervertebral foramen by reactive changes. This drawing is of a specimen of the lumbar spine. The reactive changes around the periphery of the foramen and the collapse of the disc have reduced the size of the canal severely. The nerve root is vulnerable to compression.

helpful in that the surgeon will be ready to meet the circumstance if it should arise. Anomalous roots may make the exposure of a nuclear protrusion very difficult.

ACQUIRED ABNORMALITIES IN THE LOWER LUMBAR REGION

These are usually in the form of ridges on the posterior margins of the vertebrae consisting of reactive bone and cartilage lying under a taut posterior longitudinal ligament. Their importance lies in their capacity to reduce the size of the spinal canal and occasionally a large osteophyte may press on a nerve root. Also, these changes together with similar changes on the margins of the posterior articular joints may narrow the lumens of the intervertebral foramina of the affected motor unit to such a degree that the contents of the foramina may be compressed (Fig. 15-2). Decompression of a foramen so affected requires excision of the articular facets (foraminotomy, facetectomy).

SURGICAL PATHOLOGY RELATED TO LUMBAR DISC LESIONS

Knowledge of the local pathology associated with lumbar disc lesions gives the surgeon a certain amount of confidence which permits him to

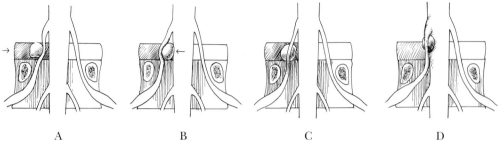

Figure 15-3   Location of protrusions in relation to the nerve roots: The protrusion lies, *A*, laterally to the nerve root; *B*, medially; *C*, directly under; *D*, in the axilla of the nerve root.

execute the various steps of the operation with precision. Much useless fumbling around in the spinal canal in search of the nuclear protrusion is avoided, and damage to the roots and dura is prevented. It was previously noted that certain characteristic lesions of the disc occur. Most of these relate to the location of the protrusion in relation to the involved nerve root. These are:

1. Lateral protrusions. These are undoubtedly the commonest. The size of the protrusion varies considerably from one patient to another. It is readily recognized as a firm mound under the taut longitudinal ligament. The nerve root may lie either lateral or medial to the protrusion. When in the lateral position, the root may be displaced far laterally into the lateral gutter of the canal and may be firmly pressed against the ligamentum flavum and the anterior margin of the lamina. If the protrusion is large, considerable difficulty may be encountered in displacing the root medially over the protrusion (Fig. 15-3). An interesting variation of this type is the protrusion located at the juncture of the dura and the sheath of the nerve root in the so-called axilla. A protrusion in this position may displace the root upward and laterally.

The root may lie medial to the protrusion; generally this type offers very little difficulty in displacing the root and making the protrusion accessible (Fig. 15-3).

2. Extruded nuclear sequestrum in the spinal canal. The nuclear material may have penetrated the posterior longitudinal ligament and lies free in the spinal canal. It appears as a shaggy, irregular mass of fibrous tissue and may be found in any position in relation to the nerve root. It may lie in the lateral recess of the canal, or it may migrate along the course of the nerve root and find its way into the intervertebral foramen. Less frequently, it may migrate upward or downward and implicate the root in relation to the disc above or the one below the disc from which it originated. It should be remembered that there may have been several sequestra extruded. In long standing cases, the sequestrum may be firmly adherent to the root sheath and the posterior longitudinal ligament, so that it may not be possible to remove it without breaking it up into smaller fragments (Fig. 3-19).

PROTRUSION LIES DIRECTLY UNDER THE NERVE ROOT

In this situation the nerve root rides the summit of the nuclear mound. If the protrusion is large, the nerve is severely stretched and flattened, appearing as a thin ribbon over and adherent to the protrusion. Great caution must be used in peeling the thin root off the protrusion. This may be very difficult to do without injuring the nerve root (Fig. 15-3).

CENTRAL PROTRUSION

The protrusion may lie close to or in the midline. It may involve one or both roots at this level. Its central position makes it difficult to visualize; this cannot be done until the root and dura are displaced far medially. As a rule, a larger exposure than usual is necessary to expose the protrusion, making injury to the root less likely (Fig. 2-14).

DISSECTING DISCS

Once the nuclear sequestrum lies under the posterior longitudinal ligament it may migrate in any direction, stripping the ligament from its underlying attachment as it proceeds onward. Not infrequently, it stays close to the midline and travels either upward or downward from its site of exit. These protrusions may be difficult to find.

THE BOGGY OR "CONCEALED" DISC

There may not be a true protrusion. In this event the disc must be exposed and inspected. If pathologic, the posterior annulus exhibits a lusterless, grayish appearance; the disc, instead of being resilient, is boggy and mushy. These features are readily demonstrable if the disc is palpated with a blunt instrument.

PLEXUS OF VEINS

Not infrequently, a large plexus of engorged veins is found on the floor and in the lateral recess of the canal. Occasionally, the tortuous veins can be seen over and around the nerve root and protrusion. In order to avoid lacerating the veins, the dura must be displaced medially very carefully and without tension. Once this is done, the area can be visualized and dealt with accordingly.

THIN INTERVERTEBRAL SPACE

In old lesions, degeneration of the disc may result in close approximation of the contiguous vertebral bodies. It may be very difficult to locate the interspace in order to evacuate it. However, close inspection often reveals some wrinkling of the posterior ligament due to collapse of the underlying annulus fibrosus. This gives a clue to the site of the interspace. Palpation with a blunt instrument locates the space.

Also, in old lesions there may be the formation of much dense fibrous tissue at the level of the intervertebral space and also in the lateral aspect of the canal. The nerve root may be bound down or enmeshed in a mass of mature fibrous tissue which may be permeated by many venous channels. This circumstance may offer considerable resistance to retraction medially of the nerve root and dura. Sometimes this can only be achieved by sharp dissection.

DEFECTS IN THE ANNULUS

From time to time small ragged defects are found in the annulus, indicating that nuclear material has been extruded. In addition, they are guides to the location of the intervertebral space. The tear may occur in the lateral or medial portions of the annulus.

MULTIPLE ROOT INVOLVEMENT

Although rare, two roots at the same level or two roots at different levels but on the same side may be involved by nuclear protrusions or extruded nuclear material; we believe they are not as common as many think. But, if there is clinical evidence of more than one root involved, these possibilities must be kept in mind and steps taken to explore the affected roots (Fig. 3-19).

TECHNICAL SURGICAL CONSIDERATIONS

THE SURGEON

At this juncture, it is almost a moral obligation on our part to point out that surgery for lumbar disc lesions should not be performed by one who is not thoroughly trained and experienced in surgery of the spine. In order to appreciate fully the detailed normal and variational anatomy of the lumbar region and the varied pathology of lumbar disc lesions, a surgeon must see and study hundreds of backs at the time of operation, as an active assistant during the execution of these operations. Only by repeated exposure and by "doing" can a surgeon perfect his surgical skills sufficiently to perform surgery for lumbar disc lesions. This type of surgery cannot be done by simply reading a description of the operation in a book or journal. Unfortunately, many backs are operated on by unqualified surgeons; the results are often catastrophic.

INSTRUMENTS

Although it may seem superfluous, mention should be made of the instruments used in surgery of the back. Every surgeon has his "pet" instruments and this is how it should be. A surgeon should get accustomed to using certain instruments of his choice; in a certain situation he may use tools which another surgeon would never think of using. With the constant use of certain instruments, a surgeon soon learns about their capabilities in specific situations. As years go by, a skillful surgeon will employ fewer and fewer instruments to perform better and better surgery. A surgeon should have available all the instruments needed to perform a smooth and expeditious operation. But beware of the surgeon whose operating table is stacked with gadgets. A gadgeteer is hopeful that the gadgets will perform the operation or will negate his own lack of skill, precision and dexterity; of course, this is an impossibility.

A good surgeon insists that his instruments be given meticulous care. Sharp instruments should be kept sharp; a knife or a scissors should cut and not tear a piece of tissue. Hemostats and other clamps should grasp, open and close with ease. Osteotomes and chisels should be sharpened after each case and then wrapped and put away so that their cutting edges are protected. It is very distressing to use a cutting tool that looks like a garden rake and performs even less effectively.

Exposure of the Lower Lumbar Spine

Regardless of the operation preferred to approach the lower lumbar disc spaces, the posterior elements of the vertebrae must be first exposed. Make the skin incision in the midline directly over the spinous processes of the lower lumbar spine and the upper sacral vertebrae. The incision from the outer surface of the skin to the tips of the spinous processes, cutting through the skin, subcutaneous layer and fascia, should be in one plane; this reduces the amount of bleeding from the sides of the incision. Next, beginning with the last lumbar vertebra, make a clean cut over each spinous process through the superspinous ligament down to the bone and, with a broad, sharp periosteal elevator, strip subperiosteally all muscle attachments from the laminae to be exposed, first on one side, then on the other. The subperiosteal stripping should extend laterally as far as the posterior articular joints. Pack tightly with tagged gauze sponges the intervals between the denuded laminae and the sides of the wound as the dissecting proceeds cephalad. Expose the base of the sacrum in the same manner. Always expose the first sacral vertebra in order to accurately identify the lumbar vertebrae. This portion of the operation should consume only a few minutes and should be bloodless. The number of laminae exposed depends on the number of disc spaces that are to be explored. If the L5-S1 disc is to be explored, expose the laminae of the L5 and L4 vertebrae and the base of the sacrum, which may include the exposure of the first two or three spinous processes of the sacrum. Remove the spinous process of the L5 vertebra at its base with a sharp, broad bone cutter. This exposure will also permit exploration of the L4-L5 interspace.

Removal of the spinous process of L5 or, if necessary, of L4 and the interspinous and supraspinous ligaments between L5 and S1, or even between L4 and L5, in no way weakens the spine. If the muscles have been stripped subperiosteally, healing in the midline by fibrous tissue is more than strong enough to meet any functional demands made on the lumbosacral spine.

HANDLING OF TISSUES

All tissues, from the skin to the dural sac, should be handled gently. Avoid tearing, lacerating and shredding of tissues with sharp toothed retractors; avoid excessive pressure and traction on tissues. Also keep tissues, especially the sides of the wound, moist and whenever possible protect them with large, warm gauze sponges. When self-retaining retractors are used on the sides of the wound, place the blades so that they are opposed to the entire thickness of the wound. If the blades are not set deeply they tend to slide out and, in so doing, they tear and macerate all tissues in their path. Occasionally release the blades to relieve the constant pressure made on the tissues. At the end of the operation, inspect the sides of the wound well and and cut away all strands of tissues, fat, muscle and fascia that appear devitalized. Thoroughly flush the wound with warm normal saline before the wound is closed. If heeded, these simple measures will reduce to a minimum the amount of blood loss, will reduce the possibility of infection and insure healing of the wound by first intention.

Exposure of the Spinal Canal

There are many methods of exposing the spinal canal. Some openings are very small, such as that produced by excising the ligamentum flavum from between two vertebrae; others are very large as produced when both laminae of the exposed vertebra are removed. The opening should be as wide as is needed to expose the nerve root, the protrusion and the affected intervertebral disc. It should be sufficiently wide to permit the work to be done without undue tension on the dural sac and the nerve root; it should permit a full view of the region of the spinal canal involved. We prefer a medium-size fenestration on the side of the affected nerve root which includes only a small portion of the lamina and the ligamentum flavum attached to it.

After the laminae are denuded of all tissues and after the interspinous and supraspinous ligaments are also removed, using a sharp beveled gouge one-half to three-quarter inches wide remove a rim of bone about one-quarter inch wide from the superior margin of the lamina. If the S1 root is to be exposed, the rim of bone is removed from the superior margin of the lamina of the first sacral vertebra and if the L5 root is to be exposed, it is removed from the superior margin of the lamina of the fifth lumbar vertebra. Tap the gouge lightly but firmly until you feel it enter the spinal canal. With a small curette, complete the separation of the rim of bone from the lamina. At this point, the ligamentum flavum is still attached to the proximal margin of the rim of bone. Grasp the rim of bone with a forceps and elevate it from the dural sac; now, with a medium-size curette or a pair of scissors cut the lateral and medial attachments of the ligamentum flavum. Finally, with a sharp, medium-size curette cut the proximal attachment of the ligament at its line of insertion into the inferior margin of the lamina of the vertebra above. This gives a surprisingly large aperture which permits adequate exposure of the nerve root and disc involved. If the fenestration is made at the L5-S1 interlaminar space and it is desirable to explore the L5 root, either a similar fenestration can be made at the L4-

L5 level, or the lamina of the fifth lumbar vertebra and a small portion of the lamina of the fourth lumbar vertebra can be nibbled away. If the opposite nerve root at the same level is to be inspected the fenestration can readily be widened to the other side of the midline by removing a portion or all of the lamina on the opposite side.

It becomes apparent that this approach to the spinal canal is very flexible and no more bone is removed than is required to adequately deal with the situation on hand. If it becomes necessary to expose the L4 nerve root, a similar but separate fenestration is made at the L3-L4 level.

We do not believe that in every case both the L5-S1 and the L4-L5 levels should be explored. Double lesions on the same side are indeed rare. Routine exploration of a normal disc does nothing more than inflict surgical trauma to a segment of the spinal canal. The reparative process following such an exposure binds down the nerve root in a mesh of scar tissue, a situation which itself is capable of producing sciatic pain. Also, having explored a disc, the temptation to puncture the annulus and evacuate the disc space is very great and is often done. It must be acknowledged that many normal discs are tampered with unnecessarily. However, if there is the slightest doubt that a second disc might be involved it should be explored.

HANDLING OF THE DURAL SAC AND THE NERVE ROOT

The dura and nerve roots are often traumatized because the lateral aspect of the spinal canal is not adequately exposed. This is particularly true if the root is bound down on the floor of the canal and to the nuclear protrusion by dense adhesions. Give yourself enough room by removing the lateral portion of the ligamentum flavum and enlarging the bony defect in the lamina. If the dura and the arachnoid membrane are inadvertently torn, repair the defect immediately using very fine silk sutures. This mishap is more likely to occur in re-explorations in which the dural sac and nerve root are enmeshed in dense, inelastic fibrous tissue. Failure to close the defect into the subarachnoid space may result in the formation of a large internal meningocele. A piece of muscle or fat, or Gelfoam will not permanently seal off the defect.

CONTROL OF BLEEDING

It is not unusual to encounter large veins in the anterolateral aspect of the spinal canal which overlay and are adherent to the dura, the root and the nuclear protrusion. As a rule, by using a slightly curved, blunt-ended dissector the vessels can be peeled off the root and protrusion; then, place a one-half inch by one-half inch pledget of soft foam rubber attached to a long thread in the lateral gutter above and below the protrusion. To prevent the foam rubber pledget from slipping out of the canal, place in front of it a small moist cotton pledget tied to a thread. (These foam rubber pledgets were first used by the late Duncan McKeever.) The foam rubber tends to expand and by so doing seals off all bleeding vessels rendering the field dry. If at the end of the operation, after removal of the pledgets, bleeding resumes, place a piece of fat tissue into the canal over the bleeding area; this invariably controls all bleeding.

Bleeding that might occur and continue from raw bony surfaces such as at the base of the removed spinous processes can readily be controlled by bone wax.

Exploration of the Spinal Canal

While exploring the spinal canal, utmost caution should be exercised in order to avert injury to the dural sac or the nerve root. If the root lies medial to the protrusion it usually can be readily displaced toward the midline to provide access to the nuclear protrusion. Occasionally a large sequestrum may be lodged in the axilla formed by the dural sac and the sheath of the nerve root. It may not be possible to displace the root medially; in this event, remove a portion or all of the nuclear material without disturbing the root. By so doing, the root will be decompressed and can be displaced medially, allowing exploration of the lateral recess of the canal for other nuclear sequestra.

The protrusion may lie inferior to the level of the intervertebral space and deep in the lateral recess. The root may be under great tension and may be adherent to the protrusion. It may be very difficult to displace the root medially without traumatizing it. Sharp dissection may be necessary to mobilize the root. A simple method of doing this is to use a medium-size curette. Hold the curette firmly against the protrusion and then slowly and gently work the root free. Always inspect the area lateral and inferior to the disc space in the lateral recess; nuclear material may be lodged at this site.

Always inspect the pathway of the root as it enters the intervertebral foramen; satisfy yourself that no nuclear material is lodged in the intervertebral canal. Explore that portion of the floor of the spinal canal immediately above and below the affected disc. Dissecting nuclear sequestra may find their way to these regions.

Occasionally a huge, more or less central protrusion is inaccessible because it is impossible to displace medially the dural sac and nerve root without injury. In such a case, a transdural approach through a full laminectomy may be necessary to remove the sequestrum.

Above the level of the L4-L5 disc, unilateral exposure and traction of the dural sac may result in injury to the cauda equina; this is not a rare occurrence. This serious complication is avoidable by making the approach to the canal as far laterally as possible, by doing a complete laminectomy and by applying as little traction as possible on the dural sac. It is very embarrassing to the surgeon for a patient to wake up with a cauda equina syndrome.

Evacuation of the Disc

Inspection of the annulus often reveals a small rent indicating the site of exit of the nuclear material. Extract all loose fragments from the disc space, using a blunt pituitary rongeur. If possible, all the nuclear material should be removed so that recurrences of extrusion of nuclear material do not occur. Though some surgeons claim that the disc space can be completely evacuated of all nuclear tissue through the posterior approach, we are of the opinion that this is rarely achieved; nevertheless, an attempt should be made to do so. Nuclear fragments still attached to the cartilaginous plates can be detached by using a sharp curette. Caution must be taken not to penetrate the anterior annulus and the anterior longitudinal ligament with the curette. In using the curette its edge must always be against the bone on either side of the disc space. No stroke of the curette must be made without feeling the underlying bone. With practice, the sensation made when the curette is in contact with bone is readily acquired. Use blunt, pituitary rongeurs of various angles to gain access to all areas within the intervertebral space. When using instruments in the disc space, always be aware of the possibility of injury to the large vessels and, on the right side, to the vena cava. If severe uncontrollable arterial bleeding occurs the possibility of injury to the abdominal vessels is real. In this event, no time should be lost to turn the patient over and explore the abdomen. Immediate and continuous replacement of blood loss is mandatory until the source of bleeding is controlled.

A sudden drop of blood pressure, shock and an increase in the white blood cell count after the completion of what appeared a routine lumbar disc operation suggests internal bleeding, most likely due to a tear in one of the abdominal vessels. Besides free bleeding resulting from tears in large vessels, injury to the vessels may be followed by an arteriovenous communication or an aneurysm.

OPERATIVE TECHNIQUE

The operative procedure about to be described has evolved over the past 30 years. Many operations and combinations of various techniques have, at one time or another, been employed by us. The procedure used currently, in our hands, has given us the best results. This technique or combination of techniques is in no way original with us.[3, 4, 6, 9, 12] We prefer it because the incidence of pseudarthrosis is practically nil, being less than one per cent in one-level fusions, it permits patients to be out of bed within a few days, and if only the L5-S1 segment is fused no external support is necessary. Spines with spondylolysis and spondylolisthesis involving the fifth lumbar vertebra are fused from L5 to S1 only. The patients can resume sedentary employment in four to six weeks and full activity in four to six months. So far in none of these spines has there been a recurrence of nuclear extrusion. With a little modification, it is an excellent operation when it is desirable to leave the dural sac uncovered, such as in spondylolisthesis after the posterior elements are removed, or in cases of exaggerated lumbosacral angle or when an extensive laminectomy has been done previously. Unless some contraindication exists to spine fusion, all spines are prepared for fusion as the operation proceeds. Essentially, after completion of the surgery concerned with the intervertebral disc, a posterolateral fusion is performed utilizing cancellous bone grafts removed from one ilium just below the posterior aspect of the iliac crest.

ANESTHESIA

Anesthesia by intratracheal intubation is to be preferred. However, the choice of the anesthetic is left entirely up to the Department of Anesthesia, whose anesthetists are very competent and accustomed to working with orthopedic patients.

POSITION OF THE PATIENT

As a rule, the prone position is used routinely; the patient lies on two long sandbags placed one on either side so that they extend from just below the shoulders to the groin; this allows ample breathing space. The anterior iliac crests lie directly over the kidney rest of the operating table. The lower end of the table is dropped so that the legs are flexed at the hips about 30 to 45 degrees; this position reduces the lumbar lordosis. By slightly elevating the kidney rest, the lumbar curve is completely obliterated or even slightly reversed (Fig. 15-4).

Incision

If one or both lower lumbar disc spaces are to be explored, a vertical skin incision is made in the midline from the tip of the spinous process of the third lumbar vertebra to approximately the tip of the third spinous process of the sacrum. At this point it curves sharply to the left and continues horizontally for two to three inches (Fig. 15-5). The horizontal extension of the incision facilitates the removal of bone from the left ilium. The vertical limb of the incision is deepened through the subcutaneous tissue and fascia down to the tips of the spinous processes of the L3, L4, L5, S1 and S2 or S3 vertebrae. For this part of the exposure, the electric cutting knife is used; this greatly reduces the amount of bleeding. Next, starting with the fifth lumbar vertebra, using a broad, sharp periosteal elevator the muscle mass is stripped subperiosteally off the left side of the spinous process and lamina. The subperiosteal dissection is carried lateral to just beyond the left apophyseal joint and then the wound is packed tightly with a narrow, long, dry sponge (tagged). The fourth and then the third lumbar vertebrae are exposed in a similar manner and finally the left side of the base of the sacrum. The entire wound is now repacked and the right side of the spine is exposed in the same manner. Next, place the blades of a self-retaining retractor deeply in the wound and spread the wound apart. Now, the surgeon should be able to visualize all the posterior elements of the vertebrae from L3 to and including the base of the sacrum (Fig. 15-6).

With a sharp angled bone cutter remove the spinous processes of the base of the sacrum and the spinous process of the fifth lumbar vertebra close to its base. If the fusion area is to include the fourth lumbar vertebra, its spinous process is also removed. Any bleeding from the raw surfaces is

Fig. 15-4

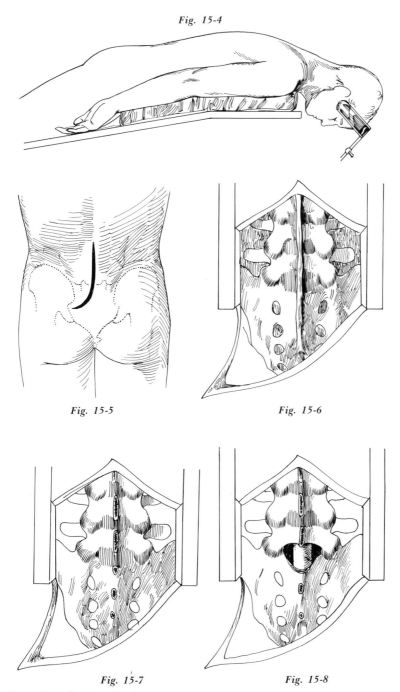

Fig. 15-5

Fig. 15-6

Fig. 15-7

Fig. 15-8

Figure 15-4 Position of patient.

Figure 15-5 Incision for exploration and posterolateral fusion.

Figure 15-6 Exposure of L3 to S3 as far as lateral to the apophyseal joints.

Figure 15-7 Ligaments and spinous processes are removed from L3 to S3.

Figure 15-8 Rim of bone has been removed from the sacrum together with the ligamentum flavum; the dura is exposed.

easily controlled with bone wax. This step also removes the supraspinous and interspinous ligaments from L3 down to the sacrum. With sharp curettes, all remaining soft tissue is removed from the base of the sacrum and the laminae of the fifth lumbar vertebrae; the only ligament remaining is the ligamentum flavum (Fig. 15-7).

The next step is to gain access to the spinal canal. If the S1 root and the L5-S1 disc are to be investigated, a rim of bone measuring approximately one-quarter inch is removed from the superior lamina of the first sacral vertebra on the side to be explored. This is achieved with a sharp beveled gouge one-half or three-quarter inches wide. Tap the gouge lightly but firmly until you feel it enter the spinal canal. With a small curette, elevate the rim of bone from the sacrum with the ligamentum flavum still attached to its anterior and proximal margin. Grasp the rim of bone with a forceps and elevate it from the dural sac; next, with a medium-size curette or a pair of scissors cut the medial and lateral attachments of the ligamentum flavum and finally cut the proximal attachments of the ligament at its line of insertion into the inferior margin of the lamina of the fifth lumbar vertebra (Fig. 15-8). If the fenestration is not large enough, a portion of the inferior aspect of the lamina of the fifth lumbar vertebra is nibbled away. This opening provides ample space to explore the S1 nerve root and the L5-S1 disc.

With a blunt-ended dissector the dura is gently displaced toward the midline and held with the least amount of traction possible. If the nerve root is normal, this maneuver brings it into view. A normal root is easily identified; it is of uniform thickness and lies free in the anterolateral aspect of the canal; its sheath is smooth, glistening and free of any evidence of inflammation such as the presence of numerous fine vessels, edema and adhesions. On the other hand, an affected root is not so readily exposed. At this stage of the operation, the surgeon proceeds with great caution. Not infrequently, upon retraction of the dura, a large mound is felt as the blunt dissector passes over the protrusion. In this event the root, as a rule, is readily located and its relationship to the protrusion noted. When this is the case, the root is carefully displaced, usually medialward, and the protrusion cleared and isolated by placing foam rubber pledgets above and below the lesion in the lateral aspect of the spinal canal; if the pledgets tend to slip out of the canal they can be secured by placing cotton pledgets in front of them (Fig. 15-9).

The root may be firmly bound down with adhesions and is not easily identifiable; in such cases the surgeon proceeds cautiously and systematically; first, the root is identified and its course noted; next, the protrusion (if present) is found and its relationship to the root established; finally, the root is mobilized and freed of the protrusion. The stretched posterior ligament over the mound is nicked and the nuclear protrusion is removed with a pituitary rongeur (Fig. 15-10). Upon nicking the ligament over the extrusion, the degenerated nuclear material, if it is a free fragment under pressure, may burst into the spinal canal, or it can be teased out with very little difficulty. If the nuclear material is bound down to the underlying tissues, when the ligament is nicked, the mound remains in situ and can only be extracted with great difficulty.

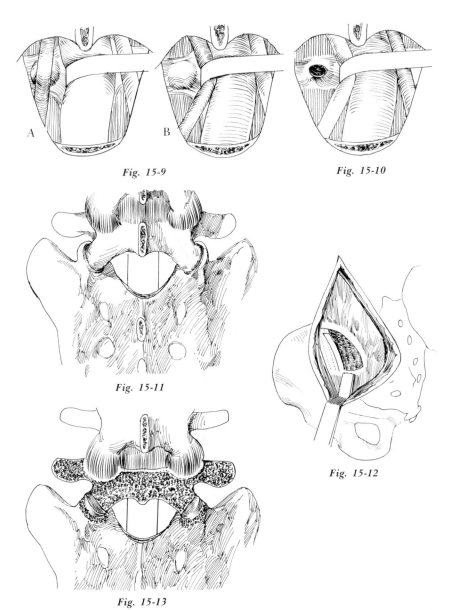

Fig. 15-9

Fig. 15-10

Fig. 15-11

Fig. 15-12

Fig. 15-13

Figure 15-9 *A*, Exposure of the spinal canal showing relation of the nerve root to the herniated disc material. *B*, The nerve root is dissected away from the disc material.

Figure 15-10 The extruded disc material is removed and the disc space curetted of all accessible nuclear fragments, leaving a hole in the annulus fibrosus.

Figure 15-11 The laminae and transverse processes of L5 and the base of the sacrum are stripped of all soft tissues; all capsular tissues are removed from the posterior joints of L5-S1.

Figure 15-12 Slivers of cancellous bone are removed from the side of the ilium.

Figure 15-13 Preparation of a raw bed to receive the cancellous grafts.

Nothing is more dramatic than to displace the dura toward the midline and have a huge, irregular mass of nuclear tissue, which is lying free in the canal, come into view; or, when a tight, tense nerve root is displaced, a large glistening mound is sighted. As previously noted, several types of lesions may be encountered; their identification and how they are dealt with has already been described. Also, the technique to locate and evacuate the affected discs and the indications and methods employed to explore bilateral lesions at the same level or double lesions at different levels has been recorded (see pages 302-304). The next stage of the operation is arthrodesis of the spine.

Technique of Arthrodesis of the Spine

PREPARATION OF THE SPINE FOR FUSION

This part of the operation should not add more than 30 to 45 minutes to the length of the combined procedure. If the fusion is to extend from L5 to the base of the sacrum, the apophyseal joint on one side between L4 and L5 is identified. Just lateral and slightly inferior to the posterior joint lies the transverse process of the fifth lumbar vertebra. Beginning at the upper level of the joint and proceeding downward, with an electric cutting knife, all the muscle attachments are severed from the lateral aspect of the L4-L5 posterior joint, the lateral aspect of the body of the fifth lumbar vertebra and the lateral aspect of the L5-S1 posterior joint down to the body of the sacrum. Next, with a broad periosteal elevator, strip all muscle attachments from the posterior surface of the transverse process of the fifth lumbar vertebra, from the lateral surface of the body of L5 and from the lateral aspect of the L5-S1 posterior joint down to the sacrum. Some bleeding may be encountered during this phase of the procedure, but this is easily controlled by a large gauze sponge packed tightly in the wound. The procedure is then repeated on the other side, the wound is packed tightly and closed temporarily with two towel clips (Fig. 15-11).

CANCELLOUS BONE GRAFTS OBTAINED FROM
THE ILIUM

Through the lower end of the incision the posterior iliac crest is exposed for a distance of three to four inches and the muscles are stripped subperiosteally from the lateral aspect of the posterior portion of the ilium down to the greater sciatic notch. A broad-toothed reverse retractor is engaged under the superior margin of the greater sciatic notch and the detached muscles are displaced laterally. Beginning just distal to the upper border of the iliac crest, with a gouge, strips of bone two to two and one-half inches long are removed from the side of the ilium; also small chips of cancellous bone are removed from the raw surface of the ilium. Cancellous bone is removed until the inner cortical table of the ilium is encountered. The bone removed from this site is more than ample. The wound is irrigated with normal saline and closed. The bone is now cut into long slivers approximately two to two and one-half inches long. Smaller pieces of cancellous bone are cut up into small chip grafts (Fig. 15-12).

PREPARATION OF THE BED TO RECEIVE THE BONE GRAFTS

The wound in the midline is reopened and self-retaining retractors are reinserted. All the sponges are removed from the wound. At this point, with the index finger, palpate all portions of the wound, especially the lateral recesses for the presence of any sponges; at this time it is wise to take a sponge count. With a sharp gouge remove a portion of the inferior and superior facets of the L5-S1 posterior joints; this increases the surface area of raw bone. Next, decorticate both laminae of L5 and the base of the sacrum (Fig. 15-13). The bone obtained is cut into small bone chips. The thin, long slivers of cancellous bone obtained from the ilium are placed longitudinally in the lateral gutter of the wound from the upper border of the transverse process of L5 to the base of the sacrum. As much bone as possible is packed into the lateral gutters; the grafts also cover the raw surfaces of the base of the facets. The remaining bone is arranged longitudinally so that it spans the interval from the upper borders of the laminae of the fifth lumbar vertebra to the sacrum as far as the second or third sacral segment (Fig. 15-14).

Before the wound is closed, it is thoroughly flushed out with normal saline solution and any devitalized tissue is cut away. Next, Hemovac drains are inserted in the wounds; one limb of the drain is placed at the bottom of the midline wound and the other between the side of the ilium which supplied the bone grafts and the detached muscles. The wound is closed in the usual manner.

If the fourth lumbar vertebra is to be included in the fusion, the fourth lumbar vertebra is exposed in a similar manner as just described. The transverse processes of the fifth lumbar vertebra lie just distal and lateral to the apophyseal joints of the third and fourth vertebrae. The facets of the posterior joints of the fourth and fifth, and those of the fifth lumbar and first sacral vertebrae, are excised at their bases.

MODIFICATION OF THE POSTEROLATERAL FUSION

It was previously recorded that it may be desirable to leave the posterior dura exposed, not making any contact with the overlying bone. This occasion arises in fusion of spines with spondylolisthesis or with an accentuated lumbosacral angle or in spines with extensive laminectomies. The procedure is exactly the same as that described above except that no bone is placed over the dural sac. All bone is placed in the lateral gutters from the transverse processes of the fifth lumbar vertebra to the sacrum. By using this technique, fusion of a spine with spondylolisthesis of the fifth vertebra need not extend beyond the fifth vertebra (Fig. 15-15). We have yet to see the patient with spondylolisthesis fused by this method that did not attain a solid fusion.

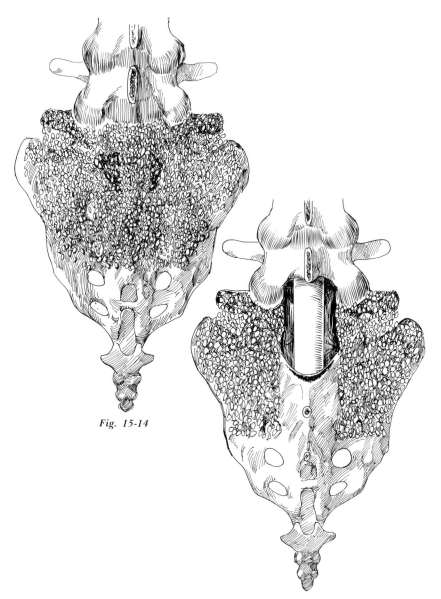

Fig. 15-14

Fig. 15-15

Figure 15-14   Cancellous bone slivers and chips span the interval from the upper borders of the transverse processes and laminae of L5 to the third sacral segment.

Figure 15-15   Modification of the posterolateral fusion, used when it is desirable to leave the dura uncovered and in spondylolisthesis requiring fusion.

POSTOPERATIVE MANAGEMENT

The postoperative course varies considerably from patient to patient and therefore its management must be fitted to the patient. Some patients complain of severe pain, whereas others have little or no complaints. Broadly speaking, the patient is kept in bed with one or two pillows as desired for the first few days and allowed to move about at his own discretion. If the patient has severe pain, narcotics are given in sufficient dosage to produce relief; as a rule, narcotics or analgesics are seldom required after the third or fourth day. Apprehensive patients are given sedatives for as long as is required. Soma (Carisoprodal), in a dosage of 350 mg. three times daily, is an excellent relaxant. Appropriate antibiotics, in adequate dosage, are administered for the first four or five days. The Hemovac tubes are withdrawn after 72 hours.

Not infrequently, patients complain of varying degrees of pain and sensory manifestations in the legs, which may last from several days to several weeks. This is undoubtedly due to surgical trauma to a nerve root producing swelling and edema. The reason for the pain must be explained to the patient lest he come to the conclusion that the operation is unsuccessful.

The patient with a fusion between the fifth lumbar vertebra and the sacrum needs no external support, but one with a fusion of more than one segment of the spine is fitted with a light corset brace. Patients are allowed out of bed as soon as they wish, usually from three to seven days after operation. They are permitted to go home seven to ten days after surgery.

While at home, the patient is allowed to move about up to his point of tolerance. He is advised against performing any activities which subject the spine to flexion strains, stair climbing and riding in an automobile. Rest periods should be taken throughout the day as needed. Patients wearing corset braces are advised to wear the support during the day only. At this time, mild radiant heat and gentle massage may be given because they produce a soothing effect and help absorb exudates in the tissues subjected to surgery. The patient's activities are gradually increased but always within the patient's tolerance. Some patients persist beyond their tolerance; they should be advised to pursue a slower course.

Within four to six weeks most patients are performing light duties, and those with sedentary employment can now return at least to part-time work. Examination of the patient is made every six weeks, and he is guided accordingly. Radiographs are taken at each examination and the status of the fusion is determined. Fusion is usually solid in four to six months; now the patients are taught mild flexion and extension exercises to restore muscle tone and flexibility of the spine (Figs. 15-16, 15-17 and 15-18). Many patients have a tendency to overexercise, believing that if an exercise performed five times is beneficial, ten times should be even more effective. They must be advised against it. Patients whose employment is doing heavy laborious work should not be allowed to return to this type of work for at least six to eight months—longer, if they can be persuaded to do so. Athletic activities, especially contact sports, should not be engaged in during the first 12 months after surgery.

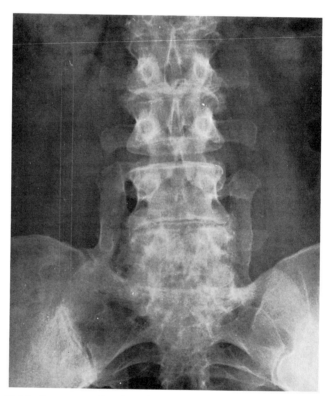

Figure 15-16   Anteroposterior view of a posterolateral spine fusion extending from L4 to S2, 18 months after the operation. Note the massive columns of bone bridging the interval from the transverse processes of L4 to the sacrum.

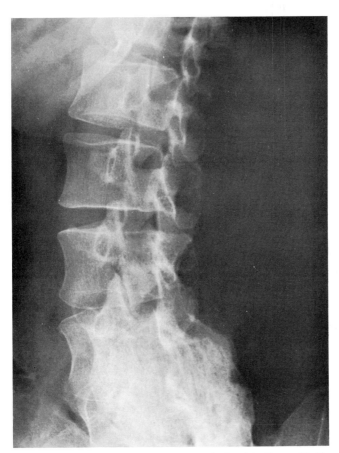

Figure 15-17 Oblique view of the spine depicted in Figure 15-16.

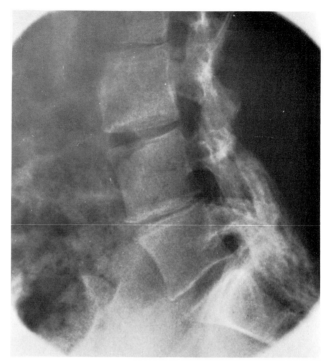

Figure 15-18   Lateral view of the spine depicted in Figures 15-16 and 15-17.

Characteristic of patients who have undergone surgery for lumbar disc lesions is the periodic recurrence of mild symptoms lasting from a few days to several weeks; usually they are not incapacitating. Undoubtedly, after surgery, adhesions form around a nerve root which restrict its normal range of movement associated with movements of the trunk and legs. Stretching of the fixed nerve roots may be responsible for the pain. A few days of rest and restricted activities for several weeks usually suffices to alleviate the pain.

Patients with long fusion areas (more than one segment) start taking the brace off when there is radiological evidence of good coalescence of the fusion mass. This usually occurs in three to four months. At this time, the brace is removed for several hours each day, and as the patient's tolerance increases the period of time without the use of the brace is increased. Usually the brace is discarded within four to six weeks. For these patients, the above program is geared to a slower pace than patients with one-level fusions.

After six to eight months, the patient is evaluated at six month periods for two years. At each examination, radiographs of the spine are taken and an evaluation is made of any residual clinical manifestations. Patients are often concerned about some of the motor and sensory manifestations such as numbness of the leg or foot, weakness of the dorsiflexors of the foot or thinning of one calf. The behavior of motor and sensory changes is very unpredictable. It may take many months for a muscle group to be restored to the power and the mass of that of the opposite, normal group. Although sensory changes have a better prognosis and return to normalcy sooner than motor deficits, we have observed many patients with residual sensory alterations which were permanent. Reflex changes are even more unpredictable; not infrequently the loss of certain reflexes is permanent, and if return does occur it may require many months. The wise and experienced surgeon explains all these possibilities to the patient and also impresses upon him the fact that mild, permanent, residual, motor, sensory or reflex changes are insignificant and will in no way interfere with the patient's normal daily activities.

ANTERIOR INTERBODY FUSION

Some surgeons are now doing anterior interbody fusions routinely for all cases in which they believe spine fusion is justified. We do not subscribe to this reasoning and perform anterior body fusions only in specific circumstances. It is our opinion that this type of fusion should be reserved for those cases which have previously been subjected to numerous operations through the posterior approach to the spine. Many of these patients exhibit profound atrophy and fibrosis of the paravertebral muscles resulting in almost complete loss of flexion of the lumbar spine. A second indication for anterior interbody fusion is found in patients with marked instability of the lumbar spine following extensive laminectomies of several vertebrae.

The operation should be performed together with an abdominal surgeon who exposes extraperitoneally the lower lumbar bodies and the promontory of the sacrum. The operation we employ is relatively simple. The level to be fused is identified and cleared of all soft tissue; the large vessels in the region are carefully retracted away from the operative field. With a sharp osteotome, two vertical cuts, one on either side of the midline, are made across the disc and the body of the vertebra above and below. The cuts span one-half the height of each body and are separated by a distance equal to one-half the width of each body. The upper and lower limbs of the vertical cuts are connected by horizontal cuts which penetrate approximately one-half the anteroposterior distance of each body. The vertical cuts are extended to the same depth and the square blocks of bone still attached to the middle portion of the intervertebral disc are elevated out of their beds, leaving a large square defect spanning the contiguous portions of the vertebrae (Fig. 15-19). The graft is rotated 90 degrees, fitted in the defect, and with an impactor and mallet it is seated deeply in the defect (Fig. 15-20). If more than one level is to be included in the fusion area the above technique is repeated at each level.

Following the operation, the vertebrae bridged by bone are locked tightly and feel very stable.

The postoperative management is the same as that described for posterior fusions. No external support is necessary.

It should be noted that occasionally it is necessary to evacuate a disc infection through the anterior route. In such an event, the entire disc space is evacuated of all debris such as remnants of disc material and articular cartilage. It is unnecessary to pack the cavity with bone, for spontaneous fusion invariably occurs. However, following this procedure the patient should be at complete rest in a plaster spica until fusion is solid.

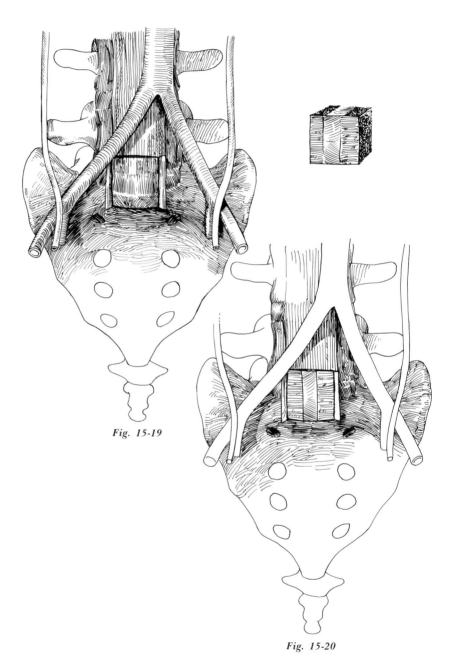

Fig. 15-19

Fig. 15-20

Figure 15-19   The graft comprises one-half of the body of L5 and one-half of the body of S1; the intervertebral disc lies between the two blocks of bone. The graft is rotated so that the disc lies in the vertical plane.

Figure 15-20   The rotated graft is countersunk into the defect.

REFERENCES

1. Armstrong, J. R.: Lumbar disc lesions. Baltimore, Williams & Wilkins, 1965.
2. Barr, J. S.: Low back and sciatic pain—results of treatment. Reference to treatment of intervertebral disc lesions. J. Bone Joint Surg. 33-A:633-649, 1951.
3. Bosworth, D. M.: Circumduction fusion of the spine. J. Bone Joint Surg. 38-A:263-9, 1956.
4. Cleveland, M. et al.: Pseudarthrosis in lumbosacral spine. J. Bone Joint Surg. 30-A:302-312, 1948.
5. Colonna, P. C. et al.: The disc syndrome. Results of the conservative care of patients with positive myelogram. J. Bone Joint Surg. 31-A:614-618, 1949.
6. DePalma, A. F. et al.: Long-term results of herniated nucleus pulposus treated by excision of the disc only. Clin. Orthop. 22:139-144, 1962.
7. DePalma, A. F. and Prabhakar, M.: Posterior-posterobilateral fusion of the lumbosacral spine. Clin. Orthop. 47:165-171, 1966.
8. Hirsch, C.: Efficiency of surgery in low-back disorders. J. Bone Joint Surg. 47-A:991-1004, 1965.
9. McElroy, K. D.: Personal communication.
10. Raaf, J.: Some observations regarding 905 patients operated upon for protruded lumbar intervertebral discs. Am. J. of Surg. 97:388-399, 1959.
11. Sarpyener, M. A.: Congenital stricture of spinal canal. J. Bone Joint Surg. 27:70-79, 1945.
12. Watkins, M. B.: Posterolateral bone-grafting for fusion of the lumbar and lumbosacral spine. J. Bone Joint Surg. 41-A:388-396, 1959.
13. Young, H. H. et al.: End results of removal of protruded lumbar intervertebral discs with and without fusion. Instruc. Course Lect. 16:213-216, 1959.
14. Ytrehus, Ø: Prognosis in medically treated sciatica (follow-up investigation of 256 patients). Acta Med. Scand. 128:452-472, 1947.

COMPLICATIONS, FAILURES AND TRAGEDIES OF OPERATIVE TREATMENT OF LUMBAR DISC DISEASE

Many complications may occur during the operative procedure or immediately after. Most of these are preventable and all, if recognized early, can be adequately treated. The most important single factor in prevention is awareness. This is particularly true of those complications that can occur during the operation. But to prevent accidents during the operation, awareness alone is not enough. It should be reenforced by caution, by skillful, exacting handling of instruments and by knowledge of the anatomy and pathology of the region.

COMPLICATIONS DURING THE OPERATION

Vascular and Visceral Injuries

Although rare, vascular and visceral injuries are more common than generally appreciated. A few cases have been reported, but many more have not been. In 1959, Desaussure[1] reported a survey which he conducted the year before: 3000 surgeons were contacted and he gathered 106 cases of vascular injuries of iatrogenic origin. Very few large surgical services

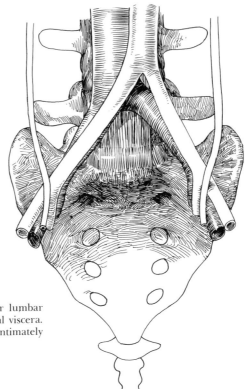

Figure 16-1 Relation of the lower lumbar discs to the large vessels and abdominal viscera. The bifurcation of the large vessels is intimately related to the L4-L5 disc.

doing back surgery have not encountered vascular accidents during surgery on the intervertebral discs. On our service, two vascular mishaps have occurred; in each instance the operation was being performed by a competent orthopedic surgeon. That these accidents carry serious implications, for both the surgeon and the patient, is self-evident. The mortality rate is almost 55 per cent.

Most of the vascular injuries occur while trying to grasp and extract an elusive fragment of degenerated nuclear material, or when attempting to determine the depth of the interspace, or when using a curette injudiciously in the disc space. The injuries that may occur are: (1) lacerations or complete avulsion of the wall of one of the large vessels lying in the prevertebral space, such as the aorta, inferior vena cava, large vessels of the extremities (the iliac arteries or veins); (2) laceration or partial avulsion of a vessel wall resulting in delayed hemorrhage or thrombosis; (3) laceration of both artery and vein resulting in an arteriovenous fistula.

Occasionally, vascular injuries are complicated by injuries to an abdominal viscus, such as the ureter, the bladder and the ileum. Visceral lesions may occur as isolated injuries.

The intimate relation of the large vessels and viscera in the prevertebral space to the lower disc spaces readily explains the ease with which one of these complications can occur. In Figure 16-1 note the relationship of the bifurcation of the large vessels to the L4-L5 disc. Most of the reported injuries have occurred while extracting nuclear material of this disc.

PREVENTION

There is no doubt that most of the vascular injuries are preventable, but we must acknowledge that some are unavoidable. Certain precautions will reduce the chances of the injuries occurring.

NEVER WORK BLINDLY IN A DISC SPACE

The operative site should always be in full vision; this is impossible if the field is obscured by blood or by inadequate retraction of the dura and nerve root. There should be ample room to retract the neural elements without tension. The field should be isolated by pledgets of foam rubber or cotton so that the aperture in the annulus is always clearly in view.

DON'T EXPLORE THE INTERVERTEBRAL SPACE
TO DETERMINE ITS DEPTH

This is a precarious procedure, usually it is performed with straight curettes which can readily penetrate a weakened anterior longitudinal ligament and pierce a vessel. There is no need for this step in disc surgery if one makes a point of not introducing an instrument into the disc space for a greater distance than one and one-eighth inches. This distance should in some way be marked on the instrument, particularly curettes and pituitary rongeurs. Some surgeons don't need these markings because they are exact and skillful enough to contain their movements well within the safe range; but for many others the markings are almost mandatory.

USE OF CURETTES AND PITUITARY RONGEURS

Curettes and rongeurs should never penetrate the disc space for more than one and one-eighth inches. But, just as important, before every stroke of the curette and every bite of the rongeur, the end of the instrument must be felt against the bony surface of the vertebra above or below. Once this little maneuver is perfected, the surgeon executes it almost reflexly and does not complete the stroke of the curette or close the jaws of the rongeur unless bone is felt at its tip.

DIAGNOSES

In some instances, the diagnosis of vascular injury is made immediately, but not infrequently it is overlooked; or, it may not manifest itself for months or years, as is the case with some arteriovenous fistulae.

DIAGNOSIS OF A VASCULAR INJURY SHOULD
BE MADE:

1. When the surgeon knows that his instrument has penetrated the

anterior confines of the joint, and the field is flooded with large amounts of blood coming from the disc space.

2. When this same type of profuse uncontrolled bleeding occurs, but the surgeon is not aware that he has penetrated the anterior aspect of the joint.

3. When the patient suddenly goes into profound vascular shock characterized by sudden hypotension, loss of the arterial pulse or the presence of a rapid, thready pulse. This state may be confused with cardiac arrest; however, the anesthesiologist can readily make the differential diagnosis by auscultation and electrocardiography. It should be remembered that evidence of vascular shock may not be associated with any external bleeding.

4. When the patient goes into vascular shock several days after the operation. If the arterial wall is contused and not avulsed, a delayed rupture of the artery with formation of a massive hematoma may occur. Secondary hemorrhage occurs when the wall eventually breaks down or an aneurysm may form.

5. When injury to a concomitant artery and vein results in the formation of an arteriovenous fistula, which may go unrecognized for months or years after the disc surgery, until the patient develops cardiac decompensation. Now the diagnosis is readily established by the clinical manifestations and arteriography. Unfortunately, almost 50 per cent of the cases of vascular injuries are not recognized at the time of surgery.

Concomitant visceral injuries may be overlooked at the time of surgery; however, within a few days manifestations of an intra-abdominal injury become apparent.

MANAGEMENT

IMMEDIATE RECOGNITION OF THE VASCULAR INJURY

Just as soon as the injury is recognized, put into motion the following steps:

1. Immediately request an abdominal surgeon with experience in vascular surgery, and request a laparotomy tray.

2. Continuously administer massive volumes of whole blood.

3. Quickly pack and close the back wound with a few through-and-through sutures and cover it with a sterile plastic drape.

4. Turn the patient to the supine position and quickly prepare the abdomen for a laparotomy.

5. If the general surgeon has arrived, turn the patient over to him; if not, proceed with the laparotomy. Upon entering the abdominal cavity massive bleeding and large quantities of blood may be present; however, the only evidence of bleeding may be the presence of a large hematoma in the retroperitoneal space. The next step is to divide the posterior peritoneum, clear the area of any blood and search for the bleeding point. Generally the site of bleeding is on the posterior aspect of the aorta, the vena cava or one of the lumbar vessels. Apply vascular clamps above and

below the site of bleeding. Bleeding having been controlled, attention is directed to restoring all the blood lost and treating the shock until the patient is stable. By this time, a general or vascular surgeon should be on the scene.

6. After the vascular injury is repaired and the vital signs are stable, the patient is turned over and attention is directed to the back wound. Further surgery on the back depends on the condition of the patient. If the condition permits, the operation is quickly completed; if not, the wound should be thoroughly irrigated, preferably with a solution containing a broad spectrum antibiotic, and closed with several through-and-through sutures.

7. Place the patient in an intensive care unit.

DELAYED RECOGNITION OF THE VASCULAR INJURY

The injury may not be recognized for several days after the operation. Usually this occurs when the arterial wall is injured but not avulsed; a hematoma forms, sealing the defect in the arterial wall; later, secondary rupture occurs.

The clinical manifestations are those of sudden vascular collapse and the management is the same as that described for lesions which are immediately recognized.

Recognition may not come for months or years after the injury. An arteriovenous fistula forms which so alters the hemodynamics that cardiac decompensation occurs. If a patient has had disc surgery and subsequently develops a palpable thrill in the lower regions of the abdomen and a continuous bruit, an arteriovenous fistula must be suspected. The management is entirely in the realm of a vascular surgeon. Another clue to the diagnosis of an arteriovenous fistula is insidious swelling of one of the lower extremities due to uncontrollable lymphedema.

Injuries to the Neural Elements

Injuries to the nerve roots, the dural sac and to the cauda equina may occur during the operation. Most injuries are avoidable if care is exercised in the handling of the structures.

TEAR OF THE DURA

The dura may be lacerated when the fenestration is being made to gain access to the spinal canal or it may be punctured while being displaced medially in order to expose the protrusion or to mobilize the nerve root. Extreme caution while unroofing the spinal canal will prevent this mishap; also when using rongeurs to remove bone, the dura should be gently picked from the bone.

The dura is more likely to be injured in cases in which there has been previous surgery. The dura may be adherent to overlying fibrous tissue, or the root and dura may be firmly adherent to the annulus, the site of previous surgery. But even in these instances, the dura can, with care, be peeled off or dissected free of the scar tissue.

Should injury occur, particularly if the rent extends into the subarachnoid space, repair of the defect is not usually difficult. It is closed with fine nylon sutures. Failure to repair the tear may result in the formation of an internal arachnoid cyst or a fistula leaking cerebrospinal fluid.

INJURY TO THE NERVE ROOT

Often the nerve root is flattened and adherent to a large nuclear protrusion making it difficult to gain access to the nuclear mass. Injuries are usually inflicted on the root while it is being peeled off the protrusion. In such cases it may be possible to partially decompress the nuclear sequestrum by extracting part of it before the root is mobilized. This is particularly applicable to large protrusions which displace the root laterally. If the area has been explored previously the root may be enmeshed in dense scar tissue, requiring sharp dissection to free it. Injury may be avoided if the fenestration is large and the root can be fully visualized.

One cause of root injury which is definitely avoidable is traction on the root while a disc space is being evacuated. The assistant making traction should be aware of this complication and should avoid excessive traction and should from time to time release all traction.

The root may be injured by thermal burns sustained when attempting to stop bleeding in the canal with a cautery; this is certainly avoidable.

Occasionally the root is fixed by anomalous nerve roots which resist traction; but even here with care enough exposure of the lesion may be attained without injuring the roots.

The residual motor and sensory deficits depend upon the extent of the root damage. If the root was severely compressed prior to or during the operation, or partly divided, the residual deficits are permanent. If the loss of root function is the result of edema and contusion, recovery can be expected, although it may require many months.

INJURY TO THE CAUDA EQUINA

This is another injury which should not occur; it is the result of excessive traction on the cauda equina during the operative procedure. Following injury recovery is often not complete, leaving the patient with motor and sensory deficits and partial or complete loss of sphincter control.

COMPLICATIONS DURING THE IMMEDIATE POSTOPERATIVE PERIOD

Although it may seem superfluous to consider this group of complications, we have seen some serious problems arise from failure to recognize or to treat them early and effectively. They are complications that are not related to the operation on the intervertebral disc and may occur after any major surgical procedure.

GASTRIC DILATATION

Gastric dilatation may occur in any age group but more frequently in the elderly patient. It comes on more or less insidiously, its earliest signs being hiccups, nausea and regurgitation of small amounts of bile-stained fluids. Later, when the distention is obvious, evidence of respiratory and cardiac embarrassment occurs, the principal signs being hypotension and tachycardia. These patients may die if not treated promptly and vigorously. Death is often the result of aspiration of gastric fluids which produce pneumonia. Radiographs will confirm the diagnosis. Essentially, the treatment is removal of the gastric fluids by intubating the stomach and applying a mechanical suction apparatus. It may also be necessary to aspirate the tracheobronchial tree. The stomach should be decompressed for several days before oral feeding is started.

INTESTINAL ILEUS

Intestinal ileus is not an infrequent complication of back surgery. The cardinal features are abdominal distention, respiratory distress and electrolyte imbalance due to the outpouring of fluids into the small bowel. Radiographs taken with the patient in the erect and lateral positions show the characteristic fluid levels in the small bowel.

Treatment should be instituted promptly; the small bowel is intubated and continuous mechanical suction maintained until there is evidence of restoration of bowel tone indicated by peristalsis and bowel function. By frequent determinations of the serum electrolytes, electrolyte imbalance is corrected by the administration of the needed solutions.

URINARY RETENTION

This complication is more frequently seen in younger patients to whom it may be very distressing. If it cannot be controlled by urecholine, catheterization of the bladder becomes necessary.

INFECTION

One of the most catastrophic complications is meningitis of staphylococcal origin. Although rare, this complication does occur, particularly if the dura has been violated while performing a myelogram or exposing the spinal canal. Symptoms pointing to infection of the meninges may not manifest themselves for several days after the surgery. But severe, continuous headaches associated with an elevated temperature, especially if it tends to spike, should make one suspicious. Later, all the signs of meningeal irritation and a systemic infection are obvious. The diagnosis is confirmed by the presence of the organisms in blood cultures and in the spinal fluid. Once the diagnosis is even suspected, heroic measures should be instituted.

Of importance is the location of the focus of infection (it may not be found). It may be in the wound and may be under pressure; therefore, the wound should be opened under sterile conditions and cultured. Periodic spinal taps may be necessary to reduce the cerebrospinal fluid pressure and, most of all, appropriate antibiotics in massive doses should be administered. It is wise to leave this part of the treatment in the hands of someone knowledgeable in infectious diseases.

WOUND INFECTION

A wound infection should always be suspected when the patient's temperature remains elevated or suddenly rises on the fifth to the seventh day. The wound should be carefully inspected; if there is any suspicion of infection the wound should be opened sufficiently to allow adequate drainage, and a culture should be made from the depth of the wound. At this time, covering the patient with a broad spectrum antibiotic is advisable until the responsible organism is identified and appropriate antibiotics administered.

THROMBOPHLEBITIS

One of the most distressing complications to contend with is thrombophlebitis of the deep veins of the extremities, usually the femoral or popliteal veins. The surgery on the back bears no relationship to thrombophlebitis; the most significant factor is immobilization. Usually the onset is insidious in nature, and indeed the first evidence of the complication may be pulmonary embolism. Generally, the first complaint is a feeling of tightness and swelling of the affected extremity, followed by pain on movements which are associated with contraction of the muscles of the calf or the thigh. There is, as a rule, little evidence of inflammation, although pain is elicited when pressure is made along the course of the vein. There may or may not be a slight rise in the temperature. Treatment is primarily directed toward prevention of pulmonary embolism. The limb should be loosely wrapped in continuous warm packs and elevated, and anti-coagulation therapy should be instituted and continued. Frequent assays of the coagulation time of the blood should be made.

CAUSES OF FAILURE FOLLOWING OPERATIVE TREATMENT

The causes of failure in operative treatment of lumbar disc lesions are many; some are due to shortcomings on the part of the surgeon, others to the nature of the disease and others are beyond the control of either. The various causes can be grouped into four categories: errors in diagnosis, errors in technique, complications directly related to the operation and causes unrelated to the operation.

Errors in Diagnosis

Most of the causes for failure following operation for lumbar disc lesions in this category have already been considered in the section on "differential diagnosis"; however, some of these need re-emphasis.

SPINAL TUMORS

These lesions undoubtedly are responsible for the greatest number of diagnostic errors. The commonest tumors of the spinal cord are: (1) gliomas which are usually intramedullary lesions, (2) neurofibromas and meningiomas which are generally intradural tumors and (3) neurofibromas and metastatic tumors which are usually extradural lesions. Although spinal tumors may mimic the symptomatology of lumbar disc lesions they are associated with certain characteristics which set them apart from disc lesions.

Back pain and sciatica are not mechanical in nature, but rather increase in intensity in the recumbent position. The pain pattern may indicate implication of more than one nerve root. Patients with neurofibromas may exhibit areas of skin pigmentation and nodules. Back pain in children should arouse one's suspicion of a tumor, especially if the child's gait and posture are abnormal. Radiological studies also convey positive information consistent with the diagnosis of spinal tumor. The vertebral bodies or posterior elements may show erosion with or without collapse, and the interpediculate distance is increased due to erosion of one or both pedicles. Myelography is most important in establishing the diagnosis and the total protein of the cerebrospinal fluid usually is markedly elevated.

ANKYLOSING SPONDYLITIS

In the early stages of ankylosing spondylitis before the characteristic radiological features are evident and before the axial skeleton loses its lumbar curve and begins to bend forward, the differential diagnosis from lumbar disc lesions may be difficult to arrive at. Many such errors have been made and many patients with ankylosing spondylitis have been subjected to disc surgery and fusion operations on the lower lumbar spine. The diffuse nature of the back pain, the bizarre vague leg pain with no particular pattern, generalized stiffness of the axial skeleton and a high sedimentation rate should suggest the presence of the disease. In the late stages of this disease, diagnosis is no problem (Fig. 16-2).

SACROILIAC JOINT DISEASE

Destructive lesions of the sacroiliac joint, such as pyogenic and tuberculous infections, pose no diagnostic dilemma. However, this is not true of ankylosing spondylitis affecting the sacroiliac joints, osteitis condensans ilii and degenerative changes in the sacroiliac joint. Ankylosing spondylitis has been considered above.

Osteitis condensans is peculiar in that it often affects young persons, usually women. It may implicate only one joint and the back pain is not that of lumbar disc lesions, but rather it is confined to the region of the sacroiliac joints. Leg pain is usually present but it has no dermatomal pattern; it radiates in the back of the legs and rarely extends beyond the knees. The radiographs reveal the typical characteristics of the disease: the bone of the ilium immediately adjacent to the joint is dense and sclerotic (Fig. 16-3 and 16-4).

(Text continued on page 336)

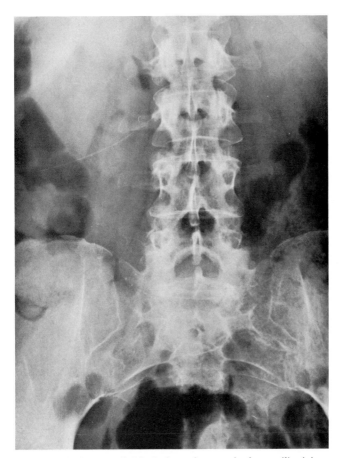

Figure 16-2 Ankylosing spondylitis. In its early stages both sacroiliac joints are involved. This patient had an exploration of the last two lumbar discs; an erroneous diagnosis of lumbar disc disease had been made.

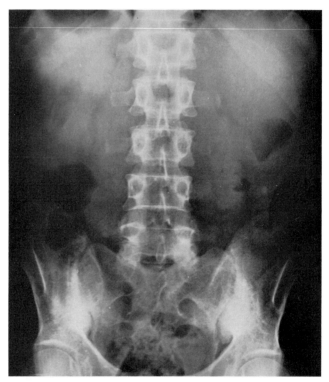

Figure 16-3   Osteitis condensans. In this radiograph of a 26-year-old woman note the sclerosis of the ilium adjacent to both sacroiliac joints.

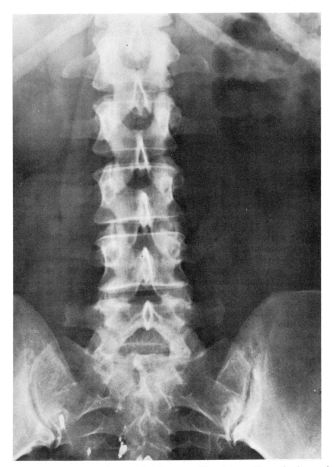

Figure 16-4 Degenerative changes in the sacroiliac joints. Note the irregular spurring at the inferior aspects of the joints. This finding may be asymptomatic. In this patient the changes produced pain which was relieved by fusion of both sacroiliac joints.

Degenerative changes in the sacroiliac joint

At one time changes in the sacroiliac joint were considered the commonest etiological factor for back pain and sciatica. Today it is hardly ever taken into consideration as a cause of back pain. Yet, we are convinced that degenerative changes in the sacroiliac joints produce back pain with or without leg pain more often than is generally realized. The pain is undoubtedly due to instability of the joint secondary to degeneration of its articular surfaces and supporting ligaments just as occurs in any other articulation afflicted with an arthrotic process. The instability we refer to is not similar to that in the peripheral joints or even in the intervertebral joints. It is more subtle, not clinically or radiologically demonstrable, but sufficient to put abnormal stress on the supporting ligaments, thereby producing pain. We have observed many patients that were subjected to disc surgery who were not relieved until one or both sacroiliac joints were fused. In the differential diagnosis of lumbar disc lesions it behooves us to give more consideration to the sacroiliac joint than was given in the past (Fig. 16-5 *a, b*).

Instability of a motor unit

Instability of a motor unit may or may not be associated with a disc lesion. Failure to appreciate the significance of the instability and to correct it has been the cause of most of the failures following surgery of the lumbar discs. It was previously noted that the structural peculiarities of certain anomalies in the lumbosacral region favor mechanical instability, such as: spondylolysis, spondylolisthesis, increase or decrease in the number of free lumbar vertebrae, acute lumbosacral angle, tropism of the apophyseal joints, incomplete lumbarization of the first sacral vertebra and partial sacralization of the fifth lumbar vertebra. In the face of these abnormalities, excision of one of the lower lumbar discs without fusion not only fails to relieve the patient of the back pain but also renders the motor unit even more unstable. These abnormalities may also be associated with leg pain; following excision of the disc alone, the leg pain persists. The same may be said of disc excision alone from an arthrotic intervertebral joint. Unfortunately some of these patients are often subjected to repeated exploratory operations. After each operation the patient is worse off than before. What these patients really need is fusion of the involved motor units. This group of patients furnishes the greatest number of candidates for re-operation.

Errors in Surgical Judgment and Technique

The second largest group of failures is the result of faulty technique and poor judgment exercised during the operation. Many decisions must be made during the course of the operation which demand astute judgment. Such judgment is the product of much surgical experience; the surgeon must be able to recognize a degenerated disc and a normal disc, and he must know how and what to do in case the lesion is not found.

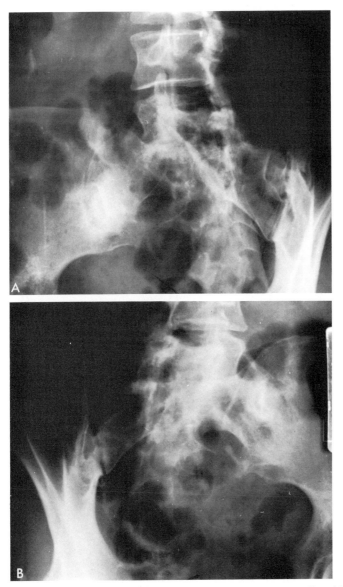

Figure 16-5 Degeneration of the sacroiliac joints; symptoms were relieved by fusion. (*A*), This patient had an excision of the L5 disc and a fusion of the lumbosacral joint but was not relieved of her back and leg pain. (*B*), Relief was obtained after both sacroiliac joints were fused.

NEGATIVE EXPLORATION

Not infrequently the surgeon explores a disc but fails to find the lesion. This poses some difficult problems which must be resolved on the spot. Provided the diagnosis is correct, what are the reasons for a negative exploration? One obvious reason is that the wrong space has been explored. Others are that the exposure of the spinal canal is inadequate, making it impossible to locate the lesion; or, because of excessive bleeding, the lesion cannot be located or recognized; or the subtle changes in the disc such as occur in the "concealed disc" are not recognized. It should be remembered that the disc protrusion may migrate up or down in the spinal canal from its site of extrusion ("dissecting disc") or it may even lodge in the intervertebral foramen. It is apparent that failure resulting from the aforementioned causes lies on the head of the surgeon and can be remedied only by another exploration.

MULTIPLE DISC LESIONS

The surgeon may fail to recognize the possibility of double lesions. Generally it is difficult to make a diagnosis of lumbar disc lesions at different levels because the symptoms produced by a lesion at one level may completely overshadow those of a different level. We are of the opinion that symptomatic double lesions are overestimated; however, if there is the slightest clue which may implicate a disc at another level, that level should be explored. On the other hand, if the clinical picture is clearly defined and correlates with a lesion at a specific level there is no reason to tamper with another disc space.

What has been said of double lesions, each at a different level, is also true of bilateral lesions which occur at the same level. There may be two protrusions at the same level, one on either side, or a large central protrusion extending to either side of the midline. These lesions increase the magnitude of the operation because both sides of the spinal canal must be explored. To remove the lesion from one side necessitates excessive traction on the dural sac; the cauda equina may be stretched and injured. If both lesions are not removed the patient will not be relieved of the symptoms.

INADEQUATE EVACUATION OF THE DISC SPACE

If loose, free sequestra or fragments of degenerated nuclear material are not removed from the disc space, extrusion of this material may occur immediately after the operation or at a later time. The aim is to remove all nuclear material from the disc space, but this is difficult to achieve. In most instances, the surgeon is successful in removing the greater part of the degenerated tissue; but we doubt that all the nuclear tissue is removed in most cases. This being so, there is always the possibility that more extrusions may occur until the intervertebral joint is stabilized completely by mature fibrous tissue.

COMPLICATIONS RELATED TO THE OPERATIVE PROCEDURE

Some of the complications about to be described can be avoided, others are unavoidable.

RECURRENT EXTRUSION OF NUCLEAR MATERIAL

Recurrent symptoms may be caused by further extrusion of nuclear material from the disc space. As previously noted, it may occur early if loose fragments are left in the disc space or later following degeneration and sequestration of what was normal nuclear tissue at the time of the first operation. In most cases, this complication is treated by re-exploration of the affected disc. We are of the opinion that if fusion has not been performed at the first operation, it should be done at the second. The incidence of recurrent extrusion of nuclear material is far greater when the first operation is disc excision alone than when the combined operation is performed.

NUCLEAR DEGENERATION AT ANOTHER LEVEL

Although rare, disc degeneration and extrusion of nuclear material may occur at a different level than the one previously subjected to surgery. There is no evidence that in the lumbar spine the operation at one level is in any way responsible for degeneration of a disc which was normal at the time of the first operation. However, there is one possibility to consider; namely, that a double lesion was missed at operation.

Treatment is essentially the same as for any other lumbar disc lesion. Surgery is indicated if, after a fair trial, conservative treatment fails.

FIBROSIS IN AND AROUND THE NERVE ROOTS

After the removal of a sequestrum of nuclear tissue adjacent to or under a nerve root, adhesions may form within and without the nerve root sheath binding the root firmly to the floor of the spinal canal. The nerve roots are no longer freely movable nor capable of moving in and out of the intervertebral foramina without tension during movements of the trunk and legs. When fixed to the floor of the spinal canal or within the foramina, the nerve roots are subjected to abnormal tension during movements of the trunk and legs, particularly those movements which require the extended leg to flex at the hip joint. Tension on the nerve roots causes radicular pain.

The management of this lesion is difficult; lysis by surgery may induce the formation of even more adhesions. Recently, steroids have been injected into the subarachnoid space with the hope of reducing the inflammatory process. The few patients in which we employed this method did not attain relief of pain. The most reasonable approach to this problem is to put the spine and pelvis at complete rest with a cast or brace, in order to avoid undue traction on the nerve roots. By so doing, the inflammatory process in and about the roots may subside and spontaneous dissolution of the adhesions may follow.

INJURY TO THE CAUDA EQUINA

It was previously recorded that injury to the cauda equina may occur by excessive traction on the dural sac during operation for lumbar disc lesions. The degree of recovery is unpredictable. Usually some residual motor and sensory deficits are permanent; there may be some loss of sphincter control. This complication carries serious implications for both the surgeon and the patient, and it can be avoided. The cauda equina syndrome may be produced by a massive posterior extrusion of nuclear material. The residual motor and sensory impairment in these cases depends on how soon the cauda equina is decompressed. Several hours may make a difference between total recovery, partial recovery or no recovery of root function.

PSEUDARTHROSIS

Pseudarthrosis is one of the dreaded complications of spine fusion. The incidence of pseudarthrosis increases as the number of vertebrae in the fusion area increases. There is no doubt that pseudarthrosis following spine fusion is capable of producing severe pain and even leg pain. When the symptoms are severe and disabling an attempt to repair the pseudarthrosis should be made. On the other hand, there are many patients with pseudarthrosis who have no complaints. In these cases, it is reasonable to assume that in spite of an area of bone dissolution across the fusion mass, sufficient stability to the spine is provided by a strong fibrous ankylosis. In the authors' series there were 39 patients with pseudarthrosis demonstrable by radiographs. Only 17 of this group were symptomatic. When the diagnosis of symptomatic pseudarthrosis is established, a trial of conservative therapy should be instituted; if the patient fails to attain relief, surgical repair is indicated (Fig. 16-6).

To us, pseudarthrosis is no longer a hazard or deterrent to spine fusion. Since the technique of posterolateral fusion has been employed, the incidence of pseudarthrosis has dropped precipitously to less than one per cent.

DISC SPACE INFECTION

Infection of a disc space following excision of a lumbar disc is relatively rare; but, since there is more awareness of the lesion, the incidence is rising. Our opinion is that the lesion occurs more frequently than generally realized. The characteristic clinical features are: (1) the sudden appearance of excruciating back pain, one to eight weeks after excision of a disc; (2) severe muscle spasm; (3) no systemic reaction; and (4) a high erythrocyte sedimentation rate. Usually the pain appears after a postoperative period in which the patient is making satisfactory progress.

The radiological examination in the early cases may give no informa-

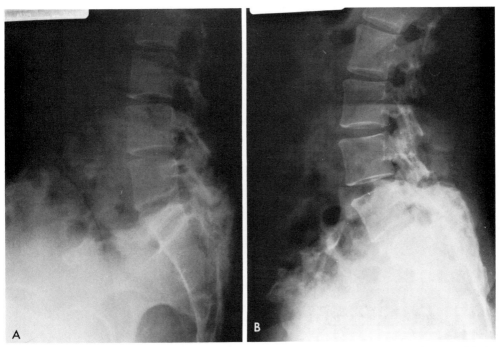

Figure 16-6 Pseudarthrosis following spine fusion. In most cases the lesion is demonstrable in lateral views, showing the lumbar spine, (*A*), in flexion and, (*B*), in extension. If these views fail to show the lesion, the lesion may be detected in anteroposterior views, taken with the spine bent to the right and to the left. This patient was asymptomatic.

tion except early collapse of the disc space. Later, the radiological findings are fairly characteristic: the disc space is narrow; there is erosion of the adjacent articular surfaces of the vertebral bodies and evidence of new bone formation at the margins of the vertebrae and between the bodies producing a bony fusion. In some cases, the destructive process is less evident and the chief radiological findings are dense, irregular sclerosis of the bodies and narrowing of the disc space. Not all cases terminate in bony fusion; in fact, it occurs in only 50 per cent of the cases[5] (Fig. 16-7).

Generally there is no clinical evidence of inflammation in the operative area; however, disc space infection may be secondary to sepsis of the wound. In these cases, there may actually be a sinus leading to the disc space.

Treatment of the early cases is total immobilization in a plaster spica extending from the lower part of the thoracic cage to just below the knees; the period of immobilization is four to six weeks. Large doses of an antibiotic with broad coverage are given for a relatively long period of time even after the cast is removed. After removal of the plaster spica the back is protected with a plaster jacket or a Taylor brace which is maintained until the spine is stabilized.

In old cases and those that do not respond to the conservative therapy, drainage of the disc space is indicated. This is best achieved through a retroperitoneal abdominal approach. The disc space is isolated and evacu-

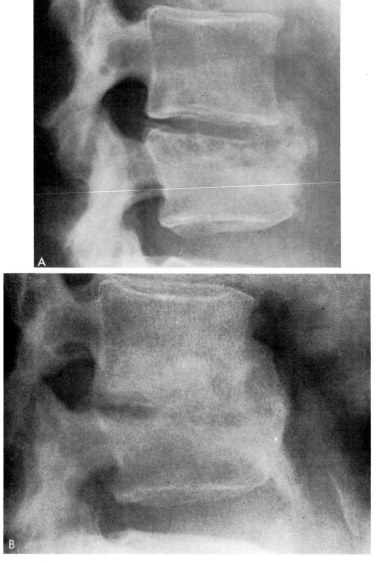

Figure 16-7   Disc space infection: (*A*), Taken three months after operation; note the narrowing of the disc space, erosion of the articular surface of the lower vertebral body and the formation of new bone along the anterior margins of the vertebra. (*B*), Taken six months after operation; the disc has disappeared and a bony fusion has occurred.

ated of all debris, granulation tissue and occasionally actual pus (frank pus is not a common finding). A polyethylene tube is inserted into the disc space and fastened to the surrounding soft tissues; its purpose is to allow the instillation of antibiotics into the disc space. The infection should be under control in four to six weeks, at which time the patient becomes ambulatory and wears a plaster jacket or a Taylor brace until the spine is stable.

ARACHNOID CYSTS

Dural tears may occur during operation for a lumbar disc lesion. Failure to repair the tear may result in the formation of an arachnoid cyst which is capable of producing low back and leg pain. The cysts are often referred to as "meningopseudo cysts."[4] The size varies considerably, but if relatively large, palpation reveals a fluctuant mass. The diagnosis is confirmed by the aspiration of the spinal fluid; also, in most instances, the cysts are readily seen in a myelogram.

The treatment of these lesions is exposure and excision of the cyst and closure of the aperture connecting it with the subarachnoid space.

INSTABILITY

Instability of a motor unit may be present before operation and made worse by excision of the disc and by removal of the posterior ligaments and some of the bony posterior elements of the vertebrae. A motor unit may be stable before surgery but is made unstable by removal of large segments of the posterior structures, especially if part or all of the pedicles are removed as occurs in decompressing an intervertebral foramen. In many instances, the instability in a motor unit can be demonstrated by radiographs taken in severe flexion and extension of the spine. When part or all of the posterior elements are removed in cases of spondylolysis and spondylolisthesis subsequent instability is a certainty. It must be remembered that instability of a motor unit not only causes back pain but may evoke either radicular or referred leg pain (Figs. 16-8 and 16-9).

Following excision of a disc, the motor unit may develop severe secondary degenerative changes consistent with arthrosis of the intervertebral and posterior articular joints. Such a joint may fail to progress to a stable fibrous fusion, but instead becomes very unstable (Fig. 16-10).

Failure of conservative therapy in these cases is an indication for spinal fusion.

IMPINGEMENT SYNDROME

Back pain after an operation, disc excision and fusion, occasionally is initiated by a mass of new bone formed at the proximal end of the fusion area abutting or impinging against the spinous process of the vertebra above the fusion. The pain comes on many months after surgery. A bursa forms at the site of contact; pressure over this region elicits considerable tenderness. Hyperextension of the spine accentuates the pain. Injection of the contact point with a local anesthetic agent brings about complete, temporary relief (Fig. 16-11).

Injection of steroids also relieves the pain. However, in most instances, a second operation is required. The bone making contact with the spinous process above is resected and a portion of the spinous process of the adjacent vertebra is removed.

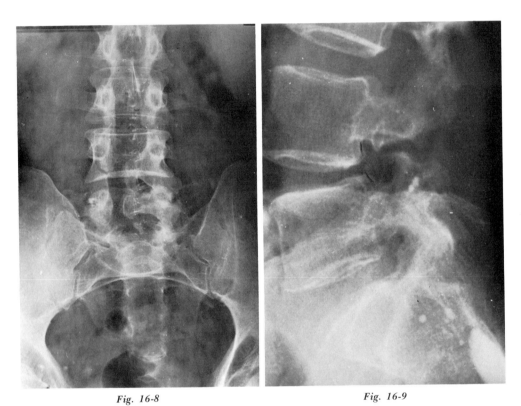

Fig. 16-8   Fig. 16-9

Figure 16-8   Unstable spine caused by extensive removal of the posterior elements of L3, L4 and L5. This patient was relieved of back pain by a spine fusion from L3 to S1.

Figure 16-9   Instability of a motor unit following extensive removal of its posterior elements. Note the narrowing of the L4-L5 disc space with forward displacement of L4 on L5.

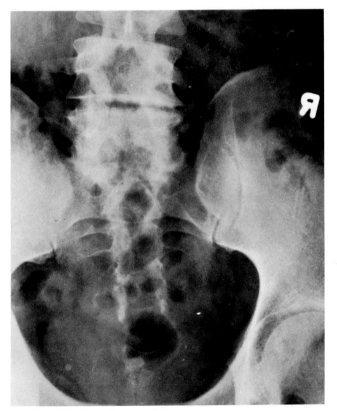

Figure 16-10 Unstable motor unit following disc excision. The L4-L5 level shows advanced degenerative changes. In this case these were not sufficient to stabilize the unit. The symptoms were relieved by fusion of the spine from L4 to S1.

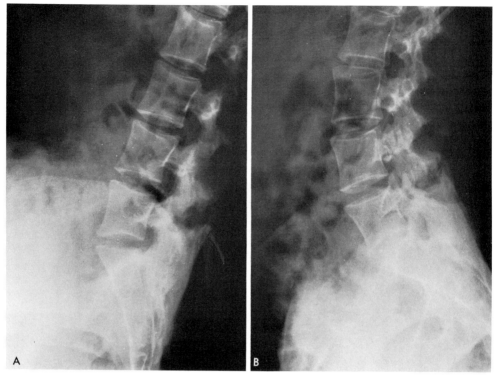

Figure 16-11 Impingement of upper end of the fusion mass against the spinous process proximal to it. (*A*), Flexion of the lumbar spine; the interval between the fusion and the spinous process of L4 opens. (*B*), Extension of the lumbar spine; the interval closes and the adjacent surfaces impinge.

FOREIGN BODIES

Although mention of this topic seems elementary, the presence of foreign bodies (sponges, bone wax, cotton pledgets) in the back may be responsible for severe pain and sepsis. Also the serious medicolegal implications are obvious.

Sponges are frequently left in the wound. During the operation this possibility should always be kept in mind; all sponges should be tagged and accounted for at the end of the operation.

Not infrequently, cotton pledgets are left in the spinal canal in the vicinity of the nerve root. We have seen several such cases. The foreign body may cause a local inflammatory condition involving the nerve root. The treatment is obvious; the area must be re-explored.

We have observed several cases of severe radicular pain following a spine fusion. Screws were used to fix the apophyseal joints. Unfortunately, one of the screws penetrated the intervertebral foramen and made pressure on the nerve root in the bony canal. The sciatica disappeared after extraction of the screws.

In one instance, the cause of drainage many months after operation was a large piece of bone wax used to control bleeding from the ilium from which bone grafts had been removed.

Causes of Pain Unrelated to Operative Treatment

Some of these causes have already been discussed such as disc degeneration and protrusion at a different level than the level previously explored. There are two other subjects to be discussed under this heading: psychogenic pain and malingering.

PSYCHOGENIC OVERLAY

Most patients with long histories of pain resulting from lumbar disc disorders develop some functional overlay. In selecting a patient for surgery, this aspect of the syndrome must be given serious consideration. If there is organic ground for pain, many of these patients will be helped immeasurably by removing the source of pain. On the other hand, if the symptomatology is based mainly on a functional basis much harm can be done to these patients. It is this group of patients that torment the surgeon after surgery. These patients need psychiatric help and it should be made available to them.

MALINGERING

Following surgery there is no doubt that some patients continue to complain of pain for reasons of financial gain. In order not to do the patient an injustice, he should be carefully evaluated by someone other than the operating surgeon and also, if the patient will agree—and this may be a problem—by a psychiatrist. The use of a differential spinal block in these cases may give some very significant information on the validity of the symptoms.

TRAGEDIES OF OPERATIVE TREATMENT OF LUMBAR DISC DISEASE

No operation in any field of surgery leaves in its wake more human wreckage than surgery on the lumbar discs. The situation becomes even more pathetic in the realization that the starting point, in most instances, is a healthy, self-sufficient individual. Many of these patients are subjected to numerous operations, and after each one the patient is worse. One patient in our practice had ten back operations and still no relief of symptoms was forthcoming. What is wrong? Is the patient at fault? Is the surgeon at fault? Or, is it the disease? Those who are called upon to salvage some of these human wrecks soon come face to face with the awful truth—that in the majority of the cases, the surgeon is at fault. In a few cases the cause of failure or recurrence of symptoms is beyond the control of the surgeon, but in most instances it is not.

Another startling fact is the reluctance of many surgeons to operate on a patient who is not relieved by a previous operation or who is relieved for a period of time and then has a recurrence of the symptoms. Many, in fact all these patients, develop a certain degree of functional overlay. The functional disorder in some reaches such proportions that it completely dominates the clinical picture making it most difficult to determine how much of the symptom-complex is functional and how much is organic. Yet there are very few of these patients who cannot be rehabilitated to a level which is tolerable and which permits the patient to be self-sufficient and economically independent.

Results of Operative Treatment in Patients With Multiple Operations

The causes of failure of operative treatment have been discussed in a previous section. In order to emphasize the fact that many of these patients can be rehabilitated, and to stimulate a more optimistic attitude toward these problems, a brief report on a group of patients who had been subjected to more than one operation follows.

In a series of 517 patients selected for postoperative evaluation, there were 150 who had undergone two or more spinal operations; of the 150, we were able to re-examine 70 patients. The average age of the patient was 43 years. This is important to record because it reveals that failures occur in the most productive period of life. The duration of symptoms ranged from one to 18 years, with an average of six years. This, too, is important to report, for it gives an indication of the length of the period of suffering. Of the 70 patients, 46 had undergone one spinal operation and 24 had been subjected to two to six operations. One case, not included in this series, had undergone ten operations.

After a careful study of the patients, the following diagnoses were made.

1. A diagnosis of an unstable motor unit associated with irritability of the intervertebral joint was made in 35 patients; all of them had disc excision without fusion. In this group there was no true radicular pain. The dominant features were those of instability and irritability of the intervertebral joints involved. Three of the 35 patients had lesions above the level of L4; all of these patients required fusion of the affected motor units. In the remaining 32 patients a fusion was performed from L4 to S1 in 25 patients and from L5 to S1 in seven patients.

2. In 18 patients the prominent clinical feature was radicular pain. A diagnosis was made of: extrusion of a disc not involved at the time of the first operation; an extrusion of nuclear material missed at the previous operation; or, extrusion of nuclear material from the previously explored interspace. In this group, extrusion of nuclear material from the interspace previously explored or from another level was encountered in 16 patients; in the remaining two, the roots were compressed within the foramina. The roots were decompressed by foraminotomies during which the pedicles were removed. In all, the affected disc was excised, and a fusion was performed from the affected motor unit to the sacrum.

3. Pseudarthrosis was observed in eight patients, and it was believed to be the responsible factor for pain. These were all repaired.

4. In four patients, it was interesting to note that the symptoms were

not related to the lower lumbar area but rather arose from an irritable sacroiliac joint. All these patients were relieved by a sacroiliac fusion. Whether involvement of the sacroiliac joint coexisted with a lumbar disc lesion or whether it was an entirely new process following the previous surgery is not clear.

5. In three patients, there was an obvious disc infection; one at L4-L5 and two at L5-S1 levels. Two of these were evacuated and fused posteriorly.

6. One patient had a low grade osteomyelitis of the fusion area. This was thoroughly debrided and packed and the wound left open. Fusion was achieved without further surgical interference.

7. One patient disclosed a sacral cyst which undoubtedly developed after a combined operation. Occasionally this occurs if the posterior sacral wall is penetrated while bone to be used for the fusion is removed. Simple curettage of the cyst and packing it with bone relieved the symptoms.

Critical subjective evaluation of these patients provided the following data. Including the last operation performed by us, excellent results were attained in 16 patients; ten of these patients had two operations, five had three operations, and one had four.

Good results were achieved in 19 patients; 15 had three operations, three had two, and one had eight.

Fair results were recorded in 24 patients; 12 of these had three operations and 12 had four.

Poor results were attained in 11 patients; these patients, as a group, had 33 spinal procedures performed, an average of three procedures per patient.

These data, based on subjective analysis, indicate that 35 or 50 per cent of the patients attained an excellent or good result and 24 patients a fair result; 11 patients were not improved.

The patients were requested to express their opinion as to whether they considered the operation worthwhile; 87 per cent considered the last operative procedure worthwhile while 13 per cent did not.

It was also significant to note that 59 per cent of the group returned to their former level of activity and 41 per cent did not do so.

From these data it becomes obvious that patients with multiple operations should not be considered incurable, and that a great number of them can be restored to a useful life. Also, it should be remembered that each patient should be considered individually, and the solution of the problems of one is not applicable to the problems of another.

Of great assistance in the evaluation of patients before submitting them to more surgery is the information as to what was found and what was done in the previous operations. It would seem that this information is readily available, but this is not the case in many instances. Such information at times is just not available, and when it is, it is often unreliable.

Technique of Reoperation

It is impossible to describe an operative procedure which would be applicable to all cases. Each case poses its own problems and, in most instances, the operative steps must be conceived to meet the situations as they arise. However, there are some surgical principles which, if adhered to, will expedite and enhance the efficacy of the procedure. In planning any reoperation, we do so with the intent that the affected spinal segments will be fused. It is our opinion that any motor unit explored for the second, third or maybe the fourth time should be stabilized by a spine fusion. Lesions of the L4-L5 level are fused from L4 to the sacrum and lesions of the L5-S1 level from L5 to the sacrum.

INCISION

At this point it should be remembered that in spines which have had previous surgery, especially those that have had several surgical procedures, the normal tissue planes are completely obliterated. Instead, a dense zone of fibrous tissue extends from the skin down to the posterior elements of the spine, then it flares out laterally on both sides and extends to the outer margins of the apophyseal joints. The tissue may be very vascular and inelastic making hemostasis difficult to achieve. When cutting through fibrous tissue in the spine it is wise to reach the depth of the wound in one plane; by so doing, bleeding will be kept to a minimum. The use of the electrocautery while making the incision also reduces the amount of bleeding.

Before the operation is started, the radiographs should be carefully studied in order to determine the exact amount of bone removed, if any, and the location of the bony defect. When only minimal bone is removed, the operation is relatively easy, but when a wide laminectomy has been performed there is much fibrous tissue which is adherent to the dural sac.

In all but a few, the incision of the previous operation is usually in the midline. Make the skin incision in the line of the previous incision. If the spinous processes are in situ, begin the incision over the spinous process rostral to the vertebra which will be the proximal vertebra in the fusion area. Extend the incision distally to the spinous process of the third sacral vertebra. Deepen the incision to the tips of the spinous processes.

WHEN THE POSTERIOR BONY ELEMENTS ARE INTACT

With a sharp periosteal elevator, strip all ligaments and muscles from the sides of the spinous processes and laminae; carry the dissection to the lateral margins of the apophyseal joints. It is most essential that the dissection be sharp dissection and in one plane, the subperiosteal plane, at all times. After the ligaments and muscles have been stripped from the vertebrae and the sacrum on one side, the wound is tightly packed to control any bleeding; the subperiosteal stripping is then performed on the opposite side. If the disc or discs had been approached through an inter-laminar fenestration or through a fenestration made in the laminae above and below the affected disc, great caution must be exercised when these areas are approached lest the dural sac be torn. By sharp dissection, a plane should be developed in the scar tissue immediately above and parallel to the laminae and extended laterally to the lateral margins of the apophyseal joints above and below the fenestration. Then with a blunt dissector, the lateral portion of the dura is exposed and the anterolateral gutter of the spinal canal is carefully developed. This last step also exposes the nerve root which may be firmly anchored by scar tissue to the floor of the canal. Once the root is identified, it is freed from the adhesions and gently displaced toward the midline. Considerable bleeding may be encountered when the nerve root is being mobilized, but it is readily controlled by placing a small foam rubber pledget in the canal above and below the nerve root. The floor of the canal can now be explored and the intervertebral space identified.

WHEN THE POSTERIOR BONY ELEMENTS HAVE BEEN REMOVED

The exploratory operation is much more difficult when a hemilaminectomy or a complete laminectomy of several contiguous vertebrae exists. The first step in exposure of the canal is to identify the intact vertebra immediately above the laminectomy. Its spinous process and laminae are then stripped subperiosteally of all ligaments and muscular attachments as far laterally as the apophyseal joints. The next step is to expose, subperiosteally, the base of the sacrum. The posterior surfaces of the laminae of the vertebra above and the posterior surface of the sacrum below can be used as guides to determine the depth of the dural sac between these two points. By sharp dissection, the center of the wound is developed, its base being immediately above the dural sac and separated from it by a thin layer of scar tissue. The dissection is carried laterally on both sides as far as the apophyseal joints. This portion of the operation must be done with meticulous care, for the dura can be torn very easily.

Beginning along the lateral aspect of the wound, by sharp dissection, the fibrous tissue is dissected away until the dural sac is exposed; now, with a blunt dissector, the dura is freed from fibrous tissue for the whole length of the wound and gently displaced toward the midline. The anterolateral gutter of the spinal canal is now explored and the nerve roots identified. These are gently mobilized from the surrounding scar tissue and with minimal traction are displaced medially. The floor of the canal can now be explored and the intervertebral disc spaces exposed.

TREATMENT OF THE INTERVERTEBRAL DISC SPACE

All disc spaces that had been previously explored should be re-explored. One is astonished at the amount of degenerated nuclear material and debris that is often removed from these disc spaces.

After all degenerated tissue is removed from the disc space, any shredded tissue and tabs of tissue on the floor of the canal are cut away. A piece of fat is placed on the floor of the canal immediately beneath the dura and nerve root. The fat controls bleeding and also acts as a temporary interposition membrane between the neural elements and the floor of the canal. When the preoperative diagnosis is an unstable or irritable intervertebral joint, all discs previously explored should be re-explored and cleaned out; however, there is no need to tamper with a disc that was not disturbed.

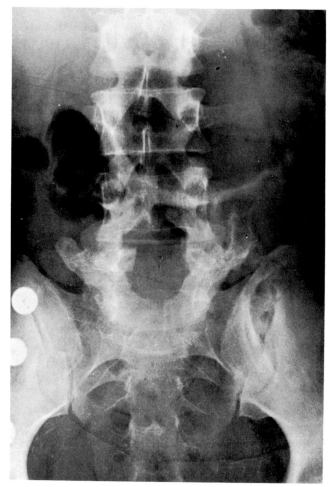

Figure 16-12 Anteroposterior view of a spine fusion two years after the operation. Observe the sturdy masses of bone extending from the transverse processes of L5 to the sacrum. Also the defect in the posterior bony elements of L5 caused by removing the laminae of L5.

FUSION OF THE AFFECTED SEGMENTS

Following reoperation a posterolateral fusion is performed in all instances unless there are special contraindications. If the lesion was confined to the L5-S1 interspace, the fusion extends from L5 to the sacrum; if the lesion implicated the L4-L5 disc or both the L4-L5 and the L5-S1 discs, the fusion extends from L4 to the sacrum. No bone is placed over the exposed dura (Fig. 16-12).

DRAINAGE OF THE WOUND

The use of the Hemovac has been found to prevent hematoma formations and remove undesirable exudates from the wound. One limb of the suction apparatus is placed deep in the wound overlying the fusion area; the other is placed immediately below the subcutaneous layer of tissue. As a rule, the tubes are withdrawn within 48 to 72 hours.

REFERENCES

1. Desaussure, R. L.: Vascular injury coincident to disc surgery. J. Neurosurg. 16:222-229, 1959.
2. Ford, L. T.: Complications of lumbar-disc surgery, prevention and treatment. Local complications. J. Bone Joint Surg. 50-A:418-428, 1968.
3. Harbison, S. P.: Major vascular complications of intervertebral disc surgery. Ann. Surg. 140:342-348, 1954.
4. Miller, P. R. and Elder, F. W., Jr.: Meningeal pseudocysts (meningocele spurius) following laminectomy. Report of ten cases. J. Bone Joint Surg. 50-A:268-276, 1968.
5. Thibodeau, A. A.: Closed space infection following removal of lumbar intervertebral disc. J. Bone Joint Surg. 50-A:400-410, 1968.

Chapter 17

RESULTS OF OPERATIVE TREATMENT OF MECHANICAL DISORDERS OF THE LUMBAR SPINE

Operative treatment for mechanical disorders of the lumbar spine which have failed to respond to conservative measures is now universally accepted. Lesion of the lumbar disc is only one causative factor which forces the patient to seek medical aid. There are many others, of which structural abnormalities and arthritic changes in the intervertebral joints are the most important. What can a surgeon achieve and what can a patient expect when the decision for operative intervention is made? The published reports on end result studies vary considerably, indeed so much so that their significance becomes questionable.[1, 2, 3, 4, 7] To the surgeon experienced in lesions of the lumbar spine, the discrepancies noted in the end result studies are comprehensible. He is keenly aware that there are many factors to be considered in postoperative evaluation of patients. None of these factors are regarded in the same light by any two surgeons. Many revolve around the surgeon himself and are very individualistic; others are related to the patient and to the disease.

Undoubtedly, the two considerations which can have the most profound effect on any study are the diagnostic acumen of the surgeon and his discriminatory skill in the selection of patients for operative treatment. These traits are not inherent qualities of a surgeon, nor does he acquire them overnight. Rather, they are the end products of a broad experience accrued over many years, often many years of trial and error. After a patient has been selected for operative treatment, the outcome will be governed in a large measure by the experience, skill and dexterity of the surgeon. These qualities too are the harvest of many years of experience. No one is more aware of this than the surgeon who is considered "the court of last resort" by his colleagues and who is flooded by cases sent for salvage.

The nature of the disease also has a bearing on the statistics of an end result study. This relates particularly to the factors initiating the disease, its duration and the absence or presence of secondary alterations such as advanced arthritic changes and motor and sensory deficits. It should be remembered that we do not treat a certain disease per se, but rather treat a patient with a specific disease. It becomes obvious that the patient's emotional make-up, motivation, age, occupation, marital status and other characteristics peculiar to the individual will have a significant bearing on operative results.

One other factor must be noted. It is difficult to determine just when the end result of any case is reached. Some patients reach this point before others and some never reach it. We noted previously that we evaluated the results in 100 patients in whom excision of the disc alone had been performed; the postoperative period ranged from one to seven years. Since the completion and reporting of this study, many patients whose results had been rated excellent or good had recurrences of symptoms necessitating a second operation. Should a re-evaluation be made now, the statistics of the two studies on the same patients would vary considerably. It becomes apparent that the surgeon's question, What can I achieve? and the patient's question, What can I expect? can only be answered by the surgeon, the answer being based on the knowledge of his own capabilities and his experience. He cannot answer these questions by referring to the statistics published by another surgeon.

In an effort to carefully and objectively evaluate the results of our surgical therapy over the past 20 years, over 1500 patients who had undergone surgery for lumbar disc degeneration, neural arch defects and mechanical instability on the authors' service from 1947 to 1965 were contacted and asked to return for complete evaluation. It is our feeling that many studies reported in the literature are based on questionnaire alone and are grossly inadequate for this reason. Only those patients who could be personally interviewed and examined were included. The figures represented below are based on 517 patients who presented for personal interview, physical examination, and radiographic examination, including flexion-extension views when fusion was performed. All pertinent information was assembled on standardized data sheets which could be easily transcribed onto punch cards for electronic data processing. Computer analysis was then performed at the Johnson Research Foundation of the University of Pennsylvania. All evaluations were performed by physicians other than the operating surgeon in order to minimize subjective bias.

Examination of the population distribution curve revealed that the average age at surgery was 40, with a normal frequency distribution above and below this level (Table 17-1). This age distribution is in keeping with the more recent pathologic concepts of disc degeneration.

The average age at follow-up evaluation was 48, the average follow-up

Table 17-1 *Decade at Surgery*

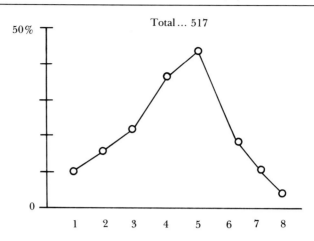

period was of eight years (Table 17-2). The range of follow-up evaluation was from a minimum of one year to a maximum of 20 years. It is our feeling that follow-up within one year is meaningless in terms of back surgery. For 195 patients, evaluation followed surgery by ten years or more.

A definitive diagnosis was reached for each patient after careful consideration of preoperative symptoms, physical findings, roentgenographic findings and the findings at operation. It is our belief that the most accurate criterion is the surgeon's careful evaluation at the operating table. The most common diagnostic category was disc degeneration, with unstable lumbosacral mechanism and neural arch defects presenting less often. In many instances the diagnostic categories overlapped and were not exclusive (Table 17-3). The diagnostic category of disc degeneration was not limited to herniations of the nucleus but included any disc which, either through inspection or palpation, showed various characteristics of degeneration such as softening, bulging, rents in the annulus or prolapse.

DISC DEGENERATION

Relief of symptoms is the most important criterion for success in terms of low back surgery. Patients were questioned about the degree and the temporal nature of their relief of back pain and leg pain. Their evaluation as to the subjective worth of their surgery was also elicited.

Table 17-2 *Population*

Mean Age Surgery	40 years
Mean Age Follow-up	48 years
Mean Follow-up	8 years
Range Follow-up	1–20 years
Ten-year or Greater Follow-up	195 patients

Table 17-3 *Diagnosis*

	%
L5-S1 Disc	42
Unstable Lumbosacral Mechanism	19
L4-5 Disc	12
L4-5, L5-S1 Disc	11
Spondylolysis	2
Spondylolisthesis	5
Unstable Lumbosacral Mechanism, L5-S1 Disc	3
Unstable Lumbosacral Mechanism, L4-5 Disc	2
Disc above L4-5	1

In individuals with L5 disc degeneration, 15 per cent had persistent back pain, seven per cent had persistent sciatica, and 14 per cent had both back pain and sciatica. The results are approximately the same with L4 disc degeneration and combined disc degeneration (Table 17-4). When questioned as to overall relief of their pain, approximately 60 per cent of individuals in each category obtained complete relief of back and leg pain, approximately 30 per cent of individuals considered themselves partially relieved, and two to three per cent were a total failure with no relief whatsoever (Table 17-5). It was interesting to note that despite the relatively long period of follow-up evaluation, temporary relief was infrequently noted. This would imply that surgical stabilization of the lumbar spine does not lead to a particularly high incidence of disc degeneration above the fusion mass during the period of time included in this study. Return of symptomatology was most often due to recurrent disc degeneration at the same or a new level. Of the patients with disc degeneration at L4 or L5 88 per cent felt their surgery was worthwhile; the percentage was less when both discs were affected (Table 17-5).

Physical findings were evaluated at follow-up and compared to preoperative findings (Table 17-6). The nonspecific findings such as muscle spasm, tenderness, limitation of motion and straight leg raising disappeared in 90 per cent of those individuals who showed these findings preoperatively. Neurologic deficits return to normal less often postoperatively. Motor and sensory deficits which had been present preoperatively disappeared in 50 per cent of the patients. Only 25 per cent of patients lost

Table 17-4 *Symptoms of Disc Degeneration*

	L5-S1	L4-5	Both
Preoperative	(%)	(%)	(%)
Back Pain	10	7	7
Leg Pain	5	0	4
Both	85	93	89
Postoperative			
Back Pain	15	17	11
Leg Pain	7	7	4
Both	14	17	20

Table 17-5   *Disc Degeneration: Subjective Relief*

	L5-S1	L4-L5	Both
	(%)	(%)	(%)
Total	62	67	59
Partial	30	24	28
Temporary	4	7	11
None	3	3	2
Surgery Worthwhile	88	88	75

Table 17-6   *Changes in Physical Findings after Surgery*

	%
Loss of all reflex change	25
Loss of all motor deficit	50
Loss of all sensory deficit	50
Loss of abnormal curve	
Muscle spasm	
Tenderness	90 or
Limited motion	more
Straight leg raising	

Table 17-7   *Diagnosis and Surgery*

	Fusion	Excision	Both
	%	%	%
L5-S1	3	8	89
L4-5	5	24	71

Table 17-8   *Type of Surgery and Relief of Symptoms (L5-S1)*

	Excision	Combined
Follup-up Symptom		
Back pain	37	32
Sciatica	27	22
Satisfactory Result	89	93
Surgery Worthwhile	74	88

Table 17-9   *Type of Surgery and Recurrence of Symptoms*

	Excision	Combined
	%	%
L5-S1	11	4
L4-5	11	5

their preoperative reflex changes. This is somewhat better than the results reported by Knutsson in which only 33 per cent of patients lost their sensory deficit, 24 per cent lost their motor deficit and two and a half per cent lost their reflex abnormalities.[5] This difference may be due to our longer period of follow-up evaluation.

Choice of Surgical Procedure

The question as to the ideal surgical procedure for a degenerated intervertebral disc is as yet unanswered. Eustace Semmes reviewed 1500 patients in whom only disc excision had been performed and found that 98 per cent considered themselves benefited by their operation.[6] Relief of back pain was complete or partial in 95 per cent, and in 96 per cent there was complete or partial relief of leg pain. Young and Love reviewed a series of 450 patients with a combined procedure and 555 patients with disc excision alone.[7] They found that the combined operation relieved both symptoms in 20 per cent more patients than were relieved with the operation for removal of the disc alone and that there were three times as many failures to the pain relief of either back or leg pain when the fusion was not performed. Barr in a ten-year series of 130 patients found eight per cent improvement and satisfactory results after the combined procedure but felt that this difference was not statistically significant.[1]

A tabulation of the type of surgical procedure performed in our series revealed that for a diagnosis of a degenerated L5 disc, the combined procedure was used in 89 per cent of the cases and a disc excision alone in eight per cent. With a degenerated L4 disc, the combined procedure was used in 71 per cent of the cases and disc excision alone in 24 per cent. This reflects the earlier hesitancy of undertaking L4 to S1 fusions before the advent of lateral fusion techniques (Table 17-7).

Examination of our results when comparing disc excision with the combined procedure revealed a five per cent increase in the relief of back pain and sciatica when the combined procedure is undertaken, as compared to disc excision alone (Table 17-8). If a satisfactory result can be considered either total or partial relief, then 93 per cent of patients with a combined procedure achieved a satisfactory result as compared with 89 per cent in individuals with disc excision alone. Of patients with disc excision, 74 per cent considered their procedure worthwhile, whereas 88 per cent with a combined procedure considered it worthwhile.

The rate of recurrence of symptoms is twice as high with disc excision alone regardless of the level of the lesion (Table 17-9).

The results expressed in Tables 17-8 and 17-9 were subjected to the Chi-square analysis, and the differences noted between the two groups were not statistically significant. Our figures are similar to those reported by Barr,[1] although our total study group is larger. Duration of follow-up is approximately the same. Our conclusions, however, are somewhat different. The words "statistically significant" and "important" are not synonymous. Although a difference of five to eight per cent when subjected to Chi-square analysis may not be statistically significant, it is extremely im-

Table 17-10   *Factors Indicative of Poor Prognosis*

Diagnosis — High disc (above L4-5)
Operation — Fusion L5-S1 with disc excision L4-5
Physical Finding — Negative straight leg raising

portant with regard to the choice of back operations for the individual patient and may not be quickly disregarded. Recurrence rate is also germane.

.Certainly those individuals with a strong history of back pain and with radiologically observed structural changes, and those engaged in vigorous activities should be considered for the combined procedure. Elderly individuals and those with a normal radiographic appearance who engage only in light activities could be considered for disc excision alone. The choice will further depend upon the training and competence of the surgeon involved. Certain general observations were noted which are also of interest. An attempt was made to select those factors which would be of poor prognostic significance for the patient undergoing back surgery (Table 17-10). In regard to diagnosis, high discs (discs above the L4-L5 level) did more poorly in regard to relief of symptomatology. One operative category appeared to fare more poorly: lumbosacral fusion combined with disc excision alone at the L4-L5 level. At one time this operation was felt to be appropriate when a degenerated L4-L5 disc was found together with evidence of an unstable lumbosacral mechanism. It is our present feeling that, in most instances, when an L4-L5 disc is present, disc excision should be combined with fusion from L4 to the sacrum.

The correlation of physical findings with quality of result revealed that a negative straight leg raising examination in the preoperative examination tended to correlate with a poor result. The explanation for this is not obvious to us. This observation, however, was also noted by Hirsch.[4] He noted that laminectomy and exploration were negative more often when the straight leg raising test and neurologic evaluation were negative. He further observed that with negative exploration, the quality of result was poor regardless of the operative procedure performed.

NEURAL ARCH DEFECTS

Individuals with a diagnosis of neural arch defect were subjected to fusion from L4 to the sacrum (Table 17-11). If combined with disc degeneration, a disc excision was also performed. Recently, with the advent of the lateral fusion technique, it has not been felt necessary to include the fourth lumbar vertebra in the fusion mass with either spondylolysis or spondylolisthesis. In spondylolisthesis, we now also excise the loose neural arch.

In follow-up evaluation, those individuals with spondylolysis noted back pain in 32 per cent, leg pain in 11 per cent, with overall subjective relief being total in 45 per cent and partial in 56 per cent. All individuals in this category felt their surgery to be worthwhile (Table 17-12).

In spondylolisthesis, back pain was noted in 12 per cent and sciatica in

Table 17-11 *Neural Arch Defects*

	No Slip	Slip
	%	%
Preoperative Symptom		
Back pain	44	36
Leg pain	0	12
Both	56	52
Postoperative Symptom		
Back pain	33	12
Leg pain	11	8
Both	0	20

eight per cent, both being present in 20 per cent of the individuals (Table 17-11). In regard to subjective overall relief, 64 per cent of the individuals with spondylolisthesis achieved total relief and 20 per cent had partial relief. Eight per cent of the individuals had temporary relief and eight per cent had no relief whatsoever. Of these patients, 88 per cent considered their surgical procedure worthwhile (Table 17-12).

UNSTABLE LUMBOSACRAL MECHANISM

This diagnostic category has been poorly defined in the past and remains poorly understood. Some individuals have back pain or leg pain, or both, which is associated with certain structural abnormalities of the lower lumbar spine and sacrum. X-ray examination may reveal an acute lumbosacral angle, tropism of the apophyseal joints, or failure of proper segmentation. There may be lumbarization of the upper part of the sacrum or sacralization of the last lumbar vertebra. Vestigial discs may be noted and are easily confused with degenerative thin discs. Stress films may reveal excessive mobility. It is our feeling that these geometric abnormalities may produce symptoms in one of three ways. The transmission of the vertical thrust of the body weight may be abnormal so that excessive stress will be placed upon the various soft tissue supporting elements of the spine. The second mechanism of pain production can be through the direct pressure of a bony structure upon the neural elements. A subluxed articular facet may migrate into the intervertebral foramen and compress a nerve root. With an acute lumbosacral angle, the lamina of L5 may compress the cauda equina. A third mechanism of pain production, closely allied to the first,

Table 17-12 *Neural Arch Defect — Subjective Relief*

	No Slip	Slip
	%	%
Total	45	64
Partial	56	20
Temporary	0	8
No relief	0	8
Surgery worthwhile	100	88

Table 17-13   *Unstable Lumbosacral Mechanism*

Preoperative Symptoms	%
Back pain only	43
Leg pain only	7
Back and leg pain	50
Postoperative Symptoms	
Back pain only	28
Leg pain only	4
Back and leg pain	18

would be the production of disc degeneration to the abnormal distribution of stress in this area. Hypermobility may or may not be present in association with this disc degeneration. It is our feeling that this last situation, in which an unstable lumbosacral mechanism has led to disc degeneration, deserves the most attention. We placed patients in this category when x-rays revealed an acute lumbosacral angle, asymmetry of the apophyseal joints, or a transitional vertebra.

The most common operation for these individuals was a posterior fusion from L5 to the sacrum. Exploration of the affected interspace was undertaken whenever suspicion was present that a degenerated disc was involved.

At follow-up evaluation back pain was noted in 28 per cent of individuals, sciatica in four per cent, and back pain and sciatica in 18 per cent (Table 17-13). Of those individuals who underwent surgery 48 per cent obtained total relief of their symptoms, 39 per cent obtained partial relief, ten per cent temporary relief, and three per cent no relief whatsoever. Of the total group 84 per cent felt their surgical procedure worthwhile (Table 17-14).

RESUMPTION OF PRIOR LEVEL OF ACTIVITY

In evaluating resumption of prior level of activity, no difference was noted by diagnostic category or type of operation performed (Table 17-15).

PSEUDARTHROSIS

The overall rate of solid fusion in our series was 92 per cent with an incidence of pseudarthrosis of eight per cent. Since the advent of the lateral

Table 17-14   *Unstable Lumbosacral Mechanism—Subjective Relief*

	%
Total	48
Partial	39
Temporary	10
None	3
Surgery worthwhile	84

Table 17-15   *Resumption of Prior Level of Activity*

	%
Unstable Lumbosacral Mechanism	73
L5-S1	76
L4-5	74
Neural Arch Defect	73

fusion technique, the incidence of pseudarthrosis in two level fusions is six per cent.[3] The incidence of pseudarthrosis in one level fusions utilizing the lateral technique is less than one per cent. In our study group, 39 patients were discovered whom we could classify as having definite pseudarthrosis. In the hope of learning in detail what the diagnosis of pseudarthrosis portends for a patient, we studied these 39 individuals in detail. They were compared with a matched group of 39 patients each having had an identical diagnosis and operation but in whom the fusion was solid. By comparing these two matched groups we can say with some degree of precision what the implication of pseudarthrosis is for the patient who has undergone a spine fusion.[3]

The duration of time from surgery to return to active employment averaged seven months in the group who developed pseudarthrosis and eight months for those with solid fusions (Table 17-16). When evaluated in regard to ability to resume preoperative level of activity, 69 per cent of patients in each group stated that at some time they had been able to resume their prior level of activity (Table 17-17).

In an overall subjective evaluation of the worth of their surgery, 82 per cent of the patients who had developed pseudarthrosis felt that their surgery was worthwhile, whereas 92 per cent of the group who had solid fusions felt that their surgery was worthwhile (Table 17-18). Little difference was found between the pseudarthrosis group and the solid fusion group when they were asked specifically about their overall relief from symptomatology. In the former group 56 per cent of patients exhibited total relief, and 61 per cent in the latter group obtained total relief. It was interesting to note that although there was a slight decrease in the number who obtained total relief in the pseudarthrosis group, three patients who achieved solid fusion obtained no relief, and all patients who developed pseudarthrosis obtained at least partial and temporary relief (Table 17-19).

When back pain alone was considered, of the 92 percent of the patients in the pseudarthrosis group who originally had back pain, 44 per cent still had the symptoms at follow-up evaluation. In the solid fusion group, of the 97 per cent of patients who originally had back pain, 38 per cent still had significant back pain at follow-up evaluation (Table 17-20).

Table 17-16   *Time to Work*

Pseudoarthrosis	Solid Fusion
7 months	8 months

Table 17-17   *Able to Resume Former Level of Activity*

Pseudoarthrosis	Solid Fusion
69%	69%

Table 17-18   *Was Surgery Worthwhile?*

	Pseudoarthrosis	Solid Fusion
Yes	82	90

Table 17-19   *Relief from Symptoms*

	Pseudoarthrosis	Solid Fusion
	%	%
Total	56	61
Partial	34	26
Temporary	10	5
None	0	8

Table 17-20   *Back Pain*

	Pseudoarthrosis	Solid Fusion
	%	%
Preoperative	92	97
Postoperative	44	38

Table 17-21   *Sciatica*

	Pseudoarthrosis	Solid Fusion
	%	%
Preoperative	79	85
Postoperative	25	20

Sciatica was eliminated more consistently than back pain at follow-up evaluation. Of the 79 per cent of patients in the pseudarthrosis group who had sciatica, only 25 per cent had their symptoms at follow-up evaluation. In the solid fusion group, of the 85 per cent of patients who originally had sciatica, only 20 per cent had their symptom at follow-up evaluation (Table 17-21). The subjective factors noted above were submitted to Chi-square analysis. In no case was a significant difference (p less than 0.05) noted between the pseudarthrosis and the solid fusion group.

It would seem justified to draw certain conclusions from the above information. One of two situations must exist: either the pseudarthrosis represents a state of fibrous stabilization which is essentially as effective as bony fusion, or the fusion component of these procedures was not essential. The former is not entirely unreasonable, as the amount of motion demonstrated on flexion-extension films of pseudarthrosis is usually minimal, often less than 2 mm. The latter conclusion, however, remains in question.

It would furthermore seem prudent to carefully observe patients with pseudarthrosis for a rather prolonged period of time before reoperating in an attempt to achieve union. There seems little rationale for submitting patients to multiple attempts at repair of pseudarthrosis when, as a group, there is little difference in the subjective result when solid fusion is obtained.

The overall picture obtained is that a certain number of patients who have undergone spinal fusion continue to have back pain and less frequently sciatica whether or not their fusion has become solid. The success rate as judged by a subjective evaluation is slightly greater in that group which has achieved solid fusion. Pseudarthrosis of itself does not appear to be the dreaded complication it is often portrayed.

SPECULATION

As noted previously, these statistics were gathered from a period of years when there was much "growing up" to be done. The pathophysiology of lesions of the lumbar spine was less understood, the role of the disc in the production of mechanical disorders of the back and sciatica was not clearly defined, and surgeons were searching for and experimenting with operative procedures designed to relieve backache with or without sciatica. We all remember the vicious attacks made on the sacroiliac joints, the lumbosacral joints and the tensor fasciae latae, all vehemently defended as the prime causes of back pain and sciatica. The goblin, pseudarthrosis, shadowed every attempt at arthrodesis of the spine, especially if more than one motor unit was fused. (This spectre is still very real to some surgeons.)

Although many areas in the realm of low back disorders are still grey, some light has filtered through, some progress has been made, and there is much evidence that the future will see even more. As for the series of cases just reported, there is reason to believe that if the patients processed in the last five years of the study period were compared with those prior to that point of time the statistics would differ markedly. More accurate diagnoses would be made, greater selectivity of patients for surgery would be exercised, and more expert surgery would be performed. All these factors would add up to a higher incidence of acceptable results and fewer failures.

REFERENCES

1. Barr, J. S. et al.: Evaluation of end results in treatment of ruptured lumbar intervertebral discs with protrusion of nucleus pulposus. Surg. Gynec. Obstet. 125:250-256, 1967.
2. DePalma, A. F. and Prabhakar, M.: Posterior-posterobilateral fusion of the lumbosacral spine. Clin. Orthop. 47:165-171, 1966.
3. DePalma, A. F. and Rothman, R. H.: The nature of pseudarthrosis. Clin. Orthop. 59:113-118, 1968.
4. Hirsch, C.: Efficiency of surgery in low-back disorders. J. Bone Joint Surg. 47-A:991-1004, 1965.
5. Knutsson, B.: How often do the neurological signs disappear after the operation of a herniated disc, Acta Orthop. Scand. 32:352-356, 1962.
6. Semmes, R. E.: Ruptures of the lumbar intervertebral disc, their mechanism, diagnosis, and treatment. Springfield, Ill., Charles C Thomas, 1964.
7. Young, H. H. et al.: End results of removal of protruded lumbar intervertebral discs with and without fusion. Instruc. Course Lect. 16:213-216, 1959.

Index

Page numbers in *italics* indicate illustrations.

Abnormalities, of lumbar spinal canal, 265
of lumbar spine, 249-276, 301
Aging, and degeneration of cervical spine, 37
and disease, biochemical changes in, 32-34
and nucleus functions, 66
process of, intervertebral disc and, 30
Alkaptonuria, 55
Ankylosing spondylitis, diagnostic error involving, 332
of lumbar spine, 274
of sacroiliac joint, *333*
Ankylosis, bony, 44
Annulus fibrosus, anatomy of, 13, *13*
calcification of, 236
defects in, surgery and, 304
degeneration of, in lumbar disc disease, 67, 76
embryological development of, 4
histochemical changes in, aging and, 36
in mechanical response of disc, 26
protrusion of, 36, 51
rupture of, thinned disc and, 48
Anomalies, acquired, of lumbosacral region, 268-274
congenital, of lumbar spine, 250-267
of lumbar nerve root, surgery and, 300
of spinal canal, 265
Apophyseal joint, changes in, in disc degeneration, 41, 42, *43*, *44*
Arachnoid cyst, following lumbar disc surgery, 343
Artery, vertebral, anatomical relations of, 24
involvement of, in cervical spondylosis, 107-109
Arthritis, degenerative, 36
Arthrodesis, in lumbar disc disease, 297
technique of, 314-316
in thoracic disc disease, 179
Arthrosis, of intervertebral joint, 232
and posterior intervertebral joint, 269
Articular facets, of lumbar vertebrae, tropism of, surgery and, 299

Atlantoaxial and atlanto-occipital joints and ligaments, 16-18
Atlas, anatomy of, 8, *8*
Auto-immune phenomena, and intervertebral disc, 34
Axis, anatomy of, 8

Ballooning, of intervertebral discs, 46, *47*
Bedrest, in cervical disc disease, 93
in lumbar disc disease, 278
Biochemical changes, in intervertebral disc, aging and disease and, 32-34
structural stresses and, 35
Blood vessels, of disc, 20
Boggy disc, surgery and, 303
Bone graft(s), cervical, absorption of, in pseudarthrosis, 163
and interbody fusion, 119
extrusion of, 164
lumbar, cancellous, from ilium, 314
Bony ankylosis, 44
Braces and corsets, for lumbar disc disease, 283-285
Brown-Séquard syndrome, incomplete, ventrolateral lesions and, 101

Calcification, of intervertebral disc, 53, 236
Cauda equina, formation of, 62
injury to, 63, 340
during surgery on lumbar spine, 329
massive nuclear extrusion and, 74, 194
surgery for, 289
Cerebrospinal fluid, cervical spondylosis and, 105
in lumbar disc syndrome, 230
Cervical disc(s), anatomy of, 14
excision of, and anterior interbody fusion, 158-161, 166
and interbody fusion, 110-122
injury to, 137-141
pathology of, 36-45
spondylosis and degeneration of, 36

367

Cervical disc disease, clinical syndrome of, 85-91
  conservative treatment of, 92-96
    results of, 156-157
  discogenic syndrome in, 97
  drug therapy in, 94
  esophageal compression and, 86
  history-taking in, 85-87
  immobilization in, 92-94
  isometric exercises and, 94-95
  neurogenic syndrome in, 100
  neurological examination in, 88
  operative treatment of, 97-133
  pain in, 85
  physical findings in, 87-88
  physical therapy in, 96
  procaine infiltration in, 95
  pupil size in, 88
  radiographic findings in, 89-91
  sleep position in, 96
Cervical disc distention test, 90
Cervical discography, 89
Cervical fusion, anterior, disc excision and, 158-161, 166
  operative technique in, 152
  anterior and posterior, 157
  disc degeneration following, 165
  disc excision and, 110-122
  osteophyte resorption following, 45
  posterior, laminectomy and, 122-126
  pseudarthrosis and, 161-166
  results of, 155
Cervical myelography, 89
Cervical myelopathy, pain in, 86
  spondylosis and, 45
  ventrolateral and midline lesions and, 101
Cervical nerves, intervertebral foramina and, 22
  sympathetic nervous system and, 24
Cervical spine, degenerative disc disease of, 36-46, 85-91
  operative treatment for, 154-170
  injuries to, 134-153
  intervertebral foramina and, 22
  radiographic examination of, 89
  soft tissue anterior to, injuries sustained by, 135-137
Cervical spondylosis, 36, 45, *105*
  cerebrospinal fluid and, 105
  myelopathy and, 44
  osseous changes in, *43*
  vertebral artery involvement in, 107-109
  vertebrobasilar ischemia in, 107
Cervical syndrome, following hyperextension, 146-148
  operative management of, 150-152
Cervical vertebrae, anatomy of, 6-9
  subluxation of, 142
Cineradiography, of cervical spine, 90
Collagen, increase of, in disc, 32
Collars, in treatment of cervical disc disease, 92, *93*
Concealed disc, surgery and, 303

Congenital abnormalities, of lumbar spine, 250-267
Coccyx, anatomy of, 12
Cord, spinal. See *Spinal cord.*
Cysts, arachnoid, following lumbar disc surgery, 343
  meningopseudo, following lumbar disc surgery, 343

Deformities, rotation, of lower lumbar vertebrae, 265
Degenerative arthritis, 36
Dermatogenous pain, in lumbar disc lesions, 183
Dermatome, in embryonic development, 1, *3*
Discs. See under specific areas, as *Cervical disc, Lumbar disc,* and *Thoracic disc.*
Disc detention test, 101
Disc excision, cervical fusion and, 110-122, 157, 158-161, 166
  lumbar fusion and, 295
Disc space, inadequate evacuation of, 338
  infection of, 54-55
    following lumbar disc surgery, 340, *342*
  narrowing of, in lumbar disc syndrome, 231
  reoperation of, 351
  thinning of, 47, 303
Discogenic syndrome, 97
Discography, cervical, 89
  in lumbar disc syndrome, 247
Disease, aging and, biochemical changes in, 32-34
Drug therapy, in cervical disc disease, 94
  in lumbar disc disease, 279-280
Dura, injury to, during surgery on lumbar spine, 328

Electromyelography, in cervical spine disease, 90
Electromyography, in lumbar disc syndrome, 230
Embryology, of spine, 1-4
Epiphyseal ring, formation of, 4
Esophageal trachea, compromise of, osteophytes and, 44
Esophagus, pressure on, in cervical disc degeneration, 86
Excision, of cervical disc, and anterior interbody fusion, failure of, 158-161, 166
  and interbody fusion, 110-122
Exercises, flexion, for lumbar disc disease, 280-282
  isometric, in cervical disc disease, 94-95
Extension, and flexion, in lumbar disc syndrome, 210
  and spine, 25
Eye, pupil size of, in cervical disc disease, 88

Fibers, Sharpey's, 13
Fibrosis, nerve roots and, 339
Flexion, and extension, in lumbar disc syndrome, 210
  and spine, 25
  exercise for, in lumbar disc disease, 280-282
  lateral, rotation and, in lumbar disc syndrome, 210
Fusion, cervical, anterior, disc excision and, 152, 158-161, 166
  anterior and posterior, evaluation of, 157
  disc degeneration following, 165
  disc excision and, 110-122
  osteophyte resorption following, 45
  posterior, laminectomy and, 122-126
  pseudarthrosis and, 161-166
  results of, 155
  lumbar, anterior, 321-322
  disc excision and, 295, 296
  following reoperation, 352
  posterolateral, modification of, 315
  preparation of spine for, 314

Gait, in lumbar disc syndrome, 207
Genetic factors, in degeneration of intervertebral disc, 34

Headache, cervical disc disease and, 87
Hemovac, use of, in draining wound, 352
Herniation, nuclear. See *Nuclear herniation.*
Histochemical changes, in intervertebral disc, 36
Horner's syndrome, cause of, 24
  in cervical disc disease, 88
Hydration, of intervertebral disc, changes in, 32
Hyperextension injuries, cervical syndrome following, 146-148
  management of, 148-149
  of neck, 134
  of soft tissues of cervical spine, 134-153
Hypermobility, of cervical disc, *152*
Hypertrophy, of ligamentum flavum, nerve compression and, 72

Immobilization, in cervical disc disease, 92-94
Impingement syndrome, 343, *346*
Infection(s), following surgery for lumbar disc disease, 330
  of disc space, 54-55
  following lumbar disc surgery, 340, *342*
Injury(ies), during operative treatment of lumbar disc disease, 324-329

Injury(ies) (*Continued*)
  hyperextension, cervical syndrome following, 146-148
  management of, 148-149
  of soft tissues of cervical spine, 134-153
  lumbar disc lesions and, 182
  to cauda equina, 340
  to cervical spine, 146
  to intervertebral disc, 137-141
  whiplash, 147
Interlaminar space, narrow, surgery and, 299
Intersegmental artery, relation of, to intervertebral disc, *3*
Intervertebral disc(s), aging and, 30, 66
  anatomy of, 12-14
  auto-immune phenomenon and degeneration of, 34
  ballooning of, 46, *47*
  biochemical changes of, aging and disease in, 32-34
    structural stresses and, 35
  blood supply of, 20
  calcification of, 53, 236
  cervical. See *Cervical disc.*
  function of, 13
  genetic factors and degeneration of, 34
  histochemical changes in, 36
  infection of space of, 54-55
  intersegmental artery and, *3*
  lumbar. See *Lumbar disc.*
  pathology of, 30-57
  posture and degeneration of, 34
  sacralization and lumbarization associated with, 235
  spinal nerves and, 22
  thin, rupture of annulus fibrosus and, 48
  thoracic. See *Thoracic disc.*
Intervertebral foramina, 6
  cervical, narrowing of, 41, *43*, 44
    relations of, 22
  lumbar, narrowing of, 240
    osteophyte formation and, 47
    relations of, 64
Intervertebral joint, arthrosis of, in lumbar disc syndrome, 232, 269, *271*
  asymmetric posterior, 267
Intervertebral space, inadequate evacuation of, 338
  infection of, 54-55
    following lumbar disc surgery, 340
  narrowing of, in lumbar disc syndrome, 231
  reoperation of, 351
  thin, surgery and, 303
Intestinal complications, following surgery for lumbar disc disease, 330
Intraforaminal lesion, 100
Intraforaminal protrusions, of nucleus, 72
Ischemia, vertebrobasilar, in cervical spondylosis, 107
Isometric exercises, and cervical disc disease, 94-95

Joint(s), apophyseal, changes in, in disc degeneration, 41, 42, *43, 44*
   atlanto-occipital and atlantoaxial, and ligaments, 16-18
   intervertebral, arthrosis of, in lumbar disc syndrome, 232, 269, *271*
      asymmetric posterior, 267
   of Luschka, *22*
      changes in, in cervical disc degeneration, 41
      formation of, 7
      vertebral discs and, 14
      vertebral artery and, 108, *109*
   sacroiliac, ankylosing spondylitis of, *333*
      degenerative changes in, *335, 336, 337*
      disease of, diagnostic errors involving, 332
Jugular compression test, in lumbar disc syndrome, 229

Kidney, complications of, following surgery for lumbar disc disease, 330

Laminae, vertebral variations in size, surgery and, 299
Laminectomy, and posterior cervical spine fusion, 122-126
   in thoracic disc disease, 178
Lasègue test, in lumbar disc syndrome 227
Leg tests, for lumbar disc syndrome, 224-229
Ligament(s), atlanto-occipital and atlantoaxial, joints and, 16, *17, 18*
   of vertebral column, 14-16
Ligamenta flava, 15
   nerve compression and, 72
Lipid, changes in, in intervertebral disc, 33
Litigation, role of, 157
Lumbar discs, anatomy of, 14
   ballooning of, 46, *47*
   calcification of, 236
   degeneration of, *68, 80*
   evacuation of, 308
   herniation of, 46, *52*
   pathology of, 46-55, 65-79
   protrusion of, 49-53
   rupture of, alkaptonuria and ochronosis and, 55
   thinned, 47-49
Lumbar disc disease, anatomical features related to, 298-301
   arthrodesis in, 297, 314-316
   back hygiene for, 282
   bedrest for, 278
   braces and corsets for, 283-285
   conservative therapy for, 277-286
   contraindications to surgery in, 293-294
   drug therapy in, 279-280
   flexion exercise for, 280-282
   operative treatment of, 287-323
      complications and failures of, 324-353
      indications for surgery in, 289-293

Lumbar disc disease (*Continued*)
   operative treatment of, objectives of, 294-298
   physical therapy for, 282
   postoperative complications, 329-331
   postoperative management of, 317-321
   pregnancy and, 285-286
   surgical errors involving, 336-338
   surgical pathology related to, 301-304
Lumbar disc lesions, anterior and lateral, 237-240
   clinical features and syndrome of, 58-84, 181-202
   injury and, 182
   level of, 190
   neural changes in, 197-201
   pain and, 183, 191-194
   recurrent attacks in, 195
   types of, 74
Lumbar disc syndrome, clinical manifestations of, 203-250
   clinical tests for, 222-230
   diagnostic tests for, 230-250
   displacement of vertebral body in, 232
   exacerbations and remissions of, 201
   flexion and extension in, 210
   gait and, 207
   motor deficits in, 197, 207, 214
      surgery and, 290
   movement and, 208
   muscle spasm in, 213
   onset of, 191-194
   pain in, 204-206
   palpation and percussion in, 213
   posture and, 208
   reflex changes in, 200, 222
   sensory disturbances in, 200, 206, 221
Lumbar fusion, anterior, 321-322
   disc excision and, 295-296
   following reoperation, 352
   posterolateral, modification of, 315
   preparation of spine for, 314
Lumbar nerve root(s), anomalies of, surgery and, 300. See also *Nerve root, lumbar.*
   relations of, 61-63
   sinuvertebral nerve and, 60-61
Lumbar spinal canal. See also *Spinal canal.*
   abnormalities of, 265
   narrowing of, surgery and, 299
   nuclear herniation and, 61
Lumbar spine, abnormalities of, 249-276, 301
   ankylosing spondylitis of, 274
   arthrodesis of, 297, 314-316
   lower, acquired abnormalities in, surgery and, 301
      exposure of, 305
   mechanical disorders of, due to operative treatment of, 354-366
   preparation of, for fusion, 314
   spina bifida and, 265
   spondylolisthesis and, 252-258
   spondylolysis and, 251, 360
Lumbar spondylosis, osteophyte formation and, 47

Lumbar vertebrae, anatomy of, 9, *11*
   free, variation in number of, 260
      surgery and, 300
   lower, rotational deformities of, 265
   lumbarization and sacralization of, 261
Lumbarization, sacralization and, in association with thin disc, 235
   of lumbar vertebrae, 261
Lumbosacral angle, exaggerated, 258
Lumbosacral mechanism, unstable, results of surgery for, 361-362
Lumbosacral region, acquired anomalies of, 268-274
Luschka, joints of. See *Joints of Luschka.*
Lymph nodes, in degeneration of intervertebral disc, 34

Malingering, 347
Meningopseudo cysts, formation of, following lumbar disc surgery, 343
Motor deficits, in lumbar disc syndrome, 197, 207, 214
   surgery and, 290
Motor unit(s), of spinal column, 59
   nerve supply of, 60-61
   instability of, 336, 343, *344, 345*
Movement, and lumbar disc syndrome, 208
   and spine, 25
Mucopolysaccharide, of disc, changes in, due to aging, 33
Muscle spasm, in lumbar disc syndrome, 213
Myelography, in cervical disc disease, 89
   in lumbar disc syndrome, 241, *242,* 244, *245, 246*
   in thoracic disc disease, 177
   in ventrolateral lesions, 105
Myeloma, multiple, ballooned discs and, 46
Myelopathy, cervical, pain in, 86
   spondylosis and, 45
   ventrolateral and midline lesions and, 101
Myotome, in embryonic development, 1, *3*

Neck, hyperextension injuries to, 134
Nerve(s), spinal, 19-20, 60. See also *Spinal nerves.*
Nerve roots, anatomy of, 21
   cervical, compression of, 100, *102, 103*
   lumbar abnormalities of, 275, 300
      compression of, in foramina, 64, *65*
      fibrosis and, 339
      injury to, during operative treatment, 329
      multiple, surgery and, 304
      nucleus protrusions and, 71, 80-83
      relations of, 61-63
Neural arch, 5
   defects of, surgery and, 360-361
Neurogenic syndrome, in cervical disc disease, 100

Nuclear herniation, 36, *38,* 49
   cauda equina syndrome and, 194
      surgery for, 289
   in lumbar disc disease, 238, 239, *242, 245, 246*
      surgery and, 303
   into vertebral body, 239
   intraspongy, 46
   lumbar spinal canal and, 61
   massive, 74, *74*
   nerve roots and, 80-83
   of thoracic disc, 172
   recurrence of, 339
   thinned disc and, 48
   types of, 69
Nucleus pulposus, anatomy of, 13
   biochemical changes in, and herniation, 35
   changes in, in lumbar disc pathology, 67, 69, 76
   disc function and, 33
   displacement of, 50
   embryological development of, 4
   function of, aging and, 66
   herniation of. See *Nuclear herniation.*
   intermittent prolapse of, 243
   structural changes and aging, 36
   trapped, 76
   vacuum phenomena in, 236
   water-binding capacity of, 32

Ochronosis, 55
Odontoid process, formation of, 8
Osteitis condensans, *334*
   diagnostic errors involving, 332
Osteitis deformans, 272
Osteopenia, ballooning discs and, 46
Osteophyte(s), anterior, in esophageal tracheal compromise, 44
   resorption of, following surgical fusion, 45, 165, *167*
Osteophyte formation, anterior, cervical disc degeneration and, 38, 41, *42*
   in lumbar vertebrae, 47
   posterior, cervical disc degeneration and, 38, *39, 40*
Osteoporosis, ballooning discs and, 46, *47*
Ovoid spinal canal, 62

Paget's disease, 272
Pain, and spina bifida, 265
   dermatogenous, in lumbar disc lesions, 183
   drug therapy for, in lumbar disc disease, 280
   in ankylosing spondylitis of lumbar spine, 274
   in arthrosis of intervertebral joints, 269
   in cervical disc disease, 85

Pain (*Continued*)
  in discogenic syndrome, 97, *98*
  in impingement syndrome, 343
  in lumbar disc lesions, 183, 191-194
  in lumbar disc syndrome, 204-206
  in lumbar spine abnormalities, 249-276
  in osteitis condensans, 332
  in Paget's disease, 273
  in sacralization and lumbarization in
      lumbosacral region, 262, 264
  in sacroiliac joint changes, 336
  in spinal tumors, 332
  in spondylolisthesis, 256
  in spondylolysis, 252
  in thoracic disc syndrome, 172, 174
  in whiplash, 148
  psychogenic, 347
  sciatic, in lumbar disc lesion, 192
  scleratogenous, in lumbar disc lesions,
      183
  source of, 19
Palpation, percussion and, in lumbar disc
    syndrome, 213
Paraplegia, massive herniation and, 74
Percussion, and palpation, in lumbar disc
    syndrome, 213
Physical therapy, in cervical disc disease, 96
  in lumbar disc disease, 282
Pneumatization phenomena, of lumbar
    disc, 236
Polysaccharide, in disc, changes in, aging
    and, 33
Posture, in degeneration of intervertebral
    disc, 34
  in lumbar disc syndrome, 208
Pregnancy, and lumbar disc disease, 285-
    286
Procaine infiltration, in cervical disc dis-
    ease, 95
Protrusion(s), annular, 36
  of disc, 49-53
  of nucleus, types of, 69
Pseudarthrosis, cervical, following anterior
    and posterior fusions, 127
  fusion results and, 161-166
  osteophytes and, 166
  repair of, 127-133
  lumbar, following spinal fusion, 340,
    341, 362
Psychogenic overlay, 347
Pupil, of eye, size of, in cervical disc disease,
    88
Pyogenic infections, of intervertebral disc
    space, 54

Radiculitis, clinical, osteophyte formation
    and, 47
Reflex changes, in lumbar disc syndrome,
    200, 222
Rotation, and lateral flexion, in lumbar disc
    syndrome, 210
  and spine, 25
Rotational deformities, of lower lumbar
    vertebrae, 265

Sacral vertebrae, 12
Sacralization, lumbarization and, in asso-
    ciation with thin disc, 235
  of lumbar vertebrae, 261
Sacroiliac joint, ankylosing spondylitis of,
    333
  degenerative changes in, *335*, 336, *337*
  disease of, diagnostic errors involving,
    332
Sacrum, anatomy of, 12
Sciatica, character of, 196
  lumbar disc excision and, 287
  lumbar disc lesion and, 192, 193
  patterns of, 197
Sciatic scoliosis, in lumbar disc syndrome,
    208
Scleratogenous pain, in lumbar disc lesions,
    183
Sclerotome, in embryonic development, 1,
    3
Senescence, aging and, 30
Sensory changes, in lumbar disc lesions,
    200, 206, 221
Sharpey's fibers, 13
Sinuvertebral nerve, 19
  origin and course of, 60, *60*
Sleep position, in cervical disc disease, 96
Somites, in development of spine, 1, *2*
Spina bifida, 265
Spinal canal, abnormalities of, 265
  disc herniation and, 61
  exploration of, 308
  exposure of, 306
  shape and size of, 61, *62*
  variations in, surgery and, 299
Spinal cord, relational anatomy of, 20
  thoracic disc disease and, 177
  vertebral canal and, 21
Spinal fusion. See *Fusion.*
Spinal nerves, 19-20
  disc and, 23
  intervertebral foramina and, 22
  relations of, 21
  sympathetic nervous system and, 24
Spinal tumors, 332
Spine, anatomy of, 1-29
  cervical. See *Cervical spine.*
  embryology of, 1-4
  function of, 27
  injuries to, 146
  kinesiology of, 25-28
  lumbar. See *Lumbar spine.*
  motions of, normal, 25
  motor unit of, 59
    nerve supply of, 60-61
  nerves of, 19-20. See also *Spinal Nerves.*
  preparation of, for lumbar fusion, 314
Spondylitis, ankylosing, diagnostic error in-
    volving, 332
  of lumbar spine, 274
  of sacroiliac joint, *333*
Spondylolisthesis, 252-258
  results of surgery for, 360
Spondylolysis, 251
  results of surgery for, 360
Spondylosis, cervical, 36, 45, *105*
  cerebrospinal fluid and, 105

Spondylosis (*Continued*)
   cervical, myelopathy and, 44
      osseous changes in, *43*
      vertebral artery involvement and, 107-109
      vertebrobasilar ischemia in, 107
   lumbar, osteophyte formation and, 47
Subluxations, of cervical vertebrae, 142
Sympathetic nervous system, relations of, to spinal nerves, 24

Thin disc, and rupture of annulus fibrosus, 48
   nuclear herniation and, 48
   sacralization and lumbarization associated with, 235
Thoracic discs, anatomy of, 14
   degeneration of, 171-175
Thoracic disc disease, operative treatment of, 176-180
Thoracic vertebrae, anatomy of, 9
Thrombophlebitis, following surgery for lumbar disc disease, 331
Tracheal compression, in cervical disc degeneration, 86
Traction, cervical, 94
Trefoil spinal canal, 62
Tuberculous infections, of intervertebral disc space, 54
Tuberculous spondylosis, 55
Tumors, spinal, 332

Urinary retention, following surgery for lumbar disc disease, 330

Vacuum phenomena, of lumbar disc, 236
Valsalva maneuver, in lumbar disc syndrome, 222
Vascular injuries, during operative treatment of lumbar disc disease, 325-327
Veins, plexus of, in lumbar disc lesions, surgery and, 303
Vertebra(e), cervical, anatomy of, 6-9
      subluxations of, 142
   embryological development of, 4, *5*
   lumbar, anatomy of, 9, *11*
      sacralization and lumbarization of, 261
   sacral, 12
   thoracic, anatomy of, 9, *10*
Vertebra prominens, 9
Vertebral artery, anatomical relations of, 24
   involvement of, in cervical spondylosis, 107-109
Vertebral body, displacement of, in lumbar disc syndrome, 232
Vertebral canal, spinal cord and, 21
Vertebral column, anatomy of, 5
   ligaments of, 14-16
Vertebral foramen, 5
Vertebrobasilar ischemia, in cervical spondylosis, 107
Vessels, blood, of disc, 20

Walk, in lumbar disc syndrome, 207
Water-binding capacity, of intervertebral disc, 32
Whiplash injury, 147